SECONDARY PREVENTION IN CORONARY ARTERY DISEASE AND MYOCARDIAL INFARCTION

DEVELOPMENTS IN CARDIOVASCULAR MEDICINE

Lancée CT, ed: Echocardiology, 1979. ISBN 90-247-2209-8.

Baan J, Arntzenius AC, Yellin EL, eds: Cardiac dynamics. 1980. ISBN 90-247-2212-8.

Thalen HJT, Meere CC, eds: Fundamentals of cardiac pacing. 1970. ISBN 90-247-2245-4.

Kulbertus HE, Wellens HJJ, eds: Sudden death. 1980. ISBN 90-247-2290-X.

Dreifus LS, Brest AN, eds: Clinical applications of cardiovascular drugs. 1980. ISBN 90-247-2295-0.

Spencer MP, Reid JM, eds: Cerebrovascular evaluation with Doppler ultrasound. 1981. ISBN 90-247-2348-1.

Zipes DP, Bailey JC, Elharrar V, eds: The slow inward current and cardiac arrhythmias. 1980. ISBN 90-247-2380-9.

Kesteloot H, Joossens JV, eds: Epidemiology of arterial blood pressure. 1980. ISBN 90-247-2386-8.

Wackers FJT, ed: Thallium-201 and technetium-99m-pyrophosphate myocardial imaging in the coronary care unit. 1980. ISBN 90-247-2396-5.

Maseri A, Marchesi C, Chierchia S, Trivella MG, eds: Coronary care units. 1981. ISBN 90-247-2456-2.

Morganroth J, Moore EN, Dreifus LS, Michelson EL, eds: The evaluation of new antiarrhythmic drugs. 1981. ISBN 90-247-2474-0.

Alboni P: Intraventricular conduction disturbances. 1981. ISBN 90-247-2484-X.

Rijsterborgh H, ed: Echocardiology. 1981. ISBN 90-247-2491-0.

Wagner GS, ed: Myocardial infarction: Measurement and intervention. 1982. ISBN 90-247-2513-5.

Meltzer RS, Roelandt J, eds: Contrast echocardiography. 1982. ISBN 90-247-2531-3.

Amery A, Fagard R, Lijnen R, Staessen J, eds: Hypertensive cardiovascular disease; pathophysiology and treatment. 1982. ISBN 90-247-2534-8.

Bouman LN, Jongsma HJ, eds: Cardiac rate and rhythm. 1982. ISBN 90-247-2626-3.

Morganroth J, Moore EN, eds: The evaluation of beta blocker and calcium antagonist drugs. 1982. ISBN 90-247-2642-5.

Rosenbaum MB, ed: Frontiers of cardiac electrophysiology. 1982. ISBN 90-247-2663-8.

Roelandt J, Hugenholtz PG, eds: Long-term ambulatory electrocardiography. 1982. ISBN 90-247-2664-8.

Adgey AAJ, ed: Acute phase of ischemic heart disease and myocardial infarction. 1982. ISBN 90-247-2675-1.

Hanrath P, Bleifeld W, Souquet, J. eds: Cardiovascular diagnosis by ultrasound. Transesophageal, computerized, contrast, Doppler echocardiography. 1982. ISBN 90-247-2692-1.

Roelandt J, ed: The practice of M-mode and two-dimensional echocardiography. 1983. ISBN 90-247-2745-6.

Meyer J, Schweizer P, Erbel R, eds: Advances in noninvasive cardiology. 1983. ISBN 0-89838-576-8.

Morganroth J, Moore EN, eds: Sudden cardiac death and congestive heart failure: Diagnosis and treatment. 1983. ISBN 0-89838-580-6.

Perry HM, ed: Lifelong management of hypertension. 1983. ISBN 0-89838-582-2.

Jaffe EA, ed: Biology of endothelial cells. 1984. ISBN 0-89838-587-3.

Surawicz B, Reddy CP, Prystowsky EN, eds: Tachycardias. ISBN 0-89838-588-1.

Spencer MP, ed: Cardiac Doppler diagnosis. 1983. ISBN 0-89838-591-1.

Villarreal H, Sambhi MP, eds: Topics in pathophysiology of hypertension. 1984. ISBN 0-89838-595-4.

Messerli FH, ed: Cardiovascular disease in the elderly. 1984. ISBN 0-89838-596-2.

Simoons ML, Reiber JHC, eds: Nuclear imaging in clinical cardiology. 1984. ISBN 0-89838-599-7.

Ter Keurs HEDJ, Schipperheyn JJ, eds: Cardiac left ventricular hypertrophy. 1983. ISBN 0-89838-612-8.

Sperelakis N, ed: Physiology and pathophysiology of the heart. ISBN 0-89838-615-2.

Messerli FH, ed: Kidney in essential hypertension. ISBN 0-89838-616-0.

Sambhi MP, ed: Fundamental fault in hypertension. ISBN 0-89838-638-1.

Marchesi C, ed: Ambulatory monitoring: Cardiovascular system and allied applications. ISBN 0-89838-642-X.

Kupper W, MacAlpin RN, Bleifeld W, eds: Coronary tone in ischemic heart disease. ISBN 0-89838-646-2.

Sperelakis N, Caulfield JB, eds: Calcium antagonists: Mechanisms of action on cardiac muscle and vascular smooth muscle. ISBN 0-89838-655-1.

Godfraind T, Herman AS, Wellens D, eds: Calcium entry blockers in cardiovascular and cerebral dysfunctions. ISBN 0-89838-658-6.

Morganroth J, Moore EN, eds: Interventions in the acute phase of myocardial infarction. ISBN 0-89838-659-4.

Abel FL, Newman WH, eds: Functional aspects of the normal, hypertrophied, and failing heart. ISBN 0-89838-665-9.

Sideman S, Beyar R, eds: Simulation and imaging of the cardiac system. ISBN 0-89838-687-X.

Van der Wall E, Lie KI, eds: Recent views on hypertrophic cardiomyopathy. ISBN 0-89838-694-2.

Mathes E, ed: Secondary prevention in coronary artery disease and myocardial infarction. 1985. ISBN 0-89838-736-1.

SECONDARY PREVENTION IN CORONARY ARTERY DISEASE AND MYOCARDIAL INFARCTION

edited by

PETER MATHES

Klinik Höhenried, Center for Cardiac Rehabilitation, Bernried (Obb.),
and Technical University of Munich
Medical School, Munich, Federal Republic of Germany

1985 **MARTINUS NIJHOFF PUBLISHERS**
a member of the KLUWER ACADEMIC PUBLISHERS GROUP
BOSTON / THE HAGUE / DORDRECHT / LANCASTER

Distributors

for the United States and Canada: Kluwer Academic Publishers, 190 Old Derby Street, Hingham, MA 02043, USA
for the UK and Ireland: Kluwer Academic Publishers, MTP Press Limited, Falcon House, Queen Square, Lancaster LA1 1RN, UK
for all other countries: Kluwer Academic Publishers Group, Distribution Center, P.O. Box 322, 3300 AH Dordrecht, The Netherlands

Library of Congress Cataloging in Publication Data

```
Main entry under title:
Secondary prevention in coronary artery disease
    and myocardial infarction.

    (Developments in cardiovascular medicine)
    Includes index.
    1. Coronary heart disease--Prevention.  2. Heart--
Infarction--Prevention.  3. Coronary heart disease--
Treatment.  4. Heart--Infarction--Treatment.  I. Mathes,
P. (Peter), 1940-    .  II. Series.  [DNLM: 1. Coronary
Disease--prevention & control.  2. Myocardial
Infarction--prevention & control.
W1 DE997VME / WG 300 S4445]
RC685.C6S42  1985      616.1'2305         85-8954
```

ISBN-13: 978-94-010-8725-4   e-ISBN-13: 978-94-009-5024-5
DOI: 10.1007/978-94-009-5024-5

Copyright

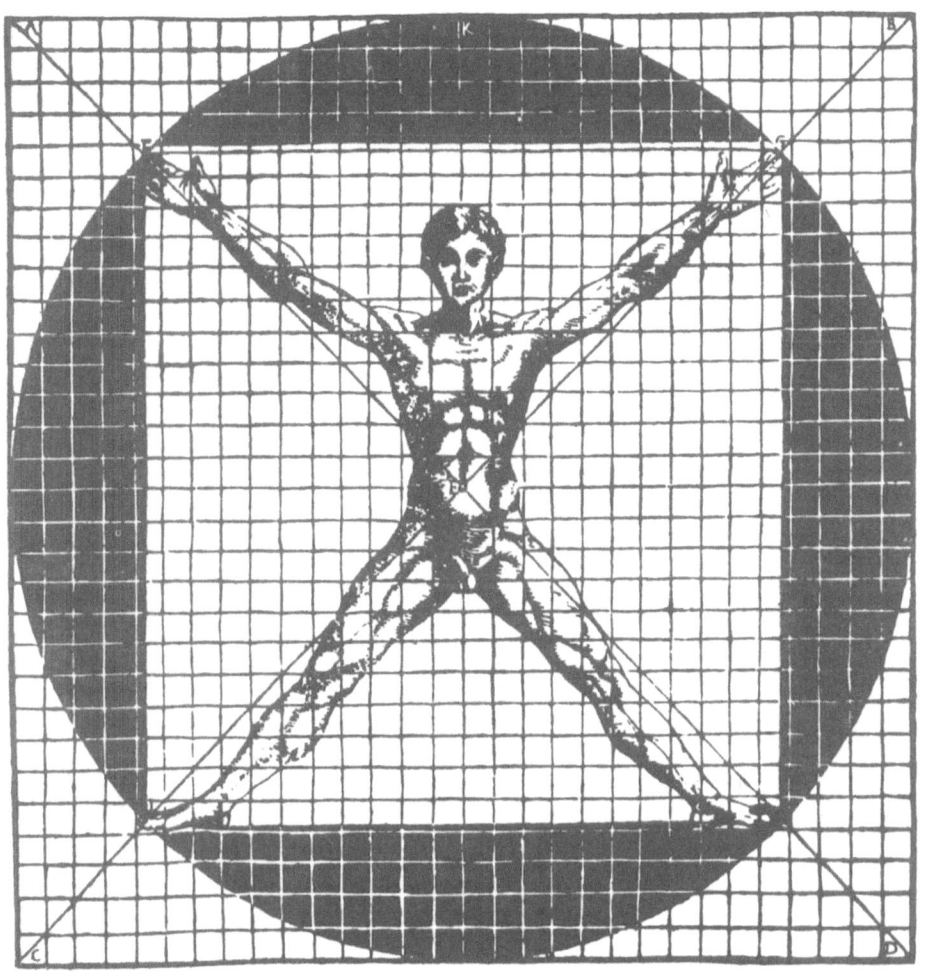

Preface

Despite considerable effort in primary prevention, coronary heart disease continues to be the leading cause of death in the industrialized nations. The patient who survives his first myocardial infarction carries approximately a tenfold risk of recurrence and sudden death when compared to the normal population. The concept of secondary prevention, therefore, has emerged as an active strategy aimed at the reduction of fatal and non-fatal recurrences of myocardial infarction. Apart from risk factors of relevance in primary prevention, secondary prevention is dependent on the extent of the disease itself; in other words the number of vessels involved, the extent of myocardial damage and the degree of electrical instability. Nonmedical aspects such as the level of education, the degree of social support and the attitude towards stress also appear to influence the prognosis.

The aim of this volume is to bring together all those factors relevant to achieving the maximal life span in patients afflicted with a disease that by its very nature is a lifelong process. However, as the late Paul Dudley White stated appropriately more than 40 years ago, it is not sufficient merely to add years to a life, one should also add life to the years. This concept truly is the nucleus of secondary prevention, sine only a life worth living generates the motivitation needed to take all the steps necessary in secondary prevention.

The authors and the editor are most grateful to Pharma Schwarz Inc. for their financial support in the publication of this book, as well as to Martinus Nijhoff Publishers, for its careful and prompt publication.

Höhenried, January 1985   P. Mathes

Contents

PART FIVE: THE ROLE OF PSYCHOSOCIAL FACTORS IN SECONDARY PREVENTION

PART SIX: THE ROLE OF REPERFUSION IN SECONDARY PREVENTION

List of Contributors

Amor M, MD, Department of Cardiology, C.H.U. de Nancy, 54500 Vandoeuvre, France

Amrein D, MD, Department of Cardiology, C.H.U. de Nancy, 54500 Vandoeuvre, France

Bergmann G, MD, Department of Internal Medicine, Medical Clinic of the University, Bergheimer Str. 58. 6900 Heidelberg, F.R.G.

Betz P, MD, Benedikt-Kreutz-Rehabilitation Center, Südring 15, 7812 Bad Krozingen, F.R.G.

Blümchen G, MD, Klinik Roderbirken of the LVA Rheinprovince, 5653 Leichlingen, F.R.G.

Borer JS, MD, Division of Cardiology, Cornell Medical Center, Cornell University, New York NY 10021, U.S.A.

Born G.V.R., FRCP, FRS, Department of Pharmacology, King's College, University of London, Strand, London WC2R 2LS, U.K.

Van den Brand M, MD, Department of Cardiology, Thorax Center, Erasmus University, P.O. Box 1738, 3000 DR Rotterdam, The Netherlands

Bruhn Th, MD, Theresienklinik, 7812 Bad Krozingen, F.R.G.

Bussmann W-D, MD, Department of Cardiology, Center of Internal Medicine, J.W. Goethe University Clinic, Theodor-Stern-Kai 7, 6000 Frankfurt a.M. 70, F.R.G.

Cherrier F, MD, Department of Cardiology, C.H.U. de Nancy, 54500 Vandoeuvre, France

Cuillière M, MD, Department of Cardiology, C.H.U. de Nancy, 54500 Vandoeuvre, France

Czerwenka-Wenkstetten G., MD, Institute of Psychology and Psychotherapy, University of Vienna, Lazarettgasse 14, 1090 Vienna, Austria

Danchin N, MD, Department of Cardiology, C.H.U. de Nancy, 54500 Vandoeuvre, France

Donat K, MD, Medical Department I, General Hospital Harburg, Eissendorfer Pferdeweg 52, 2100 Hamburg 90, F.R.G.

Duivenvoorden HJ, PhD, Department of Medical Psychology and Psychotherapy, Erasmus University, P.O. Box 1738, 3000 DR Rotterdam, The Netherlands

Eder A, MD, Institute of Sociology, University of Vienna, Alser Str. 33, 1080 Vienna, Austria

Ehsani AA, MD, Department of Internal Medicine, Cardiac Rehabilitation, Washington University School of Medicine, P.O. Box 8113, St. Louis MO 63110, U.S.A.

Erbel R, MD, Medical Clinic II, Johannes Gutenberg University, Langenbeckstr. 1, 6500 Mainz, F.R.G.

Erdman RAM, PhD, Thorax Center 1600, Erasmus University, P.O. Box 1738, 3000DR Rotterdam, The Netherlands

Ethevenot G, MD, Department of Cardiology, C.H.U. de Nancy, 54500 Vandoeuvre, France

De Feyter PJ, MD, Department of Cardiology, Thorax Center, Erasmus University, P.O. Box 1738, 3000 DR Rotterdam, The Netherlands

Fioretti P, MD, Department of Cardiology, Thorax Center, Erasmus University, P.O. Box 1738, 3000 DR Rotterdam, The Netherlands

Fleckenstein A, MD, Physiological Institute, Hermann-Herder-Str. 7, 7800 Freiburg i.Br., F.R.G.

Fleckenstein-Grün G, MD, Physiological Institute, Hermann-Herder-Str. 7, 7800 Freiburg i.Br., F.R.G.

Frey M, MD, Physiological Institute, Hermann-Herder-Str. 7, 7800 Freiburg I.Br., F.R.G.

Friedman M, MD., Harold Brunn Institute, Mount Zion Hospital and Medical Center, P.O. Box 7921, San Francisco CA 94120, U.S.A.

Gau GT, MD, Cardiovascular Disease and Internal Medicine, Mayo Clinic, Rochester Minn. 55905, U.S.A.

Gehring J, MD, Klinik Höhenried für Herz- und Kreislaufkrankheiten der LVA Oberbayern, 8139 Bernried, F.R.G.

Gill JL, MD, Harvard University Health Services, Cambridge MA 02138, U.S.A.

Godenir J-Ph, MD, Department of Cardiology, C.H.U. de Nancy, 54500 Vandoeuvre, France

Gohlke H, MD, Benedikt-Kreutz-Rehabilitation Center, Südring 15, 7812 Bad Krozingen, F.R.G.

Grodzinski E, MD, Klinik Roderbirken der LVA Rheinprovinz, Leichlingen /Rhld. 1, F.R.G.

Grossmann P, MD, Medical Clinic B, University of Düsseldorf, Moorenstr. 5, 4000 Düsseldorf, F.R.G.

Henkel B, MD, Medical Clinic II, Johannes Gutenberg University, Langenbeckstr. 1, 6500 Mainz, F.R.G.

Henrichs K, MD, Medical Clinic II, Johannes Gutenberg University, Langenbeckstr. 1, 6500 Mainz, F.R.G.

Hickey N, MD, FRCPI, FFCMI, Departments of Epidemiology and Preventive Medicine, St. Vincent's Hospital, University College, Elm Park, Dublin 4, Republic of Ireland

Hjalmarson A, MD, Department of Medicine I, Sahlgrenska Hospital, University of Göteborg, 41 41345 Göteborg, Sweden

Hopf R, MD, Department of Radiology, Center of Internal Medicine, J.W. Goethe University Clinic, Theodor-Stern-Kai 7, 6000 Frankfurt a.M. 70, F.R.G.

Hugenholtz PG, MD, Thorax Center, Erasmus University, P.O. Box 1738, 3000 DR Rotterdam, The Netherlands

Hundeshagen H, MD, Department of Nuclear Medicine, Medical School Hannover, Konstanty-Gutschow-Str. 8, 3000 Hannover 61, F.R.G.

Ivans K, MD, Medical Department I, General Hospital Harburg, Eissendorfer Pferdeweg 52, 2100 Hamburg 90, F.R.G.

Jehle J, MD, Medical Clinic B, University of Düsseldorf, Moorenstr. 5, 4000 Düsseldorf, F.R.G.

Jordan J, MD, Department of Psychosomatic Medicine and Psychotherapy, J.W. Goethe University Clinic, Theodor-Stern-Kai 7, 6000 Frankfurt a.M. 70, F.R.G.

Kallio V, MD, The Rehabilitation Research Center of the Social Insurance Institution, Peltolantie 3, 20720 Turku 72, Finland

Kaltenbach M, MD, Department of Cardiology, Center of Internal Medicine, J.W. Goethe University Clinic, Theodor-Stern-Kai 7, 6000 Frankfurt a.M. 70, F.R.G.

Kammermeier H, MD, Department of Physiology, Medical Faculty, Rheinisch-Westfalische Technical University Aachen, 5100 Aachen, F.R.G.

Kampa L, MD, Medical Clinic B, University of Düsseldorf, Moorenstr. 5, 4000 Düsseldorf, F.R.G.

Karcher G, MD, Department of Cardiology, C.H.U. de Nancy, 54500 Vandoeuvre, France

Kazemier M, MD, Thorax Center 1600, Erasmus University, P.O. Box 1738, 3000 DR Rotterdam, The Netherlands

Kellermann JJ, MD, Herman Meyer Cardiac Rehabilitation Institute, The Chaim Sheba Medical Center, Sackler School of Medicine, Tel Aviv University, Tel-Hashomer 52621, Israel

Keul J, MD, Department of Sports and Performance Medicine, Center of Internal Medicine, University of Freiburg, Hugstetter Str. 55, 7800 Freiburg i.Br., F.R.G.

Kloke M, MD, Medical Clinic B, University of Düsseldorf, Moorenstr. 5, 4000 Düsseldorf, F.R.G.

Kober G, MD, Department of Cardiology, Center of Internal Medicine, J.W. Goethe University Clinic, Theodor-Stern-Kai 7, 6000 Frankfurt a.M. 70, F.R.G.

Koenig W, MD, Klinik Höhenried für Herz- und Kreislaufkrankheiten der LVA Oberbayern, 8139 Bernried, F.R.G.

Kopp H, MD, Medical Clinic II, Johannes Gutenberg University, Langenbeckstr. 1, 6500 Mainz, F.R.G.

Kunkel B, MD, Department of Cardiology, Center of Internal Medicine, J.W. Goethe University Clinic, Theodor-Stern-Kai 7, 6000 Frankfurt a.M. 70, F.R.G.

Lehmann M, MD, Department of Sports and Performance Medicine, Center of Internal Medicine, University of Freiburg, Hugstetter Str. 55, 7800 Freiburg i.Br., F.R.G.

Lichtlen PR, MD, Department of Cardiology, Medical School Hannover, Konstanty-Gutschow-Str. 8, 3000 Hannover 61, F.R.G.

Loogen F, MD, Medical Clinic B, University of Düsseldorf, Moorenstr. 5, 4000 Düsseldorf, F.R.G.

Mathes P, MD, Klinik Höhenried für Herz- und Kreislaufkrankheiten der LVA Oberbayern, 8139 Bernried, F.R.G.

Mayer D, MD, Department of Thorax Surgery, University Clinic of Heidelberg, Im Neuenheimer Feld 110, 6900 Heidelberg, F.R.G.

Mehmel HC, MD, Department of Internal Medicine III, University Medical Clinic, Bergheimer Str. 58, 6900 Heidelberg, F.R.G.

Meyer J, MD, Medical Clinic II, Johannes Gutenberg University, Langenbeckstr. 1, 6500 Mainz, F.R.G.

Mulcahy R, MD, FRCP, FRCPI, Cardiac Department, The Sisters of Charity, St. Vincent's Hospital and University College, Elm Park, Dublin 4, Republic of Ireland

Niederberger M, MD, Herz-Kreislauf-Sonderkrankenanstalt der Sozialversicherungsanstalt der gewerblichen Wirtschaft, 4820 Bad Ischl, Austria

Pop T, MD, Medical Clinic II, Johannes Gutenberg University, Langenbeckstr. 1, 6500 Mainz, F.R.G.

Pretscher P, MD, Department of Cardiology, Medical School Hannover, Konstanty-Gutschow-Str. 8, 3000 Hannover 61, F.R.G.

Roskamm H, MD, Benedikt-Kreutz-Rehabilitation Center, Südring 15, 7812 Bad Krozingen, F.R.G.

Rothlin M, MD, Clinic of Surgery A, University Hospital Zürich, Rämistr. 100, 8091 Zürich, Switzerland

Rubermann W, MD, Health Insurance Plan of Greater New York, 220 West 58th Street, New York NY 10019, U.S.A.

Rupprecht HJ, MD, Medical Clinic II, Johannes Gutenberg University, Langenbeckstr. 1, 6500 Mainz, F.R.G.

Saggau W, MD, Department of Thorax Surgery, University Clinic of Heidelberg, Im Neuenheimer Feld 110, 6900 Heidelberg, F.R.G.

Schlief G, MD, Klinisches Institut für Herzinfarktforschung, University Medical Clinic, Bergheimer Str. 58, 6800 Heidelberg, F.R.G.

Schmitz W, MD, Department of Thorax Surgery, University Clinic Heidelberg, Im Neuenheimer Feld 110, 6900 Heidelberg, F.R.G.

Schreiner G, MD, Medical Clinic II, Johannes Gutenberg University, Langenbeckstr. 1, 6500 Mainz, F.R.G.

Schuchart J, MD, Department of Medicine I, General Hospital Harburg, Eissendorfer Pferdeweg 52, 2100 Hamburg 90, F.R.G.

Schwarz F, MD, Department of Internal Medicine III, University Medical Clinic, Bergheimer Str. 58, 6900 Heidelberg, F.R.G.

Seer P, MD, Theresienklinik, 7812 Bad Krozingen, F.R.G.

Serruys PW, MD, Department of Cardiology, Thorax Center, Erasmus University, P.O. Box 1738, 3000 DR Rotterdam, The Netherlands

Simoons ML, MD, Department of Cardiology, Thorax Center, Erasmus University, P.O. Box 1738, 3000 DR Rotterdam, The Netherlands

Thoresen CE, PhD, School of Education, Stanford University, Stanford CA 74305, U.S.A.

Ulmer D, MS, School of Education, Stanford University, Stanford CA 94305, U.S.A.

Vallbracht C, MD, Department of Cardiology, Center of Internal Medicine, J.W. Goethe University Clinic, Theodor-Stern-Kai 7, 6000 Frankfurt a.M. 70, F.R.G.

Varnauskas E, MD, Departmant of Cardiology, Sahlgrenska Hospital, 41345 Göteborg, Sweden

Weidemann H, MD, Theresienklinik, 7812 Bad Krozingen, F.R.G.

Weinblatt E, MD, Health Insurance Plan of Greater New York, 220 West 58th Street, New York NY 10019, U.S.A.

Weiss B, MD, Department of Medicine I, General Hospital Harburg, Eissendorfer Pferdeweg 52, 2100 Hamburg 90, F.R.G.

Welsch M, MD, Department of Thorax Surgery, University Clinic Heidelberg, Im Neuenheimer Feld 110, 6900 Heidelberg, F.R.G.

Wilhelmsen L, MD, Department of Medicine, Östra Hospital, CK Plan 2, 41685 Göteborg, Sweden

Wolf R, MD, Bevensen Cardiac Rehabilitation Center, 3118 Bad Bevensen, F.R.G.

Wrana N, Klinik Höhenried für Herz- und Kreislaufkrankheiten der LVA Oberbayern, 8139 Bernried, F.R.G.

Ziegler WJ, MD, Department of Medicine I, General Hospital Harburg, Eissendorfer Pferdeweg 52, 2100 Hamburg 90, F.R.G.

I. The Role of Risk Factors in Secondary Prevention

1. Cessation of Smoking

R. MULCAHY

Abstract

Cessation of cigarette smoking after myocardial infarction brings substantial benefits in terms of a reduced incidence of further fatal and non-fatal myocardial infarction, sudden death and total mortality. The evidence in favour of these benefits is overwhelming with many publications now showing a halving in mortality in survivors of myocardial infarction who stop smoking compared to those who continue. It is also evident that the benefits of stopping smoking continue over at least 15 years following the initial infarct.

Reducing the amount of smoking substantially after infarction is effective in reducing mortality, but stopping smoking achieves the best results. Cessation of cigarette smoking is by far the single most effective form of intervention available to us to reduce morbidity and mortality in survivors of myocardial infarction and in patients with angina of effort.

Stopping smoking also reduces the risk of post-infarction angina of effort and will prevent or alleviate other cigarette smoking diseases, including chronic bronchitis, peripheral vascular disease and duodenal ulcer. Successful rehabilitation and secondary prevention measures following myocardial infarction demand that patients with coronary heart disease who are smokers should be induced to eschew the habit.

Although there is less evidence to implicate pipe and cigar tobacco as harmful agents, it is probably wise to discourage all forms of smoking in coronary patients. There is conflicting evidence about the value of smoking low tar, low nicotine cigarettes and of the place of filter cigarettes in terms of reduced mortality.

Success in achieving smoking cessation depends on a dedicated approach by the physician and cardiac team. It requires a full understanding by patients and relatives of the effects of smoking on the heart, the vascular system and general health. Patients need to appreciate the physical, psychological and economic benefits of stopping smoking. Social support by family and friends is an important source of encouragement. Various techniques in achieving successful cessation of smoking and in preventing recidivism are discussed. These include regular counselling and follow-up, social support, various relaxation, aversion and rewarding techniques, smoking substitutes, the avoidance of vulnerable situations, the recognition and correction of susceptible psychological states, and the management of smoking withdrawal symptoms.

Introduction

It is now clearly established that cigarette smoking is a major and causative risk factor for coronary heart disease. A vast literature is now available to confirm the association. The degree of risk from cigarette smoking is best appreciated by referring to the most recent reports from the Surgeon General of the USA (1983) and from Framingham (Kannel et al., 1984). The Framingham report confirms that over a 26-year period the risk of myocardial infarction in middel-aged males who smoked cigarettes increased about fourfold. There was also a significant increase in women but to a lesser extent than in men. The risk of sudden death increased tenfold in men and fivefold in women.

The effect of cigarette smoking was greatest in causing peripheral vascular disease while the risk of stroke was doubled in men and the risk of congestive heart failure doubled in women. Deaths from atherosclerotic aneurysm and from subarachnoid haemorrhage were five times more frequent in smokers compared to non-smokers (Pettitii and Wingerd, 1978).

There is now evidence from Framingham and other primary prevention studies that risk is dose-realted, being greater with increased numbers of cigarettes smoked, with increased duration of smoking and with increased inhalation (Kannel, 1976). Those who stop smoking in primary prevention studies reduce the risk of myocardial infarction and sudden death substantially and increasingly over time (Kannel, 1984).

Risk factor intervention forms an integral part of secondary prevention of coronary heart disease. Successful control of hypertension, smoking and possibly hyperlipidaemia may reduce the risk of further attacks of myocardial infarction and sudden death. Such intervention may also reduce the risk of other non-coronary events such as stroke, peripheral vascular disease, bronchitis and respiratory failure. It behoves us therefore to carry out a careful evaluation of risk factors in survivors of myocardial infarction or in those with angina of effort, and to do everything possible to ensure their elimination. Apart from the anticipated medical benefits of such an approach, the patients psychological rehabilitation will be assisted by the knowledge that everything possible is being done to eliminate factors which may lead to recurrence of the illness.

The evidence in favour of stopping smoking after myocardial infarction is now overwheleming and we should be obliged to do everything in our power to help our patients to quit the habit. No other single procedure, be it surgery, drugs or lifestyle change, has been shown to confer the same benefit as stopping smoking.

It has now been shown in several studies that subsequent mortality in survivors of myocardial infarction who continue smoking is twice that of smokers who stop (Mulcahy, 1983).

Results

Our own experience of a longterm follow-up of patients shows that the 15-year mortality of initial smokers who stopped was 37% compared to a mortality of 82% in those who continued (Daly et al., 1983a). Initial non-smokers had an intermediate mortality of 62%, a finding with may be attributed to a greater incidence of hyperlipidaemia and hypertension in the initial non-smokers and to the fact that they were older. The benefits of stopping smoking were independent of other prognostic factors such as the extent of the initial infarct and age (Fig. 1).

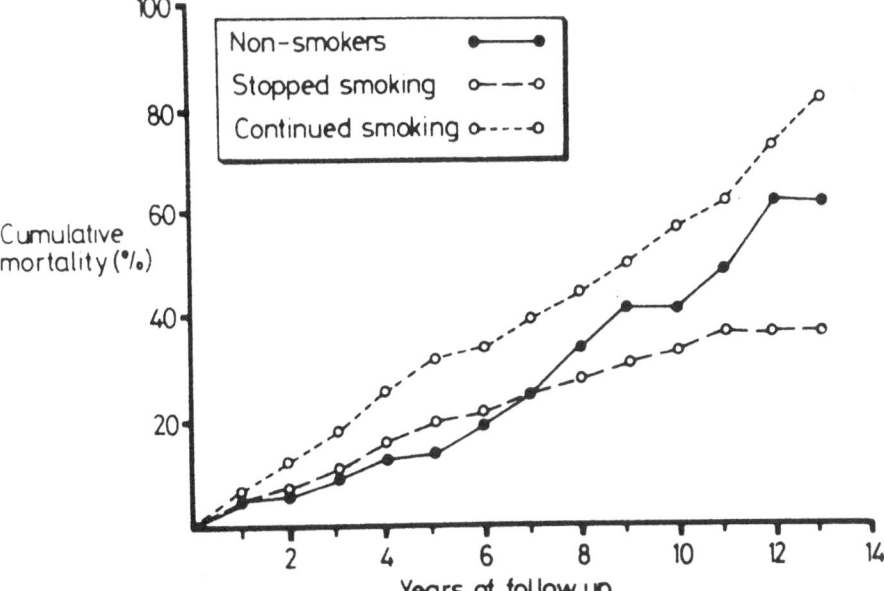

Figure 1. Cumulative mortality for 498 survivors of a coronary attack by smoking habit. Life table curves start two years after attack. Average annual mortality was 6.6% in non-Smokers, 3.7% in those who stopped smoking, and 10.2% in those who continued smoking.

Table 1. Percentage with angina pectoris at two years in 496 male survivors of myocardial infarction by anginal status prior to the coronary attack and by two-year cigarette smoking status [a]

Pre-infarction angina	Two-year smoking status		
	Continued	Stopped	Non
Present [+]	21/40 (52.5%)	24/51 (47.1%)	16/32 (50.0%)
Absent [ø]	31/117 (26.5%)	23/165 (13.9%)	16/91 (17.6%)

Two-year angina by smoking status: [+]: NS
                                       [ø]: $p<0.05$

[a]   Daly et al., 1983b.

There is also evidence that reducing smoking substantially after myocardial infarction reduces the risk of further events (Meinert et al., 1979).

In our experience subsequent smoking habits do not influence mode of death. For instance, those who stop and those who continue have the same proportion of sudden death to deaths from fresh myocardial infarction, although the total number of deaths is substantially lower in the former group (Mulcahy et al., 1982). However, the frequency of post-infarction angina is reduced in those who stop smoking (Daly et al., 1983b) (Table 1).

Recent work has shown that patients with coronary heart disease who are submitted to coronary artery bypass surgery have a higher mortality during and immediately after surgery than non-smokers (Gersh et al., 1983). Also graft patency has been shown to be adversely affected by continuing smoking after surgery (Proudfit et al., 1983). It has already been established that continuing to smoke after vascular surgery in patients with peripheral vascular disease will have an adverse effect on future claudication and the risk of amputation (Faulkner et al., 1983). It is also likely that stopping smoking will reduce the risk of stroke.

There is no reliable information about the vascular risks of pipe or cigar smoking in primary preventive studies nor has much work been done in this area of secondary prevention. However, in a previous study (Ronan et al., 1981) we showed that cigarette smokers who changed to pipe or cigar smoking following myocardial infarction had unacceptably high carboxyhaemoglobin levels and may therefore have been at continued risk of further vascular episodes.

In a recent study (Hickey et al., 1983) we showed that cigar smoking after myocardial infarction appeared to be associated with the same risk of recurrence and of high mortality as was found among continued cigarette smokers (Table 2). Pipe smokers showed the same mortality experience as those who stopped smoking. More research needs to be done to elucidate the role of pipe and cigar smoking in secondary prevention.

In evaluating the advantages of stopping smoking after myocardial infarction, it is important to identify the various benefits to be achieved, apart from reducing morbidity and mortality from coronary heart disease. Non-progression of the symptoms and consequences of peripheral vascular disease, a favourable influence on the symptoms of bronchitis and chronic obstructive lung disease, reduced risk of pulmonary insufficiency and frequent healing of duodenal ulcer are among some of these benefits. In discussing the advantages of stopping smoking, all these benefits should be emphasised as well as the sense of pride and achievement experienced by those who successfully rid themselves of a harmful and expensive addictive habit.

We have been advising survivors of myocardial infarction to stop smoking since 1961. It has been a vital part of our rehabilitation and secondary prevention programme since that time. Table 3 shows the cessation rate over the 21 year period, 1961 to 1981 (Hickey et al., 1981). An initial cessation rate of 47% has now increased to 70%.

This we can attribute to the increasing experience of a dedicated rehabilitation team on the one hand and to changes in patient attitudes based on expanding public knowledge of the harmful effects of smoking on the other.

Table 2. Four year mortality related to smoking status at last follow-up

Smoking habit at last follow-up	No	Mortality	
		No	%
Cigarettes	223	31	13.9
Cigars	33	5	15.1
Pipe	116	11	9.4
Non-smokers	299	28	9.4

Table 3. Response to cigarette smoking advice during six three year periods from 1961 to 1980

Time interval	Number of initial cigarettes smokers	Stopped smokers during follow-up period
1961–1963	63	29 (46.0%)
1964–1966	99	41 (41.4%)
1967–1969	101	57 (56.4%)
1970–1972	123	80 (65.0%)
1973–1975	129	75 (58.1%)
1978–1980	142	98 (70.0%)
Total	657	380 (58.5%)

All members of the hospital cardiac and rehabilitation teams have a responsiblity to encourage patients to stop smoking, including nurses, doctors, social workers, dietitians, physiotherapists and psychologists.

Discussion

Various methods have been advocated to encourage smokers to quit the habit. All have had some limited success but none are likely to succeed as well as the face to face approach between the patient and the dedicated and well-informed medical professional. It is essential to provide the patient with detailed and authoritative information about the adverse health effects of smoking and to stress the benefits to be derived by eschewing the habit. Advice may require to be reinforced and hence repeat visits to the rehabilitation and secondary prevention clinic are invaluable. The repeated contact with the cardiac rehabilitation team reinforces the patients motivation and improves longterm compliance. The use of printed material is also essential in achieving successful results. Patients are encouraged to read this material frequently to enhance their motivation.

Other techniques used to help patients to stop smoking include hypnotism, acupuncture, smoking substitutes, nicotine chewing gum, smoking clinics and videotapes.

These can be useful aids in a minority of cases but they are unlikely to succeed unless the subject is well motivated to quit the habit and has the confidence and will to do so. It is important to stress that motivation is best assured by having a full knowledge of the health implications of smoking and that this knowledge can only be derived from contact with health professionals or with appropriate literature.

In a minority of cases we are unsuccessful in having patients stop smoking. These patients need a compassionate and understanding approach. Any sense of impatience or criticism on the part of the health professional is counterproductive. In these cases we maintain an encouraging line and we emphasise the value of reducing smoking both on medical grounds and because substantial reductions in smoking may facilitate eventual cessation. We give the following advice to our patients:

1. Smoke a cigarette which has a low tar and nicotine content.
2. Smoke less of each cigarette so that the butt becomes progressively longer.
3. Gradually reduce the intake of tar and nicotine by cutting down on your inhaling.
4. Avoid inhaling every second puff at the beginning and gradually decrease the frequency and depth of inhalation.
5. Set out non-smoking periods for yourself each day.

6. Set out non-smoking locations for yourself such as the car, your bedroom or in the presence of your children.
7. Never offer or accept a cigarette.
8. Expect a boost to your morale and self-esteem as well as health benefits when you free yourself of this addictive habit.

Social support is an important adjunct to compliance. The spouse, family and relatives should be advised to take a sympathetic line if the patient cannot stop smoking. Impressions of criticism or resentment should be avoided at all costs. Family support can be very useful and the best contribution by members of the family is that all smoking members should stop and that those who do smoke should not do so in the presence of the patient. It is important to emphasise this point, particularly on occasions associated with smoking, such as family parties, reunions and when alcohol is being consumed.

It is important to anticipate the withdrawal or side-effects of stopping smoking. Depression, irritability, insomina and feelings of boredom are common. They usually respond to simple reassurance and reinforcement of advice and to a reminder of the value of stopping smoking. Exercise in various forms may be a valuable substitute and other leisure occupations and activities may reduce the side-effects. Occasionally a mild sedative during the day and on retiring may be helpful during the early acute withdrawal phase.

Increase in weight following cessation of smoking is common and is invariably the result of substituting food for the smoking habit. Patients may prolong meals in the absence of the highly favoured post-prandial cigarette. We have shown that weight increase after stopping smoking will not occur in post-infarction patients if they receive appropriate advice from the rehabilitation team and particularly from the dietitian (Hickey & Mulcahy, 1973). The substitution of low calorie foods such as raw vegetables and of low calorie drinks at times of risk, such as at the end of a meal or between meals, will prevent excessive weight gain. The use of chewing gum has been found helpful in a few patients, and regular and vigorous exercise will also help. The tendency to overeat after stopping smoking tends to resolve with-in weeks or months if patients are properly instructed.

In summary, most cigarette smoking patients following myocardial infarction can be induced to stop by an experienced and dedicated rehabilitation team. It is important that the members of such a team should be familiar with the proper approach to the patient and to the patient's family, and that repeated counselling should be provided where necessary. It should be emphasised that a committed family physician can be as effective in influencing smoking habits as a special hospital team. Stopping smoking after infarction not only confers important medical benefits, but also confers major psychological and economic advantages.

References

1. Surgeon General of the USA Health consequences of smoking - cardiovascular diseases, 1983. US Department of HHS, Rockville, Maryland.
2. Kannel WB, McGee DL, Castelli WP: Latest perspectives on cigarette smoking and cardiovascular disease: The Frmingham Study. J Card Rehab 4:267-277, 1984.
3. Petitti DB, Wingerd J: Use of oral contraceptives, cigarette smoking and risk of subarachnoid haemorrhage. Lancet 2:234-236, 1978.
4. Kannel WB: Some lessons in cardiovascular epidemiology from Framingham. Am J Card 37:269-282, 1976.
5. Mulcahy R: Influence of cigarette smoking on morbidity and mortality after myocardial infarction. Br Heart J 49:410-415, 1983.
6. Daly LE, Mulcahy R, Graham IM, et al.: Longterm affect on mortality of stopping smoking after unstable angina and myocardial infarction. Br Med J 287:324-326, 1983a.
7. Meinert C, Forman S, Jacobs DR. et al.: (Coronary drug Project Research Group): Cigarette smoking as a risk factor in men with a prior history of myocardial infarction. J Chron Dis 32:415-425, 1979.
8. Mulcahy R, Hickey N, Graham IM et al.: The influence of subsequent cigarette smoking habits on causes and mode of death in survivors of unstable angina or myocardial infarction. Eur Heart J 3:142-145, 1982.
9. Daly L, Graham I, Hickey N, et al.: Angina pectoris and smoking in post coronary survivors: a fifteen year mortality study. Eur Heart J 4 (Suppl E): 81 (abstract), 1983b.
10. Gersh BJ, Kronmal RA, Frye RL, et al.: Coronary arteriography and coronary artery bypass surgery: morbidity and mortality in patients aged 65 years or over. A report from the Coronary Artery Surgery Study. Circulation 67:483-490, 1983.
11. Proudfit WJ, Bruschke AVG, MacMillan JP, et al.: Fifteen year survival study of patients with obstructive coronary artery disease. Circulation 68:986-997, 1983.
12. Faulkner KW, House AK, Kastleden WM: The effect of cessation of smoking on the accumulative survival rates of patients with symptomatic peripheral vascular disease. Med J Aust 1:217-219, 1983.
13. Ronan G, Ruane P, Graham IM, et al.: The reliability of smoking history amongst survivors of myocardial infarction. Br J Addict 76:425-428, 1981.
14. Hickey N, Mulcahy R, Daly L, et al.: Cigar and pipe smoking related to four year survival of coronary patients. Br Heart J 49:423-426, 1983.
15. Hickey N, Graham I, Kennedy C, et al.: Trends in response to anti-smoking advice in patients with coronary heart disease between 1961-1975. Ir J Med Sci 150:262-264, 1981.
16. Hickey N, Mulcahy R: Effect of cessation of smoking on body weight after myocardial infarction. Am J Clin Nutr 26:385-386, 1973.

2. The Importance of the Cessation of Cigarette Smoking in the Tertiary Prevention of Coronary Heart Disease

P. SEER, H. WEIDEMANN, Th. BRUHN

Abstract

According to Brengelmann (1984) there is a relationship between personality type, psychosocial stress and smoking behavior. Persons smoking less than 20 cigarettes per day are more extroverted and tend to be social smokers; stress appears to have little effect on the number of cigarettes they smoke per day. On the other hand, persons who smoke more than 20 cigarettes per day seem to be more stress-prone, i.e. their rate of smoking increases under conditions of stress.

In male myocardial infarction (MI) patients approximately 60–70% fall into the category of stress smokers, while in female patients this percentage is between 20–30%. 73% of the males and 83% of the females who smoked before their MI stopped smoking on their own accord during their stay at a rehabilitation clinic and still were nonsmokers at a 3-year follow-up (Weidemann et al., 1983).

Those MI patients who find themselves unable to stop smoking are in need of psychological support to quit smoking. Unfortunately the status of smoking cessation programs in cardiological rehabilitation clinics in the FRG is rather poor (Seer et al., 1984). We found that only 16 out of 52 clinics offer systematic training courses to modify smoking behavior.

To treat the hard core of MI-patients who still smoke, we use in our clinic a systematic training program which was adapted from a more comprehensive treatment program developed by Brengelmann (1979). The results show that such a behavioral self-control program can be successfully adapted to the special needs of a cardiological rehabilitation clinic achieving comparable results: immediately after the training course 70% of the smokers had stopped smoking. At 8-month follow-up 50% were still nonsmokers.

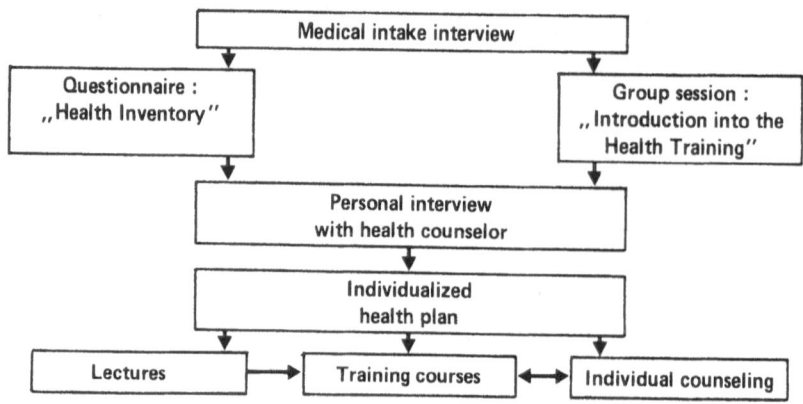

Figure 1. Procedural steps of the health training program at the Theresien Klinik.

Method

The smoking cessation program is an integral part of the clinic's more comprehensive health training program. The clinic treats some 210 patients and is divided into a department of cardiology and internal medicine and into an orthopedic-rheumatological department. The health training program is carried out by a health team consisting of the medical director, a psychologist, a health counselor, a dietary advisor, four physical therapists and an arts and crafts therapist (Fig. 1).

In the medical history interview the patient is informed about the health training program and his respective risk factors are recorded and discussed with him. He is asked to attend an introductory group session and 10 lectures. He is further asked to complete a questionnaire ('health inventory'). The health counselor then invites the patient to a personal interview in which his health behaviors are discussed and an individualized health plan, consisting of lectures, training courses and individual counseling sessions, is set up. Thus the patient becomes repeatedly involved in a discussion of his smoking behavior and is thereby motivated to attend the smoking cessation program on a voluntary basis.

The smoking cessation program used at our clinic was originally developed by Brengelmann (1979) and has been offered to the general public by the 'Bundeszentrale für gesundheitliche Aufklärung" under the name of 'Nonsmoker in 10 weeks'. The program uses information, motivation, group dynamics and, as the essential ingredient, various behavioral self-control strategies. We use the program in a condensed and adapted version of 8 sessions over a 2-week period. The first training session is preceded by a general lecture on the medical risks of cigarette smoking. The program

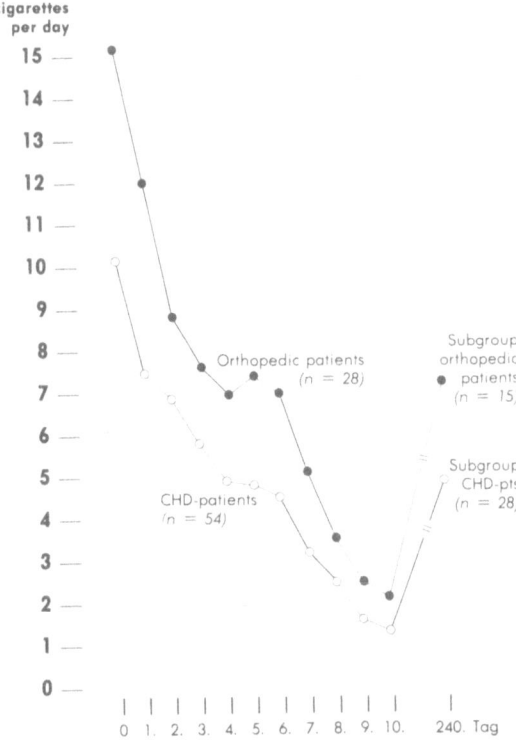

Figure 2. Average smoking rates of CHD and orthopedic patients before and after smoking cessation program and average smoking rates of a subgroup at 8-month follow up.

is scheduled in the main therapy time from 9 to 10am and is carried out by the health counselor.

Results and Conclusions

The smoking cessation program led to significant reductions in the number of cigarettes smoked per day. CHD and orthopedic patients showed comparable results immediately after training and at 8-month follow up.

Table 1. Characteristics of CHD and orthopedic patients

	CHD-patients n = 54	Orthopedic patients n = 28
Age ($\bar{x}$, SD)	47.6 (9.5)	42.5 (8.6)
Males	n = 49 (91%)	n = 9 (32%)
Females	n = 5 (9%)	n = 19 (68%)

Table 2. Means and standard deviations of average number of cigarettes smoked per day before and after training in CHD and orthopedic patients

	CHD patients n = 54	Orthopedic patients n = 28
Average no. cigarettes/day before hospitalization	$\bar{x} = 29.3$ SD = 16.1	$\bar{x} = 21.3$ SD = 14.6
Average no. cigarettes/day before training	$\bar{x} = 10.2$ SD = 6.8	$\bar{x} = 15.2$ SD = 9.3
Average no. cigarettes/day after training	$\bar{x} = 1.3$ SD = 2.4	$\bar{x} = 2.2$ SD = 4.7
% Nonsmokers after training	70%	75%

Table 3. Means and standard deviations of average number of cigarettes smoked per day in a subgroup of CHD and orthopedic patients at 8-month follow up

	Subgroup	
	CHD patients n = 28	Orthopedic patients n = 15
Average no. cigarettes/day 8 months after training	$\bar{x} = 4.9$ SD = 6.2	$\bar{x} = 7.3$ SD = 11.2
% Nonsmokers 8 months after training	50%	60%

The results of this study are practically identical with those reported by the 'Bundeszentrale für gesundheitliche Aufklärung' which uses the original 10-weeks version with subjects free of CHD. Our trials shows that this 10-week program can be administered in a condensed and adapted form to patients at a rehabilitation clinic achieving comparable results.

It is therefore strongly recommended that rehabilitation clinics offer systematic smoking cessation programs as integral part of their health training program, to help the hard core of stress smokers to quit their smoking habit.

References

1. Brengelmann JC: Informationen und Anleitungen zur Behandlung des Rauchens. Schriftenreihe des Bundesministeriums für Jugend, Familie und Gesundheit, Bd. 27. Kohlhammer Verlag Stuttgart, 1979.
2. Brengelmann JC: Status der psychologischen Methoden der Raucherentwöhnung. In: Brengelman JC (Hsrg.): Grundlagen und Praxis der Raucherentwöhnung. Röttger München (1984).

3. Seer P u H Weidemann: Raucherentwöhnung bei Koronarpatienten. Herz + Gefäße 8:462–469, 1984.

4. Weidemann H u J Finberg: Mehrjährige Verlaufsbeobachtung der medizinischen und beruflichen Rehabilitation nach Herzinfarkt bei Fauen im Vergleich zu Männern. Herz/Kreislauf 3:83, 1983.

3. Control of Hypertension

L. WILHELMSEN

Abstract

Hypertension known before myocardial infarction or detected after it has in several studies been associated with a worse prognosis after the infarction. This influence on prognosis has been found even among patients who have been treated for their hypertension, but there is no study available giving any clear evidence as to an effect on prognosis of treatment after an infarction.

Several large intervention trials such as the Australian Therapeutic Trial in mild hypertension, the Oslo Trial, the Hypertension Detection and Follow-up Programme and the Multiple Risk Factor Intervention Trial have reported their results. All these data have emerged from studies in hypertensive subjects without prior myocardial infarction. The knowledge of the benefits of antihypertensive treatment in the population as a whole has, to many, established a general justification for treating hypertensive infarction patients as well.

However, the data reported from the Multiple Risk Factor Intervention Trial indicated that subjects with organ damage at entry experienced higher mortality when their mild hypertension was treated – mostly by thiazides – than in their controls. The post-infarct patient is definitely a patient who has suffered organ damage, and it seems advisable, but far from proved, that we have to be cautious about giving drugs which might influence the electrolyte balance (especially potassium and probably also magnesium). A major reason for this is the increased risk of arrhythmias associated with myocardial damage, and probably deteriorated with electrolyte imbalance.

Thus, caution with all drugs influencing the above-mentioned variables seems advisable, but we have no scientific proof of any superior effect of one drug versus the other. However, beta-blocking drugs have been shown to be beneficial in the long-term treatment after a myocardial infarction, and they seem to have the first priority in hypertensive post-infarct patients.

Cardiac decompensation might be a relative contraindication, but could be treated with vasodilating agents.

Both the starting levels for treatment and the goal levels of blood pressure in post-infarct patients have to be established. The intervention limits in patients after an infarct could probably be more conservative than in the general population. Non-drug antihypertensive treatment may be sufficient in many cases and could be more advisable if risks of side-effects are suspected.

Introduction

Elevated blood pressure has been shown to be a risk factor for myocardial infarction (MI) in practically all populations in which it has been studied. No threshold for risk increase has been found – the risk increases gradually with increasing blood pressure level. For stroke there is a different blood pressure-risk curve among middle-aged men at least; the risk does not increase appreciably until at rather high levels, but then rather sharply.

Clinically significant hypertension, however not always in need for pharmacological treatment, was found in 38 % of 1271 non-selected male patients having suffered an MI in Göteborg, Sweden (Ulvenstam et al., 1984). Thus hypertension is an important disturbance among post-MI patients, and it is the third most important risk factor according to multivariate analysis in population studies in Göteborg, Table 1 (Wilhelmsen et al., 1984).

Recent results from clinical trials in hypertension point towards possibilities to prevent some cardiovascular complications by anti-hypertensive treatment (The Australian Trial in Mild Hypertension 1980; The Hypertension Detection and Follow-Up Program, 1979), whereas others have been less encouraging (Helgeland, 1980; The Multiple Risk Factor Intervention

Table 1. Ranking order in multivariate analysis of significant risk factors for coronary heart disease in middle-aged men. According to Wilhelmsen et al. (1984)

Variable	Direction of association
1. Serum cholesterol	+
2. Smoking	+
3. Blood pressure	+
4. Diabetes	+
5. Relative body weight	+
6. Reg. alcohol intemperance	+
7. Psychological stress	+
8. Phys. act. leisure	−

Trial, 1982). Results from our own Primary Preventive Trial (Wilhelmsen et al., 1972) indicate that antihypertensive treatment (which was given with betablockers in 78% of the treated patients) effectively prevents cardiovascular complications and reduces total mortality among those with high blood pressure (Berglund et al., 1978).

Results from controlled trials among post-MI patients are, however, not available today. Some data even cause concern regarding the advisability of extending results from studies in otherwise healthy hypertensives to post-MI hypertensives.

Hypertension as a risk factor after a myocardial infarction

Mortality rates have been high among hypertensive post-MI patients both during short-term (Frank et al., 1968; Rabkin et al., 1977), and long-term follow-up (Frank et al., 1968; Rabkin et al., 1977; Graham et al., 1978; Kannel et al., 1980).

In a recently completed 10-year follow-up in Göteborg it was shown that both mortality and non-fatal recurrence rate were related to presence of hypertension either treated after the infarction or not (Ulvenstam et al., 1984).

In several previous studies it has not been found that the post-MI blood pressure level has been significantly associated with future prognosis (Richards et al., 1956, Honey & Truelove, 1957, Hughes et al., 1963, Sievers, 1964; Henning & Wedel, 1981).

The inconsistencies seem mainly to stem from the fact that one has not taken into account the drop in blood pressure that occurs as a result of the MI (McCall et al., 1979; Kannel et al., 1980). In the first of these studies we found a positive relationship between indirect indices of a large infarct and fall in blood pressure. As large infarction is associated with increased mortality risk during several years after an MI, the blood pressure drop associated with the MI will be an important confounding factor. Analyses of the Framingham data (Kannel et al., 1980) have shed more light on the problem. In men with angina pectoris a clear relation of blood pressure to subsequent mortality was evident. Subjects who had hypertension both before and after angina became clinically manifest had higher mortality than normotensives and borderline hypertensives. A change in blood pressure after interim development of angina pectoris was not significantly related to mortality.

However, blood pressure after recovery from an MI was not related to 5-year survival. Blood pressure status *before* the MI was, however, related to survival. Hypertensive men had almost three times the mortality of normotensive men. When related to the change in blood pressure associated with the infarction it was found that a hypertensive man who normalized his blood pressure at the MI had twice the mortality risk of a hypertensive man who showed no change in hypertensive status.

The decrease in blood pressure due to an MI is sustained and amounted to 10.0 mm Hg systolic in Framingham. However, men who did not sustain an MI had a mean increase of 1.6 mm Hg during the same time period. If those MI men who were receiving anti-hypertensive medication were omitted the decrease with interim MI was 7.2 mm Hg. These data compare quite well with our data (McCall et al., 1979). One year after the infarct the decrease was 14/10 mm Hg systolic and diastolic, respectively, and after two years 10/10 mm Hg.

When an adjustment for blood pressure change after the MI was performed in the Framingham data a relationship between post-MI blood pressure status and subsequent mortality was found. To conclude: there is strong evidence for blood pressure status being of importance after an MI. The question is whether *treatment* can improve prognosis after an MI.

Treatment of hypertension in post-MI patients

Connolly et al. (1983) published retrospective data, which might be taken as some indication for a beneficial effect of antihypertensive treatment in post-MI patients, but the study was not based on prior randomization to treatment groups, and no strong case can be made from it.

Data from the Multiple Risk Factor Intervention Trial (1982) indicate that subjects with organ damage at entry to the trial experienced higher mortality when their mild hypertension was treated than their controls. Most patients were treated with rather high doses of thiazides, and it is possible that the untoward effects on the electrolyte balance might have been especially deleterious in patients with already existing signs of myocardial damage. The post-infarct patient is definitely a patient who has suffered myocardial damage, and it seems advisable, but far from proved, that we have to be cautious about giving drugs which might influence the electrolyte balance and especially potassium and magnesium. The major reason is the increased risk of arrhythmias associated with myocardial damage, and probably deteriorated with electrolyte imbalance.

There are no data from controlled trials available which do either prove or disprove the hypothesis. Beevers et al. (1983) have, however, published results which support this view. They looked upon recurrent heart attacks and strokes among patients who had received treatment with beta-blocking drugs either alone or in combination with other drugs (416 patients), and compared the incidence in those who never had received beta-blockers (504 patients). In spite of very similar characteristics at the start of the study and similar follow-up blood pressure reduction, there was a significantly lower incidence of cardiovascular complications in those receiving beta-blockers and this was found both in patients who initially presented with and without vascular complications. It must be emphasized that these results are not derived from a randomized trial, but they might still be taken as supportive of a hypothesis.

The increased risk of further complications among hypertensive post-MI patients although treatment has been given, may be taken as a contra-indication against active blood pressure reduction among them. It is, however, logical to assume that the pathological process is promoted by increased blood pressure also after the MI, and would be beneficially influenced by lowering of the pressure. Special emphasis should, however, but put on the risk of untoward side effects, and these seem primarily to be associated with thiazides. The betablocking drugs may be additionally indicated because of their special protective effects on the myocardium and against arrhythmias. We do not so far have similar indications that calcium-blockers and other antihypertensive drugs have similar cardioprotective effects.

Though drug treatment may be required to correct blood pressure in most cases, general hygienic measures should be applied first, wherever possible. These include:
1. Reduction of overweight through caloric restriction.
2. Limitation of alcohol consumption.
3. Limitation of salt intake.
4. A program of regular moderate daily exercise.
In case of need, drug(s) may later supplement – but not replace – these measures.

Summary

1. Hypertension is an important risk factor for MI.
2. Hypertension – treated or untreated continuous to be a risk factor also after an MI.
3. Antihypertensive treatment should be given after an MI.
4. Arrhythmias are of special concern in post-MI patients, and electrolyte abnormalities have to be avoided if possible.
5. The type of antihypertensive treatment may be important.
    a. Caution with diuretics.
    b. Beta-blocking drugs may have special advantages.
    c. Calcium-blockers may also be advantageous, but no clinical scientific data are so far available to support that.
    d. Non-pharmacologic measures are safe, and may be sufficient in several patients.

References

1. Beevers DG, Johnston JH, Larkin H, Davies P: Clinical Evidence that β-Adrenoceptor Blockers prevent more Cardiovascular Complications than Other Antihypertensive Drugs. Drugs 25 (Suppl 1):326–330, 1983.
2. Berglund G, Wilhelmsen L, Sannerstedt R et al.: Coronary heart-disease after treatment of hypertension. Lancet 1:1–5, 1978.
3. Connolly DC, Elveback LR, Oxman HA: Coronary Heart Disease in Residents of Rochester, Minnesota, 1950–1975. III. Effect of Hypertension and Its Treatment on Survival of Patients With Coronary Artery Disease. Mayo Clin Proc, Vol 58, p 249–254, 1983.
4. Frank CW, Weinblatt E, Shapiro S, Sager RV: Prognosis of men with coronary heart disease as related to blood pressure. Circulation 38:432–438, 1978.
5. Graham IM, Mulcahy R, Hickey N, Daly L: The effect of hypertenison and its treatment on prognosis after myocardial infarction. In: Acute and long-term medical management of myocardial ischemia. Eds Hjalmarson A, Wilhelmsen L. Lindgren & Söner, Mölndal, Sweden, p 279–284, 1978.
6. Helgeland A: Treatment of Mild Hypertension: A Five Year Controlled Drug Trial. The Oslo Study. Am J Med, Vol 69:725–732, 1980.
7. Henning R, Wedel H: The long-term prognosis after myocardial infarction: a five year follow-up study. Eur Heart J, Vol 2:65–74, 1981.
8. Honey GE, Truelove SC: Prognostic factors in myocardial infarction. Lancet, Vol 2:1155–1161, 1957.
9. Hughes WL, Kalbfleisch JM, Brandt EN Jr, Costiloe JP: Myocardial infarction prognosis by discriminant analysis. Arch Intern Med 111:338–345.
10. Hypertension Detection and Follow-up Program Cooperative Group: Five-year findings of the hypertension detection and follow-up program I. Reduction in mortality of persons with high blood pressure, including mild hypertension. JAMA 1979, 242:2562–2571.
11. Kannel WB, Sorlie P, Castelli WP, McGee D: Blood pressure and survival after myocardial infarction: The Framingham Study. Am J Cardiol 45:326–330, 1980.
12. McCall M, Elmfeltdt D, Vedin A, Wilhelmsson C, Wedel H, Wilhelmsen L: Influence of a myocardial infarction on blood pressure and serum cholesterol. Acta Med Scand 206:477–481, 1979.
13. Multiple Risk Factor Intervention Trial Research Group. Multiple risk factor intervention trial. Risk factor changes and mortality results. JAMA 1982, 248:1465–1477.
14. Rabkin SW, Mathewson FAL, Tate RB: Prognosis after acute myocardial infarction: Relation to blood pressure values before infarction in a prospective cardiovascular study. Am J Cardiol 40:604–610, 1977.
15. Report by The Management Committee: The Australian therapeutic trial in mild hypertension. Lancet 1980, 1:1261–1267.
16. Richards DW, Bland EF, White RD: A completed 25-year follow-up of 200 patients with myocardial infarction. J Chronic Dis 4:415–422, 1956.
17. Sievers J: Myocardial infarction: clinical features and outcome in three thousand thirty-six cases. Acta Med Scand 175 Suppl 406:1–123, 1964.
18. Ulvenstam G, Åberg A, Bergstrand R, Johansson S, Pennert K, Vedin A, Wilhelmsen L, Wilhelmsson C: Prognostic importance of hypertension and chronic angina pectoris in survivors of myocardial infarction. Subm for publ 1984.
19. Wilhelmsen L, Tibblin G, Werkö L: A primary preventive study in Gothenburg, Sweden. Prev Med 1:153–160, 1972.
20. Wilhelmsen L, Berglund g, Elmfeldt D, Pennert K, Johansson S, Wedel H: Multivariate analysis of risk for myocardial infarction, stroke, cancer and total mortality among middle-aged men in Göteborg, Sweden. To be publ 1984.

4. Lipid Lowering Regimens in Secondary Prevention of Coronary Heart Disease

G. SCHLIERF

Abstract

The level of plasma cholesterol is related to long-term prognosis in patients with coronary heart disease. Lowering of plasma lipid levels and normalization of lipoprotein profiles, therefore, is an integral part of secondary prevention. Evidence for its efficacy comes from epidemiological and clinical intervention studies and from well controlled clinical trials aimed at demonstrating regression of atherosclerosis.

Measures to normalize plasma lipoproteins include diet, exercise and drugs if needed. A working group of the International Society and Federation of Cardiology recommends the following:
1. Reduction of saturated fat intake of no more than 8–10% of calories; total fat no more than 25–30% of energy intake.
2. Cholesterol intake of no more than 200–250 mg/day for adults.
3. Ratio of polyunsaturated fatty acids to saturated fatty acids of 0.75–1.0.
4. Dietary fibre intake of up to 30 g/day, derived chiefly from legumes, other vegetables and fruits.
5. Gradual reduction of elevated body weight by restriction of energy intake (with attention to the qualitative recommendations above) and by physical exercise.

Although advice as above has been formulated over and over again, it is only realized in a minority of patients.

Introduction

In October 1983 several scientific councils of the International Society and Federation of Cardiology met in Titisee to update recommendations which have been issued in 1978, on secondary prevention of coronary heart disease. These 1983-recommendations [1] on diet, plasma lipids and obesity contain the following statements:

'Hypercholesterolemia, due to elevated levels of low density lipoproteins should be treated and there is evidence that effective control decreases progression of coronary and peripheral arteriosclerosis. Reduction of plasma cholesterol levels can be achieved in most patients by

1. gradual reduction of elevated body weight by energy restriction and by appropriate physical exercise, together with
2. a halving of saturated fat intake to 8–10% dietary energy and of cholesterol intake to 200–250 mg/day; total dietary fat should contribute 25–30% energy;
3. a ratio of polyunsaturated fatty acids to saturated fatty acids of 0.75–1.0,
4. a dietary fiber intake of up to 50 g/day chiefly derived from vegetables and fruit. Such a diet is both pleasant and widely used.

Familial hyperlipoproteinemias may require additional drug treatment and vigorous attention to associated risk factors.'

It is my intention in the minutes available to me to review briefly evidence underlying these recommendations which in a similar way have also been issued by a WHO expert committee [2].

Results and conclusions

Table 1 is taken from a paper by Hulley [3]. It shows that while the relative risk from hypercholesterolemia, comparing bottom and top quin-

Table 1. Relevance of serum cholesterol to preventing Coronary Heart Disease (CHD)

Serum cholesterol Quintile	CHD rate, deaths/1,000/yr	Relative risk [a]	Attributable risk [b] deaths/1,000/yr
Healthy men (aged 30–59 yr) [c]			
Bottom	6	...	...
Top	14	2.3	8
Men after myocardial infarction (aged 30–64 yr) [d]			
Bottom	38	...	...
Top	47	1.4	11

[a] Relative risk is the ratio of the rates, the proportion by which the risk in the top quintile exceeds that in the bottom quintile. It is calculated in cohort studies by dividing one rate by another.

[b] Attributable risk is the difference of the rates, the absolute magnitude by which risk in the top quintile exceeds that in the bottom quintile. It is calculated in cohort studies by subtracting one rate from another.

[c] Data from the Pooling Project.

[d] Data from the Coronary Drug Project.

Table 2. Coronary drug project

	Clofibrate	P	Placebo	P	Nicotinic acid
Deaths					
All	26%	ns	25%	ns	25%
Coronary heart disease	22%	ns	23%	ns	21%
Myocardial infarction	18%	ns	19%	ns	18%
Sudden death	11%	ns	11%	ns	12%
Recurrences					
Non-fatal myocardial infarction	13%	ns	14%	<0.001	10%
All myocardial infarct.	28%	ns	30%	<0.01	26%
Cerebrovascular	12%	ns	11%	<0.02	9%
Pulmonary embolism	2%	<0.01	1%	ns	1%

tiles of cholesterol levels is higher before myocardial infarction, then after the event, the absolute risk, i.e. deaths per thousand may be similar or even greater after the first myocardial infarction. It is this finding which forms the scientific basis for recommendations to treat hypercholesterolemia in survivors of myocardial infarction. It is not possible to review here all secondary prevention studies using diet alone or diet and drugs. Such reviews are available e.g. by Klose and Greten [4], by Hoffmeister et al. [5] or by Buchwald and coworkers [6]. Table 2 is taken from the Coronary Drug Project [7], which is usually cited as showing that lipid lowering chemotherapy was ineffective. It can be seen that for nicotinic acid, the drug which in this study produced the most pronounced lowering of plasma cholesterol levels, there was significance regarding non-fatal re-infarctions and all infarctions.

As an example of the number of epidemiologic studies on secondary prevention through management of hypercholesterolemia table 3 shows prelim-

Table 3. Rate per 100 man-years of ischeamic heart disease [8]

	Deaths IHD	Non-fatal infarcts	Combined 'major' new IHD
Controls	4.0	4.6	8.6
Drug treated	2.6	2.5 [a]	5.2 [b]

[a] p<0.05
[b] P<0.01

26

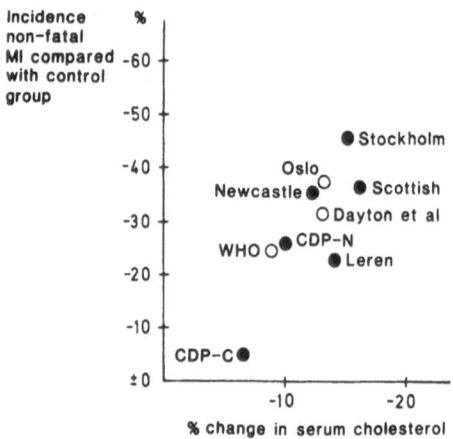

Figure 1. Intervention Trials. (Vessby (1981)).

inary data by Rosenhammer and Carlson [8] of their study comprising initially about 500 men after myocardial infarction. Lowering of plasma cholesterol concentration was 14%. In this preliminary report the drug group fared better than the control group with regard to recurrences of myocardial infarction. Dr. Rosenhammer reported one year ago at the Symposium of the European Atherosclerosis Group that with further follow up there was also a significant difference of total mortality between the groups.

Figure 1 is a summary of several studies by Vessby [9], trying to relate changes of serum cholesterol concentrations with reductions of incidence of non-fatal myocardial infarction. It is a compilation of primary and secondary prevention studies, using diet and/or drugs. One can see that if one compiles the different studies there is a reasonable dose and effect relationship regarding cholesterol lowering and lowering of recurrences.

I would like to turn now to studies which aim to look at the diseased vessels. Dr. Blankenhorn [10] pioneered in trying to standardize observa-

Table 4. Mean serum lipid (TG = triglycerides, Chol = cholesterol) and lipoprotein concentrations ($\pm$SEM) before the study, during six months of dietary treatment and during one year of treatment with fenofibrate and nicotinic acid in 8 asymptomatic men

	Total TG	Total Chol	VLDL TG	LDL Chol	HDL Chol
Before	3.26±0.93	10.10±0.16	2.93±0.64	7.15±0.37	1.47±0.11
Diet	2.74±0.58	9.49±0.32	1.57±0.42 [b]	6.92±0.48	1.60±0.08
Drugs	1.18±0.14 [a]	6.17±0.29 [c]	0.53±0.11 [c]	3.93±0.23 [c]	1.93±0.17 [c]

[a] $p < 0.05$
[b] $p < 0.01$
[c] $p < 0.001$

tions that, in the femoral artery, regression may occur. Subsequent studies tried to approach this problem in controlled experiments and at the International Symposium on Atherosclerosis in Berlin Dr. Erikson[1] showed preliminary results of a ranzomized study which intends to include 60 patients with early femoral atherosclerosis, 30 being treated and 30 not being treated for hyperlipidemia. Using a combined drug regimen he produced marked lowering of cholesterol levels in addition to that achieved by diet (Table 4). The results of this study are due to be reported in early 1985. In the meantime, Dr. Lewis' group[12] published a randomized study where they had 24 patients with peripheral arterial disease, half of them being submitted to aggressive lipid lowering treatment. In this controlled trial angiograms of the femoral arteries were performed before the experiment and 1½-2 years thereafter. Table 5 from their paper shows less progression in the treatment group as compared to the usual care group. The increase in the plaque area was also significantly different and also the changes in the edge irregularity index. The problem with the coronary arteries is much more difficult in particular with regard to quantitation of coronary arteriosclerosis. It is, therefore no surprise that Arntzenius[13] reported, at the Symposium in Berlin, negative results of dietary intervention in 22 patients with regard to demonstrable changes of coronary artery disease by repeated coronary angiography. In the meantime, 3 positive studies have been reported. Nash, in 1980 [14] studied 42 patients with angiographically documented coronary heart disease. He had 25 responders to colesti-

Table 5. Visual assessment and image analysis of arteriograms

	Treatment	Usual care
Visual assessment		
Number of assessed segments	144	156
Segments showing progression (n)	10	27
% segments showing progression	6.9	17.3
Mean increase in plaque area (mm^2 per year per segment) (range)	0.58 (0.12)	1.72 [b] (0.14)
Computerised image analysis		
Change in edge irregularity index		
Mean	0.019	0.047 [c]
Range	−0.180 to 0.116	−0.144 to 0.183
% of segments showing decrease in edge irregularity	33	15 [d]

[a] <0.01 $(\chi^2 = 7.44)$.
[b] $p = 0.06$ (Mann-Whitney U test).
[c] $p<0.05$ (Mann-Whitney U test).
[d] $p = 0.05$ $(\chi^2 = 3.82)$

pol and 17 non-responders, and compared the angiograms after 2 years. The drug treated patients as compared to the placebo-treated patients showed less progression, and fewer significantly diseased vessels.

The second relevant study was performed by Nikkilä [15]. He had 28 patients and 20 controls, and by all criteria which he used, coronary lesions progressed significantly less in the patients than in the controls. Finally, as the largest study of this kind, a randomized double blind intervention study with angiograms in 116 patients before and after 5 years of colestipol treatment was reported early this year, about the same time as the coronary drug project by the NIH group [16]. There was a general trend of less progression being found in the treated than in the non-treated patients.

Thus, we have evidence from epidemiologic and from clinical trials, that at least progression may be inhibited by vigorous – I underline – vigorous treatment of the risk factor hyperlipidemia, usually by lipid lowering chemotherapy.

It would be of interest to look at what can be achieved by life style intervention without drugs. In our hands the combination of lipid lowering diet and physical exercise leads to reductions of risk factors comparable to or exceeding those achieved by drugs [17]. Preliminary results of this ongoing study are presented at this meeting by Schuler et al.

In conclusion, lowering of plasma lipid concentrations should be part of the comprehensive package of secondary prevention. Secondary prevention, in turn, must be part of general prevention. Successful changes of faulty living habits lead to marked reduction of risk factors which raise hopes to inhibit progression and probably effect regression of coronary atherosclerosis.

References

1. Pyörälä EdK, Rapaport E, König K, Schettler G, Diehm C: Secondary prevention of coronary heart Disease. Workshop of the International Society and Federation of Cardiology, Titisee, 21–24 October 1983. Georg Thieme Verlag, Stuttgart/New York, 1983.
2. Report of a WHO Expert Committee: Prevention of coronary heart disease, Technical Report Series 678, 1982, World Health Organization, Geneva, 1982.
3. Hulley St B, Lo B: Choice and use of blood lipid tests. Arch Intern Med 143:667–673, 1983.
4. Klose G, Greten H: Risiko und Nutzen in der Behandlung von Hyperlipoproteinämien. In: Hyperlipoproteinämie. Hrsg. H. Kaffarnik/J Schneide perimed Fachbuch-Verlagsges. Erlangen, 1983, S. 160–167.
5. Hoffmeister h, Junge B, Schön D: Prävention von Herz-Kreislaufkrankheiten: Bewertung des Erfolgs von Interventionsstudien, Bundesgesundheitsblatt 27 Nr. 5, 1984.
6. Buchwald H, Fitch L, Moore RB: Overview of randomized clinical trials of lipid intervention for atherosclerotic disease. Controlled Clinical Trials 3:271–283, 1982.
7. Coronary Drug Project Research Group: Clofibrate and niacin in coronary heart disease. J Am Med Assoc 321–360, 1975.

8. Rosenhammer G, Carlson LA: Effect of combined clofibrate – nicotinic acid treatment in ischemic heart disease. Atherosclerosis 37:129–138, 1980.

9. Vessby B, Lithell H, Boberg J: Will serum lipid lowering treatment reduce the incidence of coronary heart disease? Artery 9:372–381, 1981.

10. Blankenhorn DH: Angiographic evidence of atherosclerosis regression in man Atherosclerosis IV, 1979, Springer-Verlag, Berlin, Heidelberg, New York, 414–421.

11. Erikson U, Helmius G, Hemmingson A, Ruhn G, Olsson AG: Measurement of atherosclerosis by arteriography and microdensitometry: Model and clinical investigations Atherosclerosis VI, 1983, Springer-Verlag Berlin, Heidelberg, New York, 197–201.

12. Duffield RGM, Lewis B, Miller NE, Jamieson CW, Brunt JNH, Colchester ACF: Treatment of hyperlipidaemia retards progression of symptomatic femoral atherosclerosis. Lancet II:639–641, 1983.

13. Arntzenius AC, Barth JD, Bruschke AVG, Buis B, van Gent CM, Houtsmuller UMT, Kempen-Voogd N, Dr Kromhour, Reiber JHC, Strikwerda S, van der Velde EA, van Wezel LA: Preliminary report on coronary lesion and serum lipids before and after 2 years dietary intervention in 22 patients. Atherosclerosis VI, Ed. Schettler et al., Springer-Verlag Berlin/Heidelberg/New York, 1983, S. 187–193.

14. Nash DT Gensini G, Esente P: Effect of lipid-lowering therapy on the progression of coronary atherosclerosis assessed by scheduled repetitive coronary arterography. International Journal of Cardiology 2:43–55, 1982.

15. Nikkilä EA, Viikinkoski P, Valle M, Frick MH: Prevention of progression of coronary atherosclerosis by treatment of hyperlipidaemia: a seven year prospective angiographic study. Brit Med J 289:220–223, 1984.

16. Brensicke JF, Levy RI, Kelsey SF, Passamani ER, Richardson JM, Loh IK, Stone NJ, Aldrich RF, Battaglini JW, Moriarty DJ, Fisher MR, Friedman L, Friedewald W, Detre KM, Epstein StE: Effects of therapy with cholestyramine on progression of coronary arteriosclerosis: results of the NHLBI type II. Circulation 69:313–324, 1984.

17. Schuler G, Wirth A, Schlierf G, Dinsenbacher A, Hofmann M, Röhrig N, Hartmann S, Kübler W: Dietary fat restriction and physical training in patients with coronary artery disease: 'ideal' plasma lipids without drugs (abstr.). Circulation Supp II:II–127, 1984.

II. The Role of Social Class in Secondary Prevention

5. Mortality After Myocardial Infarction
Role of Social and Behavioral Factors

E. WEINBLATT and W. RUBERMAN

Abstract

Prospective epidemiologic studies of coronary heart disease, carried out at the Health Insurance Plan of Greater New York (HIP) during the past 25 years, are reviewed to examine the extent to which social or psychosocial factors influence the mortality of men after myocardial infarction (MI). Follow-up of a cohort of 882 men with first MI diagnosed in the years 1961–65 and of a second cohort of 1739 men with acute MI experienced in 1972–75 provided the observations used to assess the prognostic role of clinical features and of personal and social characteristics of the patients.

Both in the 1960's and the 1970's, men with little education showed a higher risk of death over five years of follow-up than better-educated, otherwise comparable men. Differences that might account for these findings could not be established from comparisons of the low- and high-education groups. We then sought ways to test the hypothesis that low education was serving here as a marker for relatively high levels of psychosocial stress which placed MI patients at excess risk of death.

Most recently, as an HIP ancillary study to the Beta Blocker Heart Attack Trial (BHAT), psychosocial interviews with 2320 male survivors of acute MI permitted definition of two variables strongly associated with increased 3-year mortality risk. With other important prognostic factors controlled, patients classified as socially isolated and at high life stress showed more than four times the risk of death found among men with low levels of both stress and isolation, as defined. High life stress and social isolation were most prevalent among the least educated men and least prevalent among the best educated. The inverse association of education with mortality in this post-MI population reflects the gradient in prevalence of the defined psychosocial characteristics.

Introduction

Prospective epidemiologic studies of coronary heart disease (CHD) have been carried out at HIP – the Health Insurance Plan of Greater New York – for almost 25 years. From a population insured for comprehensive medical services, defined groups of patients have participated in a number of studies of prognosis after myocardial infarction (MI). Throughout these years, we sought to assess the role both of clinical features and of personal and social characteristics of the patients, and the opportunity to sum up is welcome.

The issue to be addressed is the extent to which social or psychosocial factors influence mortality of men after MI. Associations between social and behavioral characteristics and CHD incidence or mortality have been examined in many published reports (Jenkins, 1971, 1976). In the U.S., years of schooling provide a stable and broadly applicable socioeconomic indicator in studies of adult mortality. Lack of education is a serious handicap that excludes individuals from achieving goals much valued in our contemporary society. Studies of population groups from the U.S. and other Western societies have reported inverse relationships between CHD mortality and education (Hinkle et al., 1968, Shekelle, 1968, Kitagawa and Hauser, 1973, Liu et al., 1982), employment grade (Marmot et al., 1978), and occupation (Koskenvuo et al., 1980). But, in contrast with comparisons of mortality rates, recent prospective studies of survival after MI have usually concentrated chiefly on clinical factors (Schulze et al., 1975, 1977; Hammermeister et al., 1979; Luria et al., 1979; Wilhelmsen et al., 1982).

Early HIP studies

At HIP, our first prognostic studies followed a cohort of 882 men who met specified criteria for a first MI in the years 1961-65 (Weinblatt et al., 1968, 1973). Within one month of onset, 36% of these men were dead. The one-month survivors were still at very high risk during the next 5 months, when the annualized mortality rate approached 9%. Thereafter, over the next 4 years, the rate dropped to an annual average of about 4%.

Our analyses assessed the role of age and of clinical features both in early (one-month) mortality and in long-term survival over a 5-year period. We also examined the influence on mortality of dichotomous variables defining race, religion, education, and occupation, controlling for age and for the distribution of important clinical factors (Shapiro et al., 1970). This analysis suggested a difference of possible importance in relation to occupation: in the later follow-up period, mortality of blue-collar workers was higher than that of white-collar men. Blue-collar survivors of acute MI also experienced more change in their way of life than comparable white-collar workers –

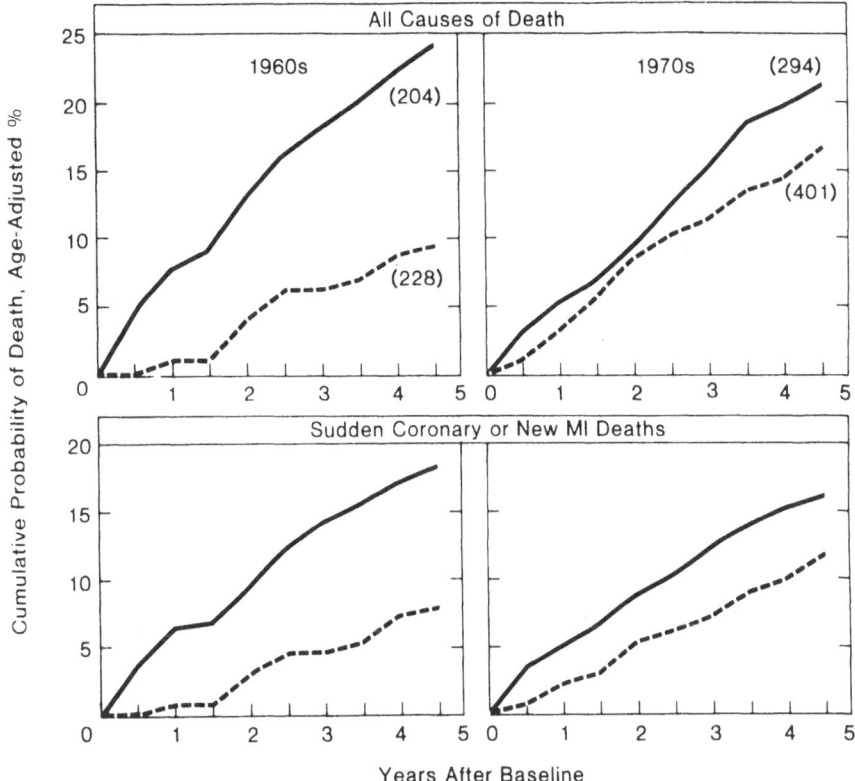

Figure 1. Mortality over 4½ years after baseline among male survivors of myocardial infarction (MI), two Health Insurance Plan coronary heart disease studies, by educational level. Solid line indicates less than 12 years of education; broken line, 12 years or more. Reprinted from Fig. 4, Weinblatt et al., 1982. JAMA 247:1576–1581. Copyright 1982, American Medical Association.

returning to work more slowly and more likely to return to a changed type of job or to exit from the labor force entirely (Weinblatt et al., 1966, Shapiro et al., 1972).

Education and post-MI prognosis.

In the early 1970's we started studies of a second cohort of HIP male MI survivors, with a major focus on the relation between post-MI ventricular arrhythmia and sudden death. On completion of these observations, interest in the possibility of illuminating the downward secular trend in CHD mortality in the U.S. led us to examine long-term prognosis in comparable age and diagnostic groups from the 1960's and 1970's HIP cohorts (Weinblatt et al., 1982). As shown in Fig. 1, this new analysis revealed a higher 4½-year mortality risk among men with less than 12 years of schooling in compari-

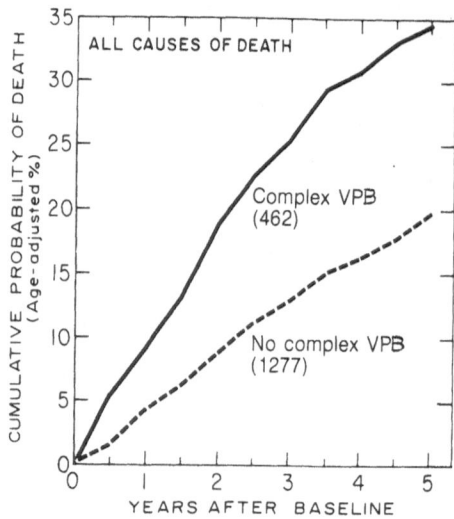

Figure 2. Mortality over 5 years in male survivors of myocardial infarction in relation to presence of complex ventricular premature beats (VPB) during 1 hour of baseline monitoring. Reprinted by permission of the American Heart Association, Inc. from Fig. 1, Ruberman et al., 1981. Ventricular premature complexes and sudden death after myocardial infarction. Circulation 64:297–305.

son with the better-educated. The differential appeared in both the 1960's and 1970's groups, but was more pronounced in the earlier period. Logrank comparisons of the 1960's survival data, with age and severity of disease controlled, showed that the low-education men had a mortality risk almost 3 times that of the better-educated ($p<0.01$).

Education again emerged as a powerful prognostic variable in our studies of the entire 1970's cohort, consisting of 1,739 male survivors of acute MI experienced during the 4 years 1972–75. These men had a baseline examination, usually within 3 months of hospital discharge, which included one hour of single-lead ECG monitoring for ventricular ectopic activity. Follow-up continued to April 1, 1978, at which time mortality status was known for all patients. We developed 3- and 5-year mortality estimates (Ruberman et al., 1977, Weinblatt et al., 1978), examining the influence on risk of death of complex ventricular beats (VPB) identified during one hour of ECG monitoring. Taking into account 16 important clinical variables in addition to age, we found that men with complex VPB had 3 times the risk of sudden coronary death and twice the risk of death from any cause shown by the men free of such arrhythmia in the monitoring hour. Fig. 2 shows cumulative probabilities for all causes of death in relation to the presence of complex VPB in the baseline monitoring hour.

Controlling for age, we next developed mortality estimates in relation to many personal and demographic features. Among these, only education discriminated between men at relatively high and low risk of death (Weinblatt et al., 1978). Patients who had completed 8 years of schooling or less showed a large disadvantage in comparison with better-educated men. The differential was especially pronounced with respect to risk of sudden coronary death, where the age-adjusted 3-year cumulative mortality risk was 13.1% for the low-education group and 5.6% for the better-educated. The difference in mortality risk between high- an low-education groups was localized among men who had demonstrated complex VPB in the monitoring hour. The excess risk for sudden death shown by the low-education men with complex VPB persisted throughout a cross-classification analysis involving many variables examined one at a time. In addition, multivariate analyses which controlled simultaneously for many factors showed that the low-education men with complex VPB had a 3-year sudden-death risk more than 3 times that of the comparable high-education men.

How explain the low education-mortality association?

Search for systematic differences between the low- and high-education groups in no case suggested even a partial explanation for these findings. We therefore reasoned that low education in our data could be serving as a marker for life circumstances characterized by high psychosocial stress, proposed by some as a trigger mechanism for converting a stable arrhythmia to lethal ventricular fibrillation (Lown and Verrier, 1976). We next explored methods to define and assess this postulated stress as a further research effort.

Thelephone interviews were used to obtain additional information on psychological, behavioral, and social characteristics of the men in the 1970's MI Cohort. Factor analysis of the questionnaire data extracted 4 psychosocial variables, but these were independent of the patients' educational level and did not account for the observed education-related difference in mortality risk (Ruberman et al., 1983). We were aware of methodologic problems that could have influenced the results of this pilot study. And, despite the negative findings, small differences in risk suggested by some of the analysis encouraged us to design a new research proposal as an ancillary study to the national β-Blocker Heart Attack Trial (BHAT).

The HIP-BHAT ancillary study

The BHAT clinical trial of propranolol was a multicenter, randomized, double-blind, and placebo-controlled research sponsored by the National Heart, Lung and Blood Institute (Beta-Blocker Heart Attack Trial Research Group 1982). Objectives of the HIP-HBAT ancillary study were to ascertain: (1) whether patients with relatively low and high levels of education showed

38

different distributions of psychosocial characteristics defined on the basis of interviews with men 6 weeks after MI; and (2) whether male MI survivors classified from the interview data as at high psychosocial stress showed an elevated risk of death when other factors influencing prognosis were controlled. A report on this study was recently published (Ruberman et al., 1984), and a summary of the main features and results is pertinent.

Candidates for enrollment in BHAT were men and women aged 30–69 years who were hospitalized with an acute MI meeting defined criteria. Exclusions appropriate to a clinical trial of propranolol were specified. The total target population for our ancillary study consisted of 2,572 males who had been randomized in the 25 BHAT centers that had agreed to cooperate in the study. HIP interviews were completed with 2,320 men, a 90% response. Trained BHAT personnel interviewed male patients face-to-face. The HIP questionnaire touched on ease and extent of communication between the patient and his family and between patient and medical personnel; on sleep patterns and traits reflecting personality and moods; on attitudes toward job and retirement, indicators of social relatedness, occurrence of and reaction to specified types of life crisis.

Four hypotheses, influencing the design of our questionnaire and analysis of the data, held that increased post-MI mortality risk would be associated with each of the following: (1) selected life circumstances producing reactions that suggest high levels of stress or difficulties in coping; (2) relatively high levels of social isolation, including difficulty in communicating with others about the illness; (3) the absence of qualities usually classified as strong Type A behavior pattern; and (4) depression. We used 20 questionnaire items to contstruct 4 dichotomous psychosocial variables corresponding to these 4 hypotheses. In addition, alternative analyses of the questionnaire data used several methods of factor analysis.

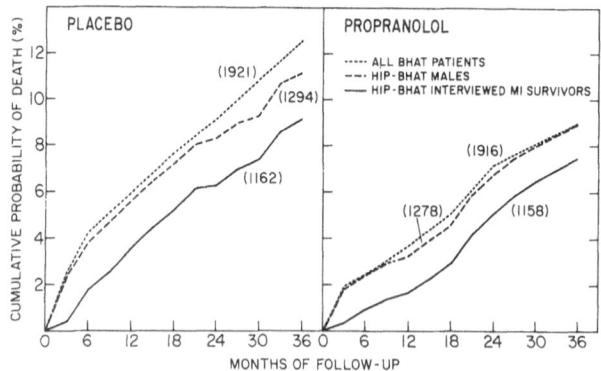

Figure 3. Life-table cumulative mortality curves for placebo and treatment groups, total Bhat and HIP-BHAT ancillary study. Reprinted by permission of The New England Journal of Medicine from Fig. 1, Ruberman et al., 1984. 311:552–559.

Target data for obtaining the HIP interview was the visit scheduled by BHAT at 6 weeks after entry, and no interviews could be obtained with patients who died before this date. Consequently, although the overall response rate for the interviews was 90%, it was only 70% of patients who died. The mortality estimates developed for the interviewed men express the experience of men who survived the acute MI by 2 to 3 months. Fig. 3 illustrates these relationships, showing cumulative 3-year mortality among treatment and placebo groups for the total BHAT study population, the total male population in the 25 ancillary study centers, and the interviewed population in those centers. The experience of the ancillary study population differs little from that of the entire trial. The lower mortality among the interviewed men reflects the absence of the early deaths.

We compared characteristics of the interviewed patients at 3 educational levels: less than 10 years, 10–12 years, and more than 12 years of schooling. As expected, the least educated were somewhat older than the best educated, and showed higher proportions of black and unmarried men and of cigarette smokers. Distribution of clinical findings varied little with education. But findings with respect to 2 of the psychosocial variables developed from the interview and defined in Table 1 were in sharp contrast. Fig. 4 shows pronounced inverse gradients in relation to education for both 'life stress' and 'social isolation' as we defined these variables from selected

Table 1. Definition of two psychosocial variables from the HIP-Bhat questionnaire

RELATIVELY HIGH LIFE STRESS — considered present if ONE OR MORE of the following statements is true:

- Patient is retired but would prefer to be working
- Last occupation before MI was relatively low-status job - clerical or sales, non-silled blue-collar, service
- Enjoyed this work 'not very much', or did not answer question
- In past year violent event (muggings/robberies/accidents) happened to patient/family/friends *and* patient's reaction was 'very upset'
- In past year divorce/break-up involving family members/friends occurred *and* patient's reaction was 'very upset'
- Major financial difficulty was experienced in preceding year

RELATIVELY HIGH LEVEL OF SOCIAL ISOLATION – considered present if TWO OR THREE of the following statements are true:

- Did not talk with medical personnel (while in hospital, or soon after discharge) about any possible need for life changes
- Around time of MI was not a member of any club, social or fraternal organization, church or synagogue
- Around the time of MI, Frequency of visiting friends of relatives in their homes was 'hardly ever'

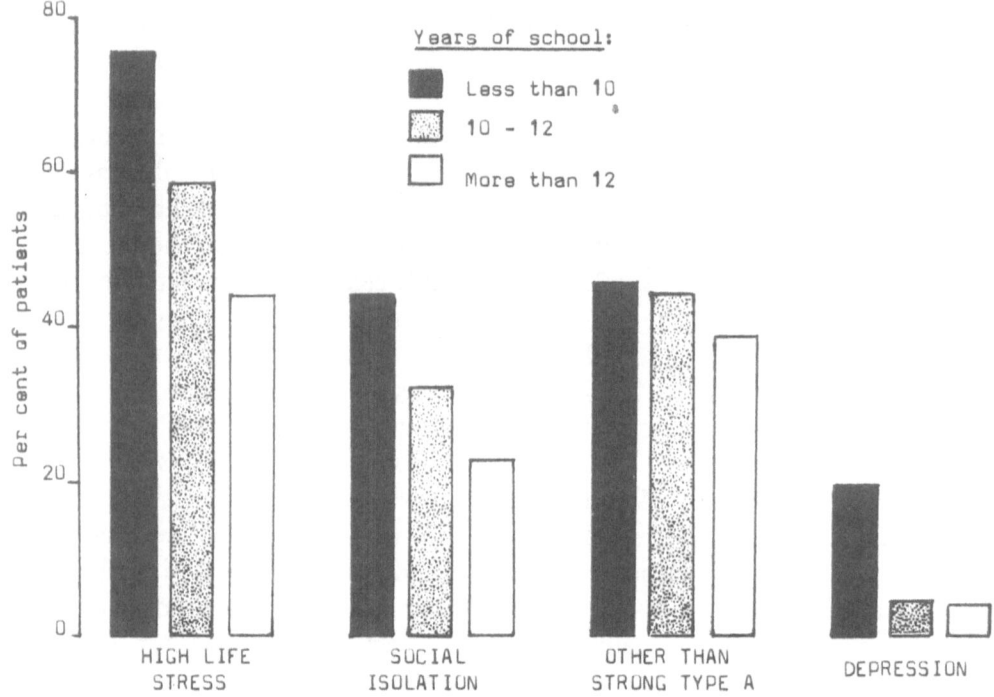

Figure 4. Prevalence of psychosocial categories defined from HIP-BHAT questionnaire in relation to educational level.

questionnaire items. No important differences in relation to education were suggested for the other 2 psychosocial variables.

Mortality in relation to education, life stress, social isolation

In Fig. 5 we examine mortality in relation to education and to the 2 psychosocial variables whose prevalence varied inversely with education. Over the 3-year period, risk of death is highest for the least educated, lowest for the best educated, and intermediate for the middle group. High life stress and high social isolation are each associated with roughly double the risk of the groups classified as low in these respects. And when the life stress and social isolation variables are combined, a large gradient in mortality risk is apparent. Logrank chi-squares to assess the statistical significance of differences among these 4 sets of curves all result in *p*-values of less than 0.001.

Fig. 6 presents life-table cumulative mortality curves in relation to both education and the combined life stress-social isolation variable. At each of

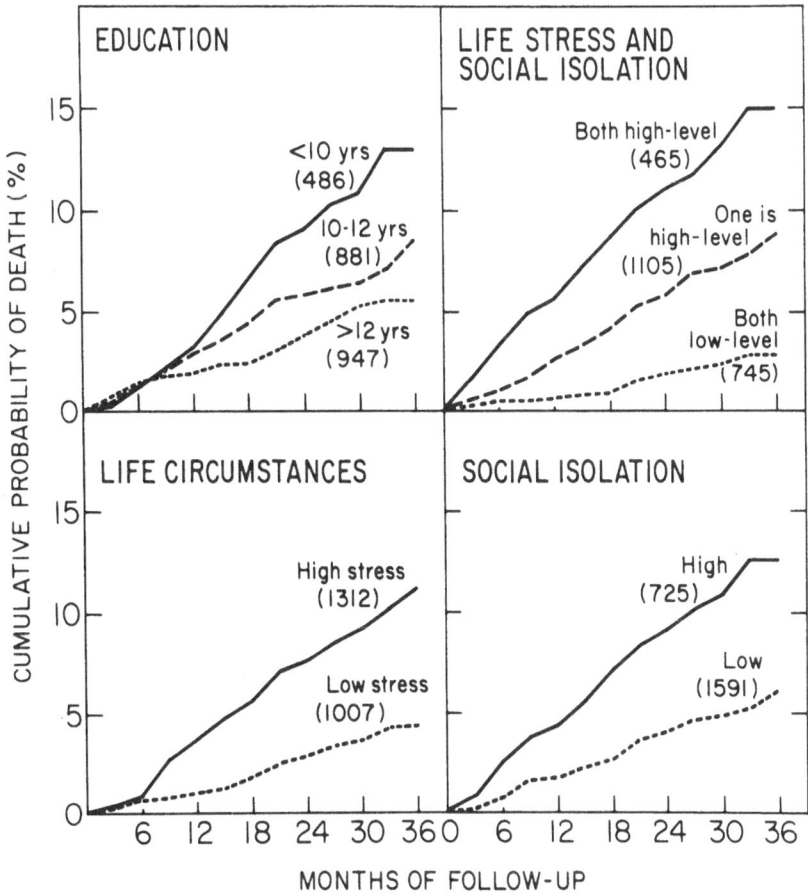

Figure 5. Life-table cumulative mortality curves for the HIP-BHAT male survivors of myocardial infarction who completed the psychosocial interview, according to levels of education, life stress (life circumstances), and social isolation. Reprinted by permission of The New England Journal of Medicine from Fig. 2, Ruberman et al., 1984. 311:552–559.

the 3 educational levels (panels A, B and C), there is a mortality gradient associated with the summary psychosocial variable. But when the curves are rearranged, on the right-hand side of the figure, no differential in mortality with respect to education is apparent, either when both life stress and isolation are low-level (D) or high-level (F). These data suggest that the high mortality risk associated with low education reflects the greater prevalence of high stress and high social isolation among the MI survivors with little schooling.

We next examined the influence on mortality of education and of psychosocial characteristics, taking into account other important prognostic variables. These multivariate analyses made extensive use of the Cox regression model, both to select appropriate non-redundant clinical, ECG, personal and psychosocial variables and to assess simultaneously the contributors of these variables to mortality risk (Cox, 1972).

42

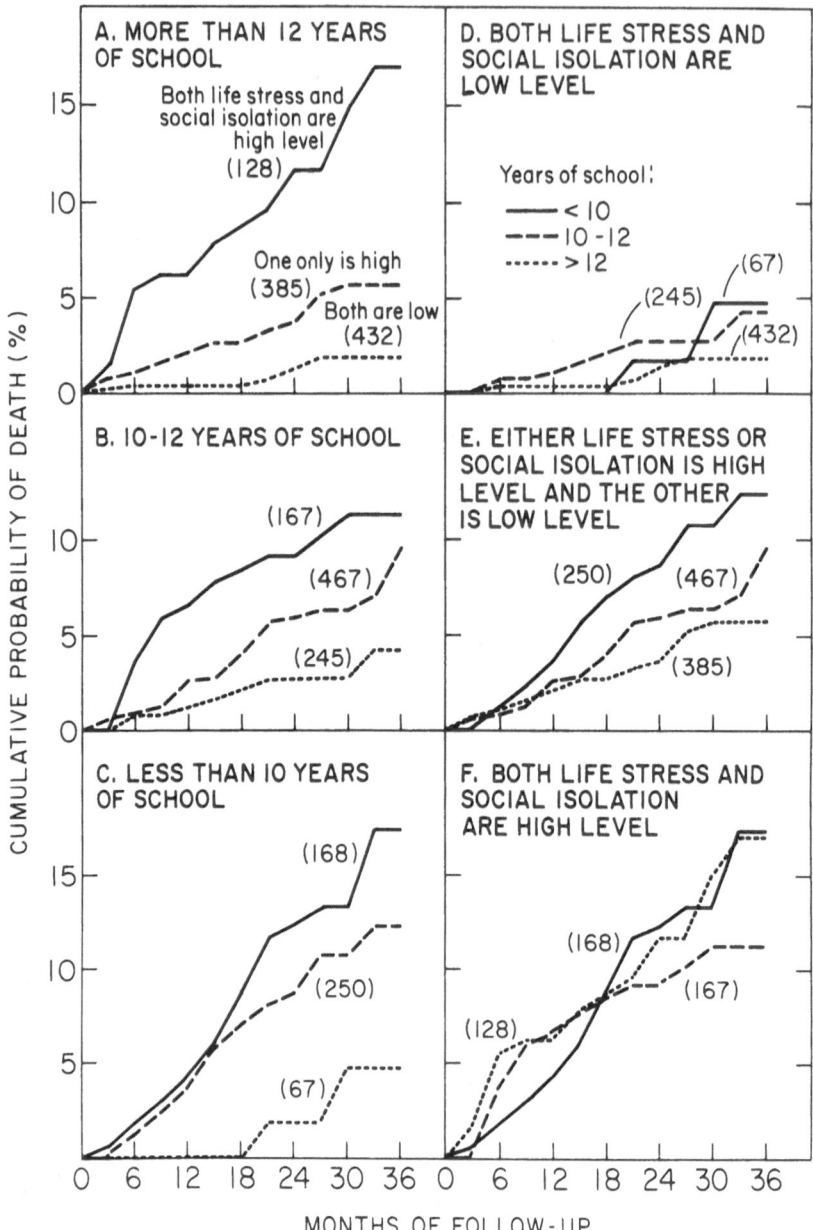

Figure 6. Life-table cumulative mortality curves according to education and specified psychosocial variables for the HIP-BHAT male survivors of myocardial infarction who completed the psychosocial interview. Reprinted by permission of The New England Journal of Medicine from Fig. 3, Ruberman et al., 1984. 311:552–559.

Table 2 summarizes the independent contributions to risk of death made by the most important variables identified in these analyses. Relative risk is computed from the estimated coefficients obtained from the Cox models. For 3-level variables this is the ratio of the class at highest risk to that at

Table 2. Estimated relative risk of death (all causes) over 3 years of follow-up (Based on Cox Multivariate Regression Models for Survival)

Variable making significant contribution to 3-year mortality risk in either patient group	Pts with psycho-social interview	Total HIP-BHAT study patients
Age: 60–69; 30–59	1.96	1.70
Myocardial function – number of positive components[b]: 2 or more; one only; none	3.05[a]	3.50[a]
Ventricular arrhythmia – % of HM hours with CPB: $\geqslant 50\%$; $\geqslant 10\%$; $<50\%$; $<10\%$	3.82[a]	3.60[a]
Cigarette smoking (at MI onset): yes; no	1.75	1.55
Angina (MD opinion): yes; no		1.36
Treatment group: placebo; propranolol		1.38
Education (years of school): <10; 10–12; >12		1.63
Psychosocial variables, life stress & social isolation: both high; one only is high; both low	4.56[a]	Not applicable
Chi-square (degrees of freedom)	132.3 (5)	159.2 (7)
P-value	<0.001	<0.001
Number of patients, known values for all variables	2062	2286
Number of deaths	128	184

[a] Indicates 3-level variable where the relative risk shown is the ratio of the class at highest risk to that at lowest risk. Other variables are dichotomous.

[b] Positive components for the myocardial function summary are: (1) prior MI; (2) heart rate exceeding 80; (3) congestive failure by baseline; (4) taking digitalis at baseline

lowest risk; for dichotomies it is the ratio of the higher-risk group to the lower. Among both interviewed patients and total study males, those in the poorest myocardial-function class and men with the highest degree of ventricular arrhythmia show between 3 and 4 times the risk of the least compromised category. In both groups older men (ages 60–69) have a risk almost twice that of the younger men, and cigarette smokers show a higher risk than non-smokers.

Education is a significant independent influence on mortality only in the total group of men, where the interview-derived variables were not available for entry into the model. Among the interviewed men, the life stress-social isolation variable substituted for education in the final model. The risk of death associated with high levels of both life stress and social isolation is 4 to 5 times that for men in whom both these categories are low, with the influence of all other variables in the model controlled.

Table 3. Estimated relative risk of sudden ASHD death over 3 years of follow-up (Based on Cox Multivariate Regression Models for Survival)

Variable making significant contribution to 3-year mortality risk in either patient group	Pts with psycho-social interview	Total HIP-BHAT study patients
Myocardial function – number of positive components: 2 or more; one only; none	3.76 [a]	3.79 [a]
Ventricular arrhythmia – % of HM hours with VPB: $\geq 50\%$; $\geq 10\%$, $< 50\%$; $< 10\%$	5.74 [a]	5.72 [a]
Education (years of school): < 10; 10–12; > 12		2.04 [a]
Psychosocial variables, life stress & social isolation: both high; one only is high; both low	5.62 [a]	Not applicable
Chi-square (degrees of freedom)	81.9 (3)	90.1 (3)
P-value	< 0.001	< 0.001
Number of patients, known values for all variables	2062	2286
Number of deaths	68	97

[a] All variables in this table are 3-level, and the relative risk shown is the ratio of the class at highest risk to that at lowest risk.

Table 3 summarizes multivariate analyses using sudden cardiac death as the end point. For the total study group the significant variables are myocardial function, ventricular arrhythmia, and education. Among the interviewed men, for sudden death as for all causes of death, education is replaced by the life stress-social isolation variable. The risk associated with the highest level of this variable relative to that for the lowest level is of the same order of magnitude as that associated with much ventricular arrhythmia.

Caution in generalizing from these data must stem from the rather crude questionnaire, from the selected nature of the BHAT study population, and from our lack of information about the psychosocial characteristics of the missed early deaths. Our findings apply to men from this population who survived the acute MI by 2–3 months. Defined in this way, the results suggest a reasonable explanation for the unfavorable experience of patients with little education, found in the earlier HIP studies and in the BHAT study. We should note that a number of studies have found bereavement (Rees and Lutkins, 1967, Parkes et al., 1969, Helsing and Szklo, 1981) and lack of social and community ties (Berkman and Syme, 1979, Blazer, 1982) to be associated with an overall increase in mortality in general populations.

Neither strength of Type A behavior pattern nor depression as defined from our questionnaire data showed any influence on mortality when we controlled for other important variables. The questionnaire is probably inadequate for identifying depressed patients. But our negative findings with respect to behavior pattern are consistent with results from some other studies (Marmot, 1982, Case et al., 1983, Shekelle et al., 1983).

Our results support 2 of the 4 hypotheses proposed at the start of this study, and we conclude that social and psychosocial factors, as well as clinical ones, exert an important independent influence on 3-year mortality among male MI survivors. Awareness of this impact on the part of physicians and other health workers can perhaps improve the counseling of post-MI patients – in particular, those with little education – to help them cope better with threats from this area of their lives.

References

1. Berkman LF, Syme L: Social networks, host resistance, and mortality: a nine-year follow-up study of Alameda County residents. Am J Epidemiol 109:186–204, 1979.
2. Beta-Blocker Heart Attack Trial Research Group: A randomized trial of propranolol in patients with acute myocardial infarction. I. Mortality results. JAMA 247:1707–1714, 1982.
3. Blazer DG: Social support and mortality in an elderly community population. Am J Epidemiol 115:684–694, 1982.
4. Case RB, Heller SS, Shamai E, MPIP Collaborators: Type A behavior and survival after myocardial infarction. Circulation 68 (Part II):III-29, 1983.
5. Cox DR: Regression models and life tables. J R Stat Soc (B) 34:187–220, 1972.
6. Hammermeister KE, DeRouen TA, Dodge HT: Variables predictive of survival in patients with coronary disease. Selection by univariate and multivariate analyses from the clinical, electrocardiographic, exercise, arteriographic and quantitative angiographic evaluations. Circulation 59:421–435, 1979.
7. Helsing KJ, Szklo M: Mortality after bereavement. Am J Epidemiol 114:41–52, 1981.
8. Helsing KJ, Szklo M: Factors associated with mortality after widowhood. Am J Publ Health 71:802–809, 1981.
9. Hinkle LE Jr, Whitney LH, Lehman EW, Dunn J, Bry B, King R, Plakun A, Flehinger B: Occupation, education, and coronary heart disease. Science 161:238–246, 1968.
10. Jenkins CD: Psychologic and social precursors of coronary disease. N Engl J Med 284:244–255, 307–317, 1971.
11. Jenkins CD: Recent evidence supporting psychologic social risk factors for coronary disease. N Engl J Med 294:987–994, 1033–1038, 1976.
12. Kitagawa EM, Hauser PM: Differential mortality in the United States. A study in socioeconomic epidemiology. Harvard University Press, Cambridge, 1973.
13. Koskenvuo M, Kaprio J, Kesäniemi A, Sarna S: Differences in mortality from ischemic heart disease by marital status and social class. J Chron Dis 33:95–105, 1980.
14. Liu K, Cedres LB, Stamler J, Dyer A, Stamler R, Nanas S, Berkson DM, Paul O, Lepper M, Lindberg HA, Marquardt J, Stevens E, Schoenberger JA, Shekelle RB, Collette P, Shekelle S, Garside D: Relationship of education to major risk factors and death from coronary heart disease, cardiovascular disease and all causes. Circulation 66:1308–1314, 1982.

15. Lown B, Verrier RL: Neural activity and ventricular fibrillation. N Engl J Med 294:1165–1170, 1976.
16. Luria MH, Knoke JD, Wachs JS, Luria MA: Survival after recovery from acute myocardial infarction. Two and five year prognostic indices. Am J Med 67:7–14, 1979.
17. Marmot MG, Rose G, Shipley M, Hamilton PJS: Employment grade and coronary heart disease in British civil servants. J Epidemiol and Community Health 32:244–249, 1978.
18. Marmot MG: Socio-economic and cultural factors in ischaemic heart disease. Adv Cardiol 29:68–76, 1982.
19. Parkes CM, Benjamin B, Fitzgerald RG: Broken heart: a statistical study of increased mortality among widowers. Br Med J 1:740–743, 1969.
20. Rees WD, Lutkins SG: Mortality of bereavement. Br Med J 4:13–16, 1967.
21. Ruberman W, Weinblatt E, Goldberg JD, Frank CW, Shapiro S: Ventricular premature beats and mortality after myocardial infarction. N Engl J Med 297:750–757, 1977.
22. Ruberman W, Weinblatt E, Goldberg JD, Frank CW, Chaudhary BS, Shapiro S: Ventricular premature complexes and sudden death after myocardial infarction. Circulation 64:297–305, 1981.
23. Ruberman W, Weinblatt E, Goldberg JD, Chaudhary BS: Education, psychosocial stress and sudden cardiac death. J Chron Dis 36:151–160, 1983.
24. Ruberman W, Weinblatt E, Goldberg JD, Chaudhary BS: Psychosocial influences on mortality after myocardial infarction. N Engl J Med 311:552–559, 1984.
25. Schulze RA Jr, Rouleau J, Rigo P, Bowers S, Strauss HW, Pitt B: Ventricular arrhythmias in the late hospital phase of acute myocardial infarction. Relation to left ventricular function detected by gated cardiac blood pool scanning. Circulation 52:1006–1011, 1975.
26. Schulze RA Jr, Strauss HW, Pitt B: Sudden death in the year following myocardial infarction: Relation to ventricular premature contractions in the late hospital phase and left ventricular ejection fraction. Am J Med 62:192–199, 1977.
27. Shapiro S, Weinblatt E, Frank CW, Sager RV: Social factors in the prognosis of men following first myocardial infarction. Milbank Memorial Fund Quarterly 48:37–50, 1970.
28. Shapiro S, Weinblatt E, Frank CW: Return to work after first myocardial infarction. Arch Envir Health 24:17–26, 1972.
29. Shekelle RB: Educational status and risk of coronary heart disease. Science 163:97–98, 1969.
30. Shekelle R, Hulley S, Neaton J et al. for the MRFIT Research Group: Type A behavior and risk of coronary death in MRFIT. Presented at the 23rd Conference on Cardiovascular Disease Epidemiology, San Diego, California, March 3-5, 1983.
31. Weinblatt e, Shapiro S, Frank CW, Sager RV: Return to work and work status following first myocardial infarction. Am J Publ Health 56:169–185, 1966.
32. Weinblatt E, Shapiro S, Frank CW, Sager RV: Prognosis of men after first myocardial infarction: mortality and first recurrence in relation to selected parameters. Am J Publ Health 58:1329–1347, 1968.
33. Weinblatt E, Shapiro S, Frank CW: Prognosis of women with newly diagnosed coronary heart disease – a comparison with course of disease among men. Am J Publ Health 63:577–593, 1973.
34. Weinblatt E, Ruberman W, Goldberg JD, Frank CW, Shapiro S, Chaudhary BS: Relation of education to sudden death after myocardial infarction. N Engl J Med 299:60–65, 1978.
35. Weinblatt E, Goldberg JD, Ruberman W, Frank CW, Monk MA, Chaudhary BS: Mortality after first myocardial infarction. Search for a secular trend. JAMA 247:1576–1581, 1982.
36. Wihelmsen L, Wilhelmsson C, Vedin A, Elmfeldt D: Effects of infarct size, smoking, Physical activity and some psychological factors on prognosis after myocardial infarction. Adv Cardiol 29:119–125, 1982.

6. The Impact of Social Level on Prognosis After Myocardial Infarction

H. GOHLKE, P. BETZ and H. ROSKAMM

Abstract

Previous studies have suggested that the prognosis after MI may be dependent on social class and the educational level of the patient. The purpose of the present study was to examine the prognostic importance of these factors in a patient cohort undergoing a comprehensive rehabilitation program.

The baseline characteristics and the longterm prognosis of 627 male patients who had survived the acute phase of a transmural MI before age 40 were analyzed.

These patients had undergone coronary angiography and ventriculography irrespective of clinical status or symptoms within 12 months after MI. In addition all patients underwent evaluation of supine exercise hemodynamics with determination of cardiac index at rest and during the highest exercise level. The mean follow-up was 4.5 years.

The 8 year survival rate was 84.5% for BC workers and 80.6% for WC workers (p = n.s.). Stratification according to the educational level failed to show differences in survival up to 8 years. Multivariate analysis (Cox model), including 17 variables relating to age, extent of CAD, left ventricular function, exercise hemodynamics, risk factors, social status and educational level, revealed that maximal cardiac index achieved during exercise was the most important variable correlating with survival.

In patients undergoing a comprehensive rehabilitation program after MI, the social situation and the educational level were of no prognostic importance. However, functional and angiographic variables were strong determinants of prognosis.

Introduction

The social class has been shown to play an important role for the prevalence of coronary heart disease and for the incidence of cardiac death (Rose and Marmot, 1981).

Whereas previously coronary heart disease was thought to be associated with those classes of society or those professionals that are subjected to excessive mental or emotional stress (Price, 1941, Friedberg, 1966), several reports in recent decades have emphasized the higher prevalence of coronary disease and its manifestations in the lower social economic strata of the society (Rose and Marmot, 1981, Antonovsky, 1968).

Studies from the United States have suggested that the prognosis of survivors of a first myocardial infarction is related to the level of education although some mitigation of this difference has occurred in the 1970ies (Weinblatt et al., 1978, 1982).

The purpose of the present investigation was to analyze the prognostic importance of the educational level and of the physical job requirements in young survivors of a transmural myocardial infarction in relation to other prognostic variables.

Methods

Patient Population

627 young (< 40 years old) male survivors of the acute phase of a transmural myocardial infarction constitute the study population. These patients had undergone coronary angiography and exercise testing with evaluation of exercise hemodynamics within 12 months after the acute event (Gohlke et al., 1983, Roskamm et al., 1984).

In addition all patients underwent a physical rehabilitation program and a teaching program with emphasis on risk factor modification.

Variables Examined

At the time of admission a history of the educational level was taken. Patients were grouped into 3 subgroups according to the length and intensity of their formal education. Group I was constituted of patients with 10 or less years of school education who were unskilled or semiskilled. Group II included skilled workers who had finished a formal job training program, and group III included patients with highschool training and a university degree.

In addition the physical job requirements were evaluated for each patient at the time of admission. Patients whose job required predominantly physical labor were labelled as 'blue collar workers', patients with predominantly non physical work such as clerical, administrative or professional work were labelled as 'white collar workers'.

Aside from these variables related to the social level, 15 other variables related to angiographic findings such as the angiographic extent of coronary disease, extent of left ventricular dysfunction, as well as variables related to exercise performance such as exercise tolerance, cardiac index at rest and during the highest work load, as well as variables related to the risk factor profile, heart size, and age, were included in the analysis.

Follow up

Follow up was obtained by a written questionnaire or by repeat visits in our outpatient department. Follow up was 98.6% complete.

Statistical Analysis

Survival curves were computed according to Cutler and Ederer (1958). The comparison of survival rates between the different groups were tested according to the method of Mantle and Haenszel (1959).

The correlation between the individual variables and subsequent death was determined by use of multivariate analysis with the proportional hazards regression model of Cox (1972). Calculations were performed on a VAX 750 computer.

Results

Of the 627 male patients 324 were classified as blue collar workers, and 233 as white collar workers. Mean age for the total group was 35.6 years. Of the baseline variables relating to extent of coronary disease, left ventricular dysfunction, functional exercise parameters, and risk factors, only cardiac index at rest and serum triglyceride levels were different between the two groups (Table 1). The 8-year survival rate was 84.5% for blue collar workers, and 80.6% for white collar workers. This slight difference in favour of blue collar workers was not significant (Fig. 1).

If patients were stratified into three groups according to the level of education, i.e. in unskilled or semiskilled workers, skilled workers and patients with a university degree, the analysis of variance of baseline variables showed only small differences for the maximal blood pressure during exercise ($p < 0.05$) and heart volume per square meters body surface area ($p < 0.005$). Because of the problem associated with multiple comparisons these differences can still be considered random variations.

Longterm prognosis of these three groups with different levels of educa-

Table 1. Baseline variables in blue and white collar workers

	Blue Collar	White Collar
Mean age	35.5±3.7	35.8±3.5
Extent of CAD		
– Kaltenbach score	20.2±12	21.2±15
– Friesinger score	6.5±3.4	6.7±3.2
LV score	6.3±3.1	6.0±3.3
LVEDP (mm Hg)	14.9±7.2	15.3±7.3
Exercise tolerance (watt)	105±37	103±37
Angina-free exercise tolerance (watt)	98±44	97±42
Pulmonary capillary wedge pressure (mmHg)		
– at rest	11.1±4.5	11.2±5.3
– at highest work load	18.6±10	19.7±10
Cardiac index $(l/min \times m^2)$		
– at rest	3.07±0.5	3.19±0.7 (p<0.02)
– at highest work load	8.0±1.8	8.0±2.0
Serum cholesterol (mg/dl)	276±61	278±65
Serum triglycerides (mg/dl)	269±144	243±112 (p<0.03)

Survival rate of Blue- and White Collar Workers after MI

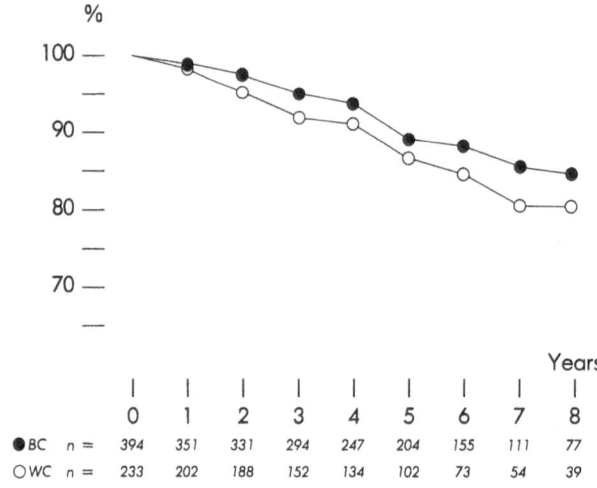

tion did not show significant differences. There was no trend for better survival of patients with better education (Fig. 2).

We also analyzed other variables which have previously been shown to be strong predictors of prognosis in different subgroups of patients with coronary disease (Gohlke et al., 1983).

Survival rate after MI in relation to the educational level

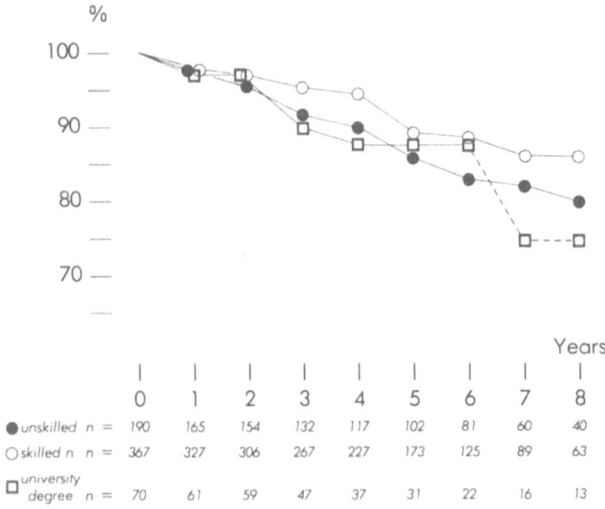

		0	1	2	3	4	5	6	7	8
● unskilled	n =	190	165	154	132	117	102	81	60	40
○ skilled n	n =	367	327	306	267	227	173	125	89	63
□ university degree	n =	70	61	59	47	37	31	22	16	13

The exercise tolerance was in this group of young myocardial infarction patients of prognostic importance: Patients with an exercise tolerance of < 100 watts had a significantly less favourable prognosis than patients with better exercise tolerance: 5 year survival 85% vs 93% ($p < 0.0002$).

Of even greater importance was the maximal cardiac index achieved during exercise. Patients able to achieve a cardiac index of more than 8 l/min and square meters body surface area had a significantly better survival with 95% at 5 years than patients who were able to achieve only a lower cardiac index; these had a 5 year survival rate of 82% ($p < 0.00001$) (Gohlke, 1983).

Uni- and multivariate analysis of 17 variables related to exercise performance, angiographic findings, risk factors, and social status revealed that the maximal cardiac index achieved during exercise is the most important variable correlating with survival. Variables related to the social status or level of education were of no prognostic importance in this patient cohort (Table 2).

Discussion

Previous studies have related the differences in survival after myocardial infarction between patient groups in different social strata largely to differences in education (Weinblatt et al., 1978, 1982). Better educated patients

Table 2. Univariate and multivariate analysis of variables correlating with death after MI ($n = 567$)

	Chi-square analysis	
	Univariate	Multivariate
Cardiac index$_{max}$	38.95	38.9
Pulm. cap. wedge pressure$_{max}$	30.36	4.8
Exercise tolerance	30.13	
Kaltenbach score	28.16	9.6
Angina free exercise tolerance	21.55	
Heart size	20.20	7.9
Pulm. cap. wedge pressure$_{rest}$	17.40	
LV-score	14.18	
Serum cholesterin	6.78	3.1
Serum triglycerides	2.56	
Blue/white collar occupation	1.24	
Educational level	0.61	
Age	0.58	
Global chi-square		85.91

may be more responsive to medical advice on diet, nicotine consumption, weight loss or exercise. If the rehabilitation program was successful in improving knowledge on the importance of risk factors and in achieving behaviour modification after myocardial infarction in the less educated patients the lack of difference in prognosis between the different social levels could be explained. The educational intervention after myocardial infarction in this group of patients was probably more intense than in any of the other reported studies. However, the success of the educational efforts in improving knowledge on risk factors and achieving behaviour modification was not assessed. Other reasons for failing to show the importance of social class for the prognosis should also be considered: The low overall mortality during follow up in this rather young age group, contrasts to markedly higher mortality in other studies (Weinblatt et al., 1978, 1982).

Because of the limited age spectrum the number of patients in our study is small; however, in contrast to previous studies, our study affords the possibility of comparing the prognostic importance of the social level with that of other non invasive and invasive parameters.

The social gradient has been shown to be of greater prognostic importance in females than in males (Rose and Marmot, 1981); females were not included in our study.

Finally, the sector of the social spectrum included in this study may be narrower than in studies from the United States, because of different socioeconomic conditions in these countries. In our study the unemployed and indigent or poor may be underrepresented.

Summary

In summary, in young male survivors of the acute phase of transmural myocardial infarction who have undergone a comprehensive cardiac rehabilitation program, the educational level and the physical job requirements do not play a significant role for longterm survival.

In asmuch as the educational level and the physical job requirements can be considered markers of the social level, the latter has lost its importance for survival.

References

Antonovsky A: Social class and the major cardiovascular diseases. J Chron Dis 21:65–106, 1960.

Cox DR: Regression models and life tables. Jr Stat Soc 22:719–726, 1972.

Cutler S, Ederer F: Maximum utilization of life table method in analyzing survival. J Chron Dis 8:34:187–219, 1958-

Friedberg CK: Diseases of the heart, 3rd edn. WB Saunders, Philadelphia, London, p 650, 1966.

Gohlke H: Der transmurale Herzinfarkt vor dem 40. Legensjahr. Anamnese, Risikofaktorenprofil, hämodynamische und angiographische Befunde, Progression der Koronarsklerose und Langzeitprognose. Habilitationsschrift, Freiburg i. Br, 1983.

Gohlke H, Samek L, Betz P, Roskamm H: Exercise testing provides additional prognostic information in angiographically defined subgroups of patients with coronary artery disease. Circulation 68:979–985, 1983.

Mantel N, Haenszel W: Statistical aspects of the analysis of data from retrospective studies. JNCJ 22:719–726, 1958.

Price FW: A textbook of the practice of medicine. 6th edn. Oxford University press, p 981, ed/1941.

Rose G, Marmot MG: Social class and coronary heart disease. Brit Heat J 45:13–19, 1981.

Roskamm H Gohlke H, Stürzenhofecker P, Droste C, Thomas H, Samek L, Schnellbacher K, Betz P: Der Herzinfarkt im jugendlichen Alter (unter 40 Jahren) Koronarmorphologie, Risikofaktoren, Langzeitprognose der Erkrankung und Progression der Koronargefäßklerose. Z Kardiol 72:1–11, 1983.

Weinblatt E, Goldberg JD, Ruberman W, Frank CW, Monk MA, Chaudhary BS: Mortality after first myocardial infarction — search for a secular trend. JAMA 247:1576–1581, 1982.

Weinblatt E, Ruberman W, Goldberg JD et al.: Relation of education to sudden death after myocardial infarction. New Engl J Med 299:60–65, 1978.

7. Social Class and Prognosis in Coronary Heart Disease

N. HICKEY

Abstract

The relationship between social class and prognosis was studied in 299 successive men under 60 years who survived a first attack of acute coronary heart disease (CHD). Indices of prognosis included risk-factors, return to work and 3-year mortality. Occupation was used as the index of social class.

Risk-factors were uniformely distributed in the different social groups at entry to the study. Over 3 years a highly significant association was noted between social class and risk-factor changes. Cigarette smoking, level of exercise and weight showed a significant improvement in the higher social classes.

90% of patients had returned to work after one year. While lower special classes were significantly slower in returning to work there was no significant relationship between social class and re-employment.

The 3-year mortality was not influenced by social class despite the difference in risk-factor changes.

It is concluded that an independent influence of social class on return to work and on mortality is not apparent. However, further study is needed to determine the effect of poor compliance on subsequent morbidity and mortality.

Introduction

There is a persisting social class difference in morbidity, mortality and health service use (Report of a research working group, London, DHSS, 1980). It has been suggested that social class is a useful description of life styles (McCarthy, 1983) which could explain the higher mortality from coronary heart disease in working class as compared to middle-class (Joint Working Party: Report, 1976).

Mulcahy et al. (1984) reported an excess of coronary risk factors among Irishmen in the lowest social classes. Because of the relationship between risk-factors and prognosis from coronary heart disease (Mulcahy et al., 1975) it might be expected that social class differences would be apparent in prognosis.

The present report examines the relationship between social class and coronary heart disease prognosis in 299 male patients.

Materials and methods

Between February 1978 and January 1982, 299 consecutive male patients under 60 years survived an acute coronary episode by at least 28 days. Details of coronary risk-factors were recorded as well as occupation, and patients were followed at a special cardiac rehabilitation clinic for at least two years. Follow-up examinations were performed at three weeks, three months, six months, one year and two years.

Risk-factors measured included: smoking habits, total serum cholesterol, blood pressure, physical activity and weight. The number of cigarettes or cigars smoked and the duration of smoking was recorded. Serum cholesterol was measured by autoanalyser. Blood pressure was measured with the mercury sphygmomanometer, the mean of several readings during the third day of admission being recorded. Diastolic pressure was recorded at phase five (disappearance of sounds). Hypertension was recorded in patients who had one or more of the following criteria:

1. In-patient diastolic pressure greater than 90 mm Hg.
2. Diastolic pressure in excess of 110 mm Hg at follow-up visits.
3. History of treated hypertension.
4. History of past hypertension with electrocardiographic evidence of left ventricular hypertrophy or hypertensive retinopathy.

Physical activity was recorded for work and for leisure. Minimal exercise during leisure was defined as non-vigorous and non-consistent exercise, such as occasional leisurely walking or its equivalent. Weight was measured in kilogrammes to the nearest half kilo and height was recorded in centimeters. Body Mass Index (BMI) was calculated as the ratio of weight in kilos to the square of height in metres.

Social class was categorised into five groups by occupation, employing the occupational grading scale of the British Registrar General.

Only patients with confirmed acute myocardial infarction and unstable angina were included in this study. Myocardial infarction was diagnosed in the presence of cardiac rest pain with fresh Q waves in the ECG and/or a greater than twofold rise in enzymes. Unstable angina was defined as rest pain, normal enzymes and serial ST-T changes in the ECG.

During their hospital stay and at each follow-up visit, patients were given advice and treatment for risk-factors. Smokers were encouraged to stop smoking. An individually planned exercise programme was outlined for patients who took minimal exercise and patients with BMI greater than 25 were encouraged to lose weight. Dietary advice was given to all patients in relation to serum cholesterol with especial interest taken in those with cholesterol levels in excess of 260 mg/dl.

All patients were encouraged to return to work early after discharge, this being considered an important component of successful management.

Prophylactic drugs were not employed in the 299 patients included in this report.

Results

Table 1 shows the number and percentage of patients with risk-factors in the five social classes. Of the 299 patients, 114 (38.1%) had serum cholesterol levels greater than 260 mg/dl and 67 (22.4%) were classed as hypertensives. 162 (54.2%) of patients were cigarette smokers, 183 (61.2%) took minimal leisure exercise and 146 (48.8%) had a BMI greater than 25.

Except for cigarette smoking, none of the other risk-categories were significantly associated with social class. A marked gradient in the percentage of smokers in the different social classes was observed from 30.8% in class II to 79.2% in class V (Tau = 0.26, $p < 0.001$).

Although no correlation was found between hypertension status and social class, a significant correlation was observed for mean inpatient blood pressure and social class.

Table 2 shows the change in risk-factor status among the five social classes after one year. Cessation of cigarette smoking was significantly correlated with social class, social classes IV and V exhibiting the poorest cessation rate. In the early weeks following discharge from hospital similar proportions of patients in each social class had stopped smoking. Of the patients initially classed as performing minimal leisure exercise, significant-

Table 1. Initial risk-factors and social class Number (%) of patients in risk categories

Social Class	Total Number	Ser. Chol. <260 mg/dl	Hypertension	Cig. Smokers	In-activity	BMI >25.
1	26	9 (34.6)	4 (15.4)	8 (30.8)	16 (61.5)	14 (53.8)
2	96	37 (38.5)	18 (18.8)	40 (41.7)	60 (62.5)	48 (50.0)
3	81	34 (41.9)	22 (27.2)	46 (56.8)	50 (61.7)	42 (51.9)
4	72	28 (38.9)	17 (23.6)	49 (68.1)	41 (56.9)	33 (45.8)
5	24	6 (25.0)	6 (25.0)	19 (79.2)	16 (66.6)	9 (37.5)
all	299	114 (38.1)	67 (22.4)	162 (54.2)	183 (61.2)	146 (48.8)

Table 2. Social class and risk factor changes at one year, Percentage Patients

Social class.	Smoking		Exercise		BMI	
	Stopped	Continued	Increase	No change	Less 25	25 & over.
1	71.4	28.6	61.5	38.5	45.5	55.5
2	82.1	17.9	61.5	38.4	35.3	64.7
3	78.9	21.1	32.4	67.5	36.7	63.3
4	52.9	47.1	42.9	57.2	22.2	77.8
5	50.0	50.0	8.3	91.7	0.0	100.0

Table 3. Return to work by social class

Social Class	% 1-Year Return to work
1	84.0
2	95.3
3	90.9
4	85.2
5	77.3

ly more patients in social classes I and II increased and maintained the increase in exercise compared with patients in the other social classes. Although overweight was not related to social class at admission, social class correlated with weight loss after 1 year. 11 (45.5) patients in social class I initially overweight, had achieved a reduction of BMI to less than 25 compared with none (0%) patients in social class V.

No significant social class differences were observed for serum cholesterol and blood pressure at 1 year.

Table 3 records the employment status at 1 year of patients who had not retired and were working prior to admission. No significant social class difference in return to work was found, although at 1 year the rate was lowest (77.3%) in social class V.

Table 4 shows the total mortality over 3 years of follow-up. No differences are apparent over the first 2 years. Because of the small numbers in social class I and V over a 3-year follow-up, the apparent excess mortality in social class V is not significant.

Discussion

Cultural and psychosocial factors are important influences on the health of the community. Many of the primary risk-factors for coronary heart disease, such as smoking, overweight, inactivity and serum cholesterol are products

Table 4. Social class and total mortality

| Social Class | Percentage deaths at follow-up | | |
	1-Year	2-Years	3-Years
1	4.1	13.4	13.4
2	7.4	7.4	11.8
3	7.6	13.0	18.0
4	7.2	11.6	18.7
5	4.3	8.7	23.9

of social and individual behaviour and are related to socio-economic class and level of education.

The present study outlines in particular the strong association between social class and response to risk-factor intervention in men following acute coronary heart disease. All patients included in the study received the same level of medical care including advice on risk-factors. The response in terms of risk-factor reduction was significantly worse in class IV and V. Although similar proportions of patients in all social classes stopped smoking for the initial weeks post coronary, significicatnly more of the lower social classes resumed smoking subsequently. Similarly, failure to maintain an exercise programme was more apparent in the lower social classes. The strong relationship between overweight, eating habits and social class (Stunkard, 1975) is supported in this study by the marked social class difference in response to overweight intervention.

The effect of social class on re-employment after coronary disease is not so apparent. Only a small number of patients were still unemployed at 1 year, confirming previous reports on different patient groups (Mulcahy & Hickey, 1970). Nevertheless, return to work rates were better among patients in the high social classes. Reasons for failure in returning to work were examined but because of small numbers no association with social class could be determined.

Mulcahy et al. (1975) have shown that in the early years following acute coronary heart disease, the presence of clinical complications at time of attack and subsequent smoking habits are important determinants of long-term survival. In particular, complications are associated with a high mortality in the first year. This may explain in this study the inability to demonstrate any relationship between social class and mortality. No social class difference was observed between patients in the three diagnostic categories, uncomplicated infarction, complicated infarction and unstable angina. In addition, the variable follow-up period of from one to three years allowed too few patients for analysis over the longest period.

The disparity in social class risk-factors following acute coronary heart disease observed in this study reflects differences in response to secondary prevention. Although no significant social class difference in mortality was found, it is likely that for the sub-group of continued smokers a strong social class difference in mortality exists. Studying a larger group of patients with longer follow-up, it is hoped to delineate social class sub-groups with variations in mortality.

Summary

299 men under 60 years who survived a coronary episode were included in a secondary prevention rehabilitation programme. The aim of this study was to examine factors influencing prognosis. The present report concerns the relationship between social class and indices of prognosis including reduction of risk-factors, return to work and mortality.

A strong association was observed between social class and risk-factor alteration one year following the acute coronary event. Significantly fewer patients in the lower social classes stopped smoking, increased their level of exercise and reduced weight. No social class difference was found for change in cholesterol and blood pressure. Approximately 90% of all patients had returned to employment at 1 year follow-up. Although social classes IV and V showed the lowest return to work rate, the differences between the social classes were not significant.

No social class difference in mortality was observed. This may be because of small numbers and an inadequate period of follow-up. A further study of larger numbers with longer follow-up is at present examining the relationship between social class and mortality.

References

1. Daly L, Hickey N, Graham I, Mulcahy R: Socio-economic factors and coronary heart disease. European Congress of Cardiology. Abstract, p 68, 1980.
2. Department of Health and Social Security. Inequalities in Health: Report of a research working group. London DHSS, 1980.
3. Joint Working Party of the Royal College of Physicians of London and the British Cardiac Society. Prevention of coronary heart disease report. Journal of the Royal College of Physicians 10:214–275, 1976.
4. McCarthy M: Epidemiology and Policies for Health Planning. Oxford University Press, UK. p 184, 1983.
5. Mulcahy R, Hickey N, Graham I, McKenzie G,: Factors influencing long-term prognosis in male patients surviving a first coronary attack. British Heart Journal, 37:158–165, 1975.
6. Mulcahy R, Hickey N: The rehabilitation of patients with coronary heart disease. Scandinaire Journal of Rehabilitation Medicine, 2:108–110, 1970.
7. Mulcahy R, Hickey N, Graham I, McAirt J: Factors affecting the 5-year survival rate of men following acute coronary heart disease. American Heart Journal, 93:556–559, 1977.
8. Stunkard AJ: Obesity and the Social Environment. In: Howard A (Ed) Recent advances in obesity research,p 178–190. Newman Publishing Ltd., London, 1975.

8. Short and Long-term Prognosis After First Myocardial Infarction. Influences of Social Class

B. WEISS, K. DONAT, W.J. ZIEGLER,
K. IVENS and J. SCHUCHART

Abstract

Retrospectively the clinical course of acute myocardial infarction (MI) was investigated in 1840 patients (1211 men and 629 women of all ages) treated in 11 hospitals (90 % of emergency capacity) at Hamburg in 1980. 71 % were older than 60 years, the average age was 69,3. 1237 patients had the first MI. There were no differences in frequency of MI in the different social classes (self-employed, employees or officials, workers) compared to the population of Hamburg. The in-hospital mortality of first MI was 23 %, mortality of reinfarction was 43 % ($p < 0.05$).

Prospectively 1019 patients under 75 years and surviving a first MI were enrolled in a cooperative, non-randomized study from July 1st, 1979 until December 31st, 1980. These patients are observed in cooperation with more than 400 practitioners in Hamburg over 3 years at least. Self-employed and employees/officials are somewhat overrepresented in this sample. The drop-out rate was 4 %. Bypass surgery was done in 49 patients. 92 patients died in the following 3 years after discharge from hospital, 10 by non-cardiac causes. The cardiac mortality was 5.1 % in the 1st year, 1.4 % in the 2nd year and 1 % in the 3rd year. 65 patients suffered non-fatal reinfarction. The frequency of all cardiac complications (fatal and non-fatal reinfarction, sudden death) rises over 60 significantly (<43 years 11 %, 46–60 years 11 %, 61–75 years 20 %, $p < 0.05$). Sudden death is more frequent in women than in men under 45 ($p < 0.05$). Cardiac complications are less, bypass surgery is more frequent in self-employed than in employees oder workers, but the differences are not statistically significant.

Introduction

The relation between social class respectively occupation and ischemic heart disease is a topic of controversial discussion. In former investigations the incidence and mortality of ischemic heart disease was higher in the upper social classes, especially in high salary groups, self-employed or physical inactive persons [2, 3, 8, 12]. But the difference was not as great as is often assumed. In contrast to these findings the Whitehall Study found a fourfold higher mortality in the lowest social class (mainly semiskilled and unskilled workers) than in administratives [10]. An unsolved problem of all investigations is the association of very heterogeneous occupations in few social classes.

The incidence of acute myocardial infarction in different social classes and the influence of these classes on short and long-term prognosis after surviving infarction are investigated using the customary German insurance-related social classification.

Patients and methods

1. In a retrospective study the clinical course of acute myocardial infarction was investigated in all patients treated in 11 hospitals in Hamburg in 1980. 90% of all cases of emergency are admitted into these hospitals. A certain myocardial infarction was found in 1840 patients (3.7% of all patients in the medical departments).

2. Prospectively 1019 patients under 75 years and discharged from hospital after surviving first acute myocardial infarction were enrolled in a cooperative non-randomized post-infarction-care-study (German: Infarkt-Nachsorge-Studei 'INS') from July 1st, 1979 until December 31st, 1980. These patients are observed in cooperation with more than 400 practitioners over three years at least. The study design was carried out in 75%. The fate of drop-out patients is known in all but 4%.

Results

The age-distribution of all patients with acute myocardial infarction treated in 11 hospitals at Hamburg, 1980, is shown in fig. 1. The average age of men is 63.5, of women 71.3 years. 71% are older than 60; 50% are older than 70 years. The men-women-ratio is 1.8:1. 1237 patients are admitted with first myocardial infarction.

The overall hospital mortality of first myocardial infarction is 23%. The mortality of reinfarction is 43% ($p<0.05$). The mortality is higher in women than in men under 60 and increases with age, especially over 60 (Fig. 2).

In the retrospective study the frequency of myocardial infarction shows in patients under 60 no differences in the three main social classes in comparison to the population of Hamburg. In the prospective non-randomized post-infarction-care-study 'INS' self-employed and employees/officials are

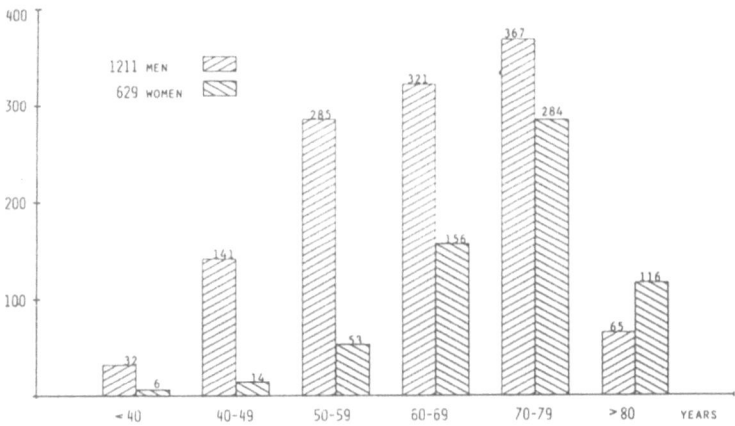

Figure 1. Age-distribution of 1840 patients with acute myocardial infarction (11 hospitals in Hamburg, 1980).

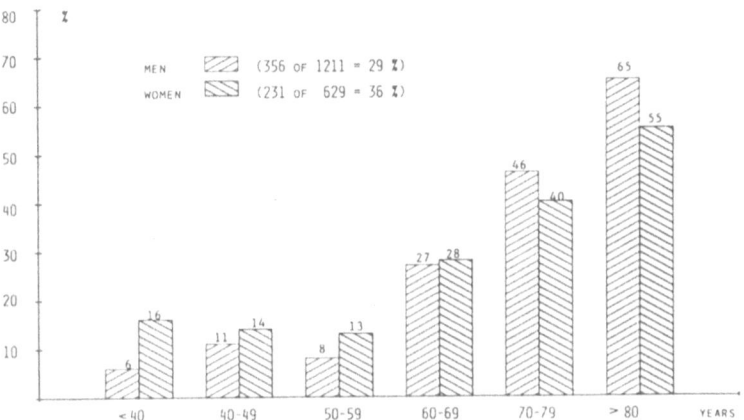

Figure 2. Hospital mortality of acute myocardial infarction.

Table 1. Social classes of patients under 60 with acute myocardial infarction

	All patients 11 hospitals 1980	Patients with first M.I. discharged	Inhabitants Hamburg 1980
Self-employed	8%	12%	9,4%
Employees/Officials	46%	57%	55,1%
Workers	34%	30%	35,5%
Retired	8%		

Table 2. Complications after surviving first myocardial infarction in the following 3 years (841 men, 178 women)

	1st year	2nd year	3rd year	Total
Non-fatal re-infartction	3,9%	1,7%	1,2%	6,8%
Fatal re-infarction	2,3%	0,7%	0,7%	3,7%
Fatal chronic heart failure	0,8%	0,3%	0,3%	1,4%
Sudden cardiac death	2,7%	0,9%	0,9%	4,5%
non-cardiac death	0,5%	0,5%	0,4%	1,4%
Bypass-surgery	3,4%	1,0%	0,9%	5,3%

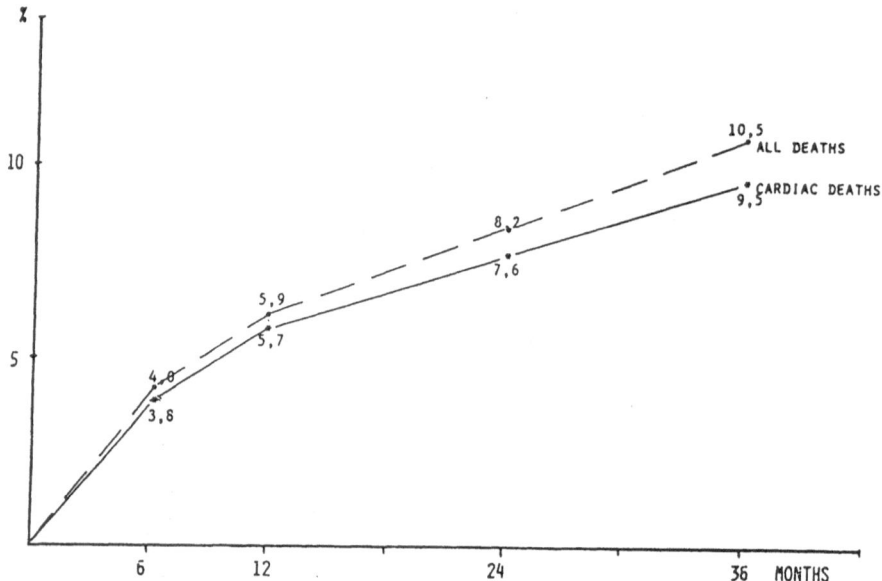

Figure 3. Cumulative three-year mortality after discharge from hospital in 1019 patients surviving a first myocardial infarction.

somewhat overrepresented, workers are somewhat underrepresented in comparison to the population of Hamburg (Table 1).

In the long-term follow-up the frequency of reinfarction and cardiac death is higher in the first year, especially in the first months after discharge from hospital than in the second and third year. But the rate of lethal complications after discharge is lower than expected (Table 2).

The cardiac mortality falls from 5.7% in the first year to 1.9% in the second and third year. 36 months after discharge the overall cardiac mortality is 9.5% (Fig. 3). After non-fatal reinfarction in the follow-up the mortality increases in the next 36 months to 19% ($p < 0.01$).

The frequency of all cardiac complications (it means reinfarctions and all

Table 3. Frequency of cardiac complications in relation to age (reinfarction and cardiac death)

	Men	Women	Total	N
Under 45 years	9%	29%	11%	135 (14 ♀)
46–60 years	13%	12%	13%	482 (52 ♀)
61–75 years	25%	16%	22%	401 (112 ♀)
# p<0,05				1019 (178 ♀)

Table 4. Cardiac complications and bypass surgery in different social classes

	Self-employed		Employee/official		Worker	
Age	<60	All	<60	All	<60	All
N	74	115	352	448	185	240
Reinfarction	2,7%	5,2%	6,8%	8,2%	7.0%	9,5%
Fatal refarction	–	2,6%	3,1%	5,3%	–	1,7%
Fatal chronic heart failure	1,4%	1,7%	0,6%	1,7%	1,1%	1,7%
Sudden cardiac death	1,4%	2,6%	3,7%	5,4%	3,2%	6,3%
Total	4 (5,4%	14 (12%)	50 (14%)	91 (20%)	21 (11%)	46 (19%)
	$p < 0.05$					
	N.S.					
Bypass surgery		9 (8%)		25 (6%)		15 (6%)

cardiac deaths) increases with age significantly. Under 45 years of age cardiac complications are more frequent in women than in men (Table 3).

In the 3-year follow-up cardiac complications occur more frequently in employees/officials and workers than in self-employed. But the differences are statistically not significant. Only self-employed under 60 suffer significantly less complications than employees and officials of this age.

Bypass-operations are carried out in equal frequency in the three social classes (Table 4).

Conclusions

Acute myocardial infarction is a disease of the older non-employed people particularly. Also younger patients under 60 with acute myocardial infarction are retired in 8% already.

66

In contrast to other findings there are no differences in the frequency of acute myocardial infarction in the three main social classes in Hamburg [2, 3, 8, 10, 12].

In our long-term follow-up study the cardiac mortality and frequency of reinfarction after surviving first infarction is lower than in former investigations [5, 6, 9, 11]. The mortality rate is in accordance with the Framingham Study and the verumgroups of intervention trials [1, 4, 7].

An essential influence of social class on the incidence of cardiac complications in the follow-up is not recognizable in our study.
deel 2 hoofdstuk 8

References

1. Aspirin myocardial infarction study research group: A randomized trial of aspirin in persons recovered from myocardial infarction. J Am Med Ass 243:661, 1980.
2. Cassel J, Heyden S, Bartel AG, Kaplan BH, Tyroler HA, Cornoni JC, Hames CC: Occupation and physical activity and coronary heart disease. Arch int Med 128:920, 1971.
3. Döring H, Loddenkämper R: Statistische Untersuchung über den Herzinfarkt. Z Kreislaufforsch 51:401, 1902.
4. Kannel WB, Sorlie P, Mc'Namara PM: Prognosis after initial myocarction: The Framingham Study. Amer J Cardiol 44:53, 1980.
5. Koch HU: Prognose nach akutem Herzinfarkt, regional Daten und Kontingenzuntersuchung zu Sterblichkeit, Todesursachen, Funktion und beruflicher Reintegration. Intensivmed 17:24, 1980.
6. Norris RM, Caughey DE, Deeming LW, Mercer CJ, Scott PJ: Coronary prognostic index for predecting survival after recovery from acute myocardial infarction. Lancet 1970, 486.
7. Norwegian Multicenter Study Group: A multicenter study on timolol in secondary prevention after myocardial infarction. Acta scand med Suppl 674, 1982.
8. Pell S, D'Alonzo CA: Acute myocardial infarction in a large industrial population. J Amer Med Ass 185:831, 1963.
9. Pohjola S, Siltanen P, Romo M: A five-year survival of 728 patients after myocardial infarction, a community study. Brit Heart J 43:176, 1980.
10. Rose G, Marmot MG: Social class and coronary heart disease. Brit Heart J 45:13, 1981.
11. Schettler G, Nüssel E: Herzinfarkt-Epidemiologie. Dtsch Med Wschr 99:2002, 1974.
12. Weidemann H, Nöcker J: Herzinfarkte in der Bevölkerung einer Industrie-Grosstadt. Münch med Wschr 107:2297, 1965.

III. The Role of Medication in Secondary Prevention

9. Beta-blocking Agents in Secondary Prevention

Å. HJALMARSON

Abstract

During the last 20 years a very large number of randomized double-blind trials have been performed to study the influence of beta-blockers on mortality and morbidity in patients who survived the acute myocardial infarction. The majority of these studies are of late entry type with start of treatment about 2 weeks after onset of infarction and with 1–3 years of follow-up. By pooling all these studies the total number of patients involved is about 20,000 and the beta-blockers reduced both mortality and incidence of a reinfraction by about 25 percent, respectively. The most convincing of these postinfarction studies of late entry type were the Norwegian timolol trial and the American propranolol trial (BHAT) published in 1981 with a 36 and 26 percent reduction in mortality, respectively. Also in 1981 the first convincing study of early entry type with start of treatment shortly after onset of infarction was published. This was the Swedish metoprolol trial which showed a reduction in total mortality by 36 percent after 3 months. With continued metropolol treatment in both groups after 3 months, the early beneficial effects were maintained over 2 years. The prophylactic instituion of metoprolol also prevented development of infarction by 35 percent during 3 months.

It can be concluded that prophylactic institution of a beta-blocker after acute myocardial infarction can prevent mortality and morbidity significantly. Most convincing results were obtained with timolol, metoprolol and propranolol. Before it has been clarified whether these effects can be generalized also to other beta-blockers, it seems justified to recommend one of the three beta-blockers in secondary prevention. In the trial on timolol, metoprolol and propranolol about 20 percent of the patients had contraindications to betablockade which means that about 80 percent of all patients after acute myocardial infarction can be safely treated with a beta-blocker. Since patients at risk for reinfarction cannot be predicted, all patients considering certain contraindications could be recommended long-term treatment for a period of 2–3 years.

Introduction

The use of betablocking agents after myocardial infarction has been extensively studied. There are about 35 prospective placebo controlled trials with more than 20,000 patients in the literature. The aim of this presentation is to give a review on the effects of betablocking agents on mortality and on morbidity after the acute myocardial infarction.

Effects on mortality

It was first reported in 1965 [1] that the institution of a betablocker in patients with acute myocardial infarction could reduce mortality. During the following 20 years a large number of non conclusive and conclusive studies on mortality were published. The first positive study after 1965 was a small study from Sweden on alprenolol 1974 [2]. In this study on 230 patients there was a significant reduction in sudden cardiac death referred to as deaths within 24 hours. A similar observation was made from the Multicenter International Study on practolol involving more than 3,000 patients reported in 1975 [3]. In 1975 another small study on alprenolol with 282 patients demonstrated a positive effect on one years survival in patients younger than 65 years of age, but there was a trend towards increased mortality by the beta blocker in patients older than 65 [4]. With exception of these three studies all the other studies on betablockers after myocardial infarction were non-conclusive without any significant effects on mortality. All but the Multicenter International Study on practolol with more than 3,000 patients involved a low number of patients and rather a few endpoints.

In 1981 three larger studies where published which convincingly demonstrated a reduction in total mortality by a betablocker after myocardial infarction. These studies were the Norwegian timolol study [5], the American BHAT study on propranolol [6] and the Swedish metoprolol study [7]. These studies included 1,400–3,800 patients with a significant reduction in mortality in each study in the order of 26–36% (Fig. 1). The Norwegian timolol study and the American BHAT study were late intervention studies with start of treatment about three weeks after onset of infarction with a mean follow up time of 17–25 months. In the Swedish metoprolol study the treatment was started with i.v. administration of metoprolol or placebo shortly after onset of acute myocardial infarction followed by oral blind treatment for three months. Thereafter all patients were given open treatment with metoprolol for two years. In this study metoprolol reduced three months mortality by 36% and the difference between treatment groups were

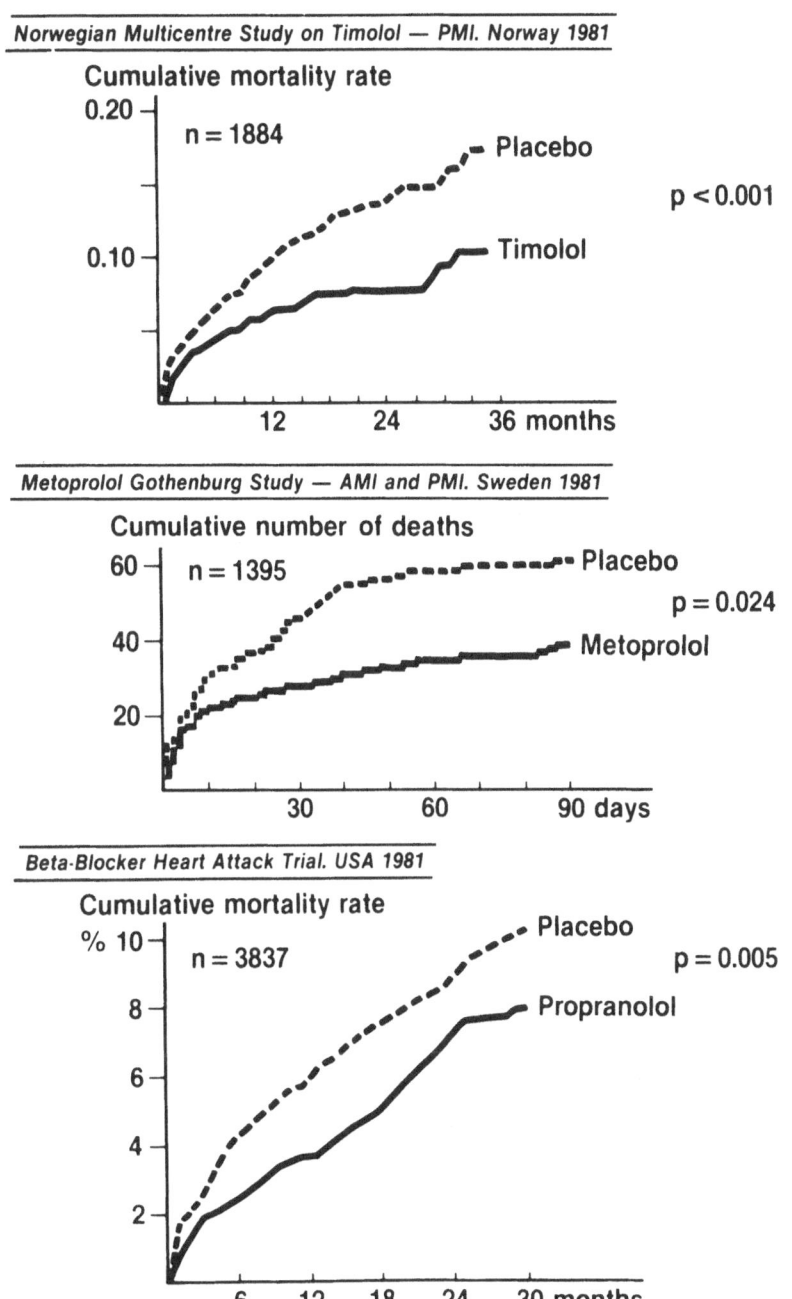

Figure 1. Mortality rate in the Norwegian timolol study (5), the Swedish metoprolol study (6) and the American BHAT trial (7). Patients were analysed according to the intention – to – treat.

maintained over two years despite the same treatment after three months [6, 8]. In 1982 two studies were reported on propranolol [9] and sotalol [10] in 560 and 1,456 patients respectively. The propranolol study from Norway included high risk patients and showed a significant reduction of sudden death. In the sotalol study the mortality after one year was 18% lower in the sotalol group although not statistically significant. In this study there was a reduction in the sum of fatal and nonfatal reinfarctions during this follow up. In 1983 the Australian-Swedish pindolol study [11] including 529 patients showed no effect on either total or sudden death. In 1984 the European infarction study group reported for one year mortality no difference in 1,741 patients treated with sustained release oxprenolol [12]. It was recently reported that metoprolol compared to placebo in a study of 301 patients during three years follow-up after myocardial infarction significantly reduced sudden death in all patients and cardiac deaths in those with large infarcts [13].

Pooling all patients from the placebo-controlled trials the average reduction in long-term mortality is in the order of 25% and highly significant. The most important and more recent trials are summarized in Table 1. One

Table 1. Reduction of total mortality by long-term beta-blockade

Trial	Year	Beta-blocker	No of pts	Reduction of total mortality (%)	Reduction of sudden deaths (%)
Wilhelmsson et al. (2)	1974	Alprenolol	230	50	72 [a]
Multicentre International Study (3)	1975	Practolol	3053	20	29 [a]
Andersen et al. (4) (≤65 yrs)	1979	Alprenolol	282	55	—
Norwegian Multicenter Study Group (5)	1981	Timolol	1884	36 [a]	49 [a]
Hjalmarson et al. (6)	1981	Metoprolol	1395	36 [a]	40 [b]
Beta Blocker Heart Attack Trial (7)	1981–1982	Propranolol	3837	26 [a]	28 [a]
Hansteen et al. (9)	1982	Propranolol	560	32 [a]	52 [a]
Julian et al. (10)	1982	Sotalol	1456	18 [a]	15
Australian Swedish Pindolol Study Group (11)	1983	Pindolol	529	3.4	9.4
European Infarction Study Group (12)	1984	Oxprenolol	1741	−30	—
Olsson et al. (13)	1984	Metoprolol	301	23	59 [a]

[a] Statistically significant
[b] Instantaneous

important question is whether the effects on mortality of betablockers can be referred to as a class action. Although the mortality reduction most likely is due to beta$_1$ receptor blockade, similar to other beneficial effects in patients with cardiovascular disease, there are other properties of betablockers that differ. It seems wise to choose a betablocker with documented and significant effect on post infarction mortality.

Effects on morbidity

It is well known since more than 20 years that betablocking agents are of value in the treatment of angina pectoris. It is also well known that many patients after their acute myocardial infarction have ischemic chest pain. From various review material it has been calculated that about 90 per cent of the patients with angina pectoris resulting from obstructive coronary artery disease demonstrate improved exercise tolerance and reduced chest pain with betablocker therapy. It was first shown by Waagstein and Hjalmarson [14, 15] that betablocking agents could also reduce the severity of chest pain during the early phase of acute myocardial infarction. This has later on been confirmed in the larger Swedish metoprolol trial [8] which showed a significant reduction in the need of morphine for the treatment of chest pain.

A larger number of the placebo-controlled postinfarction trials on betablockers have reported a beneficial effect on the development of a reinfarction (see table 2). Pooling the results from all published studies gives an average reduction of reinfarction rate by about 25 per cent, which is statistically highly significant. The fact that the development of an infarction can

Table 2. Reduction of non-fatal reinfarctions by long-term beta-blockade

Trial	Year	Beta-blocker	No of pts	Reduction of reinfarctions (%)
Wilhelmsson et al. (2)	1974	Alprenolol	230	11
Multicentre International Study (3)	1975	Practolol	3053	23
Norwegian Multicentre Study Group (5)	1981	Timolol	1884	28 [a]
Hjalmarson et al. (6)	1982	Metoprolol	782	40 (35 [a])
Beta Blocker Heart Attack Trial (7)	1981–1982	Propranolol	3837	16
Hansteen et al. (9)	1982	Propranolol	560	24
Julian et al. (10)	1982	Sotalol	1456	29 (41 [a])
Olsson et al. (13)	1984	Metoprolol	301	45 [b]

[a] Fatal and non-fatal reinfarctions and statistically significant.
[b] Non-fatal and statistically significant.

be prevented by prophylactic betablockade is in agreement with the observations that early administration to patients with suspected acute myocardial infarction could limit the infarct size [8, 16]. The exact mechanism for the antiischemic action of betablockers is not fully clear, but action is multifactorial including a reduction of heart rate, contractility, ventricular pressure development, ventricular wall stiffness of ischemic myocardium and lengtening of diastolic perfusion period and also possible effects on platelet function and the oxyhemoglobin equilibrium curve.

It is generally believed that the majority of deaths among patients surviving the acute phase of myocardial infarction occurs rather suddenly and are due to ventricular fibrillation. The prophylactic institution of betablocking agents has reduced mortality and most drastically the incidence of sudden cardiac death (Table 1). In contrast to the positive findings with betablocking agents, class I-antiarrhythmic agents have failed to show any reduction of mortality in patients after myocardial infarction. Most of the larger placebo-controlled trials designed to study mortality have also involved analyses of ventricular arrhythmias. Thus, a reduction of ventricular arrhythmias has been reported from the Norwegian timolol study [17] the American BHAT study [18] and the Swedish metoprolol study [8, 19]. In all these studies there was also a significant reduction of supraventricular tachyarrhythmias by prophylactic institution of a betablocker. In view of the results of these controlled trials and from other smaller studies [20] it can be stated that betablocking agents can prevent and reduce the frequency of ventricular and supraventricular tachyarrhythmias in patients after acute myocardial infarction.

In the Swedish metoprolol study [8, 19] there was a marked prevention of ventricular fibrillation as well as ventricular tachycardia by the betablocker. As can be seen from Fig. 2, there was a significantly lower number of patients in the metoprolol group who developed ventricular fibrillation compared to the placebo group. Even more impressive was the difference in the number of episodes of ventricular fibrillation. Lidocaine was used only after conversion of ventricular fibrillation and in patients with sustained ventricular tachycardia (> 1 minute). A similar observation of a prevention of ventricular fibrillation during the early phase of acute myocardial infarction was demonstrated by prophylactic institution of propranolol in a study by Norris and co-worker [21]. The mechanism of the antifibrillatory action of betablockade is not clear. There might be a direct antiarrhythmic effect, but also an indirect antiischemic influence on ventricular fibrillation.

When should treatment start and for how long to continue

Most of the studies referred to in this review are of late entry type with start of treatment 1–2 weeks after onset of myocardial infarction. The first larger

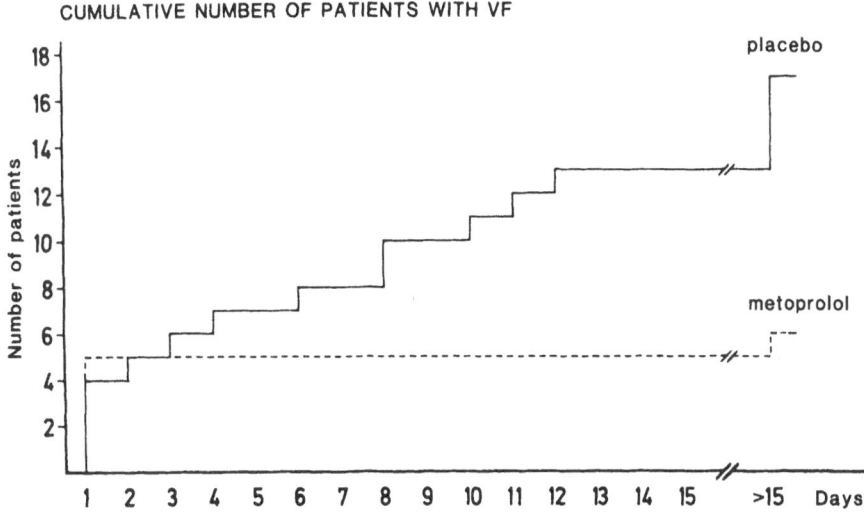

CUMULATIVE NUMBER OF PATIENTS WITH VF

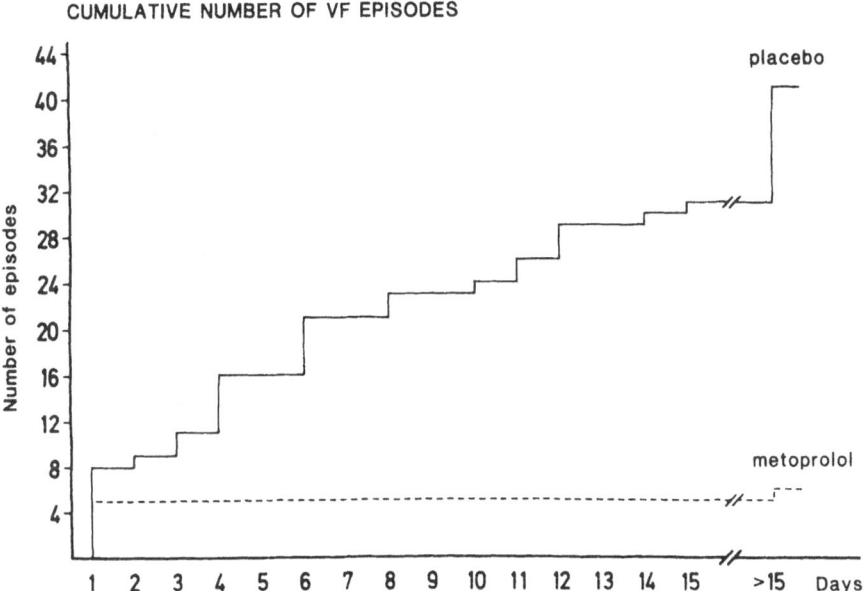

CUMULATIVE NUMBER OF VF EPISODES

Figure 2. The upper part of the figure shows number of patients who developed ventricular fibrillation and the lower part, number of epidoses of ventricular fibrillation in patients treated with metoprolol and placebo in the Swedish metoprolol study (8, 19).

study with convincing results from early treatment with start shortly after onset of symptoms of suspected acute myocardial infarction was the Swedish metoprolol study [6, 8, 19]. Conclusions from this study are summarized in table 3. This study showed a significant reduction in both short-term and long-term mortality when metoprolol treatment was started intravenously followed by oral treatment in patients with suspected acute myo-

Table 3. Conclusions from the Swedish metoprolol study

---

1. *In all patients given metoprolol*
   - Reduction of 3-month (and 2-year) mortality
   - Prevention of late myocardial infarction (first and recurrent)
   - Prevention of ventricular fibrillation and tachycardia
   - Reduction and prevention of chest pain
   - Lower use of lidocaine and morphine
   - Well tolerated

2. *In patients given metoprolol within 12 hours after onset of symptoms*
   - Limitation of 'infarct size'
   - Lower use of diuretics for congestive heart failure
   - Lower number of days in hospital
   - Well tolerated

(From References 6, 8, 19)

cardial infarction with start of treatment a few hours after onset of symptoms. There were positive effects also on infarct development, ventricular fibrillation and tachycardia, chest pain and congestive heart failure. As an overall measure of the positive influence the patients who started treatment within 12 hours could be sent home from hospital significantly earlier than the placebo treated patients. Beneficial effects on the initial infarct development and on early infarct complications have been reported also in a number of other smaller studies on e.g. propranolol, atenolol and timolol [21–23].

Since the Swedish metoprolol study was the first one to report very positive effects of a betablocker during the early phase, there was a need to try to confirm these findings in a larger trial. Therefore, the MIAMI trial (metoprolol in acute myocardial infarction) was performed with the primary objective to test whether early institution of metoprolol could reduce mortality, already within 15 days after onset of infarction. The results of the MIAMI trial were recently announced [24]. In this study 15 mg of metoprolol or placebo was given intravenously as soon as possible in the coronary care unit and this was followed by oral treatment with 200 mg daily or placebo for at least 15 days. 5,778 patients were included in 104 hospitals around the world. For all randomised patients the difference in mortality after 15 days was 13 per cent and not statistically significant. It was calculated based upon the experience from the Swedish metoprolol study [4], that the 15 days' placebo mortality should be 7 per cent and it was hypothesized that metoprolol could reduce this mortality by 35 per cent. However, the results of the MIAMI trial showed that a higher number than calculated of low risk patients were included and the placebo mortality after 15 days was less than 5 per cent. In a retrospective analysis it was found that in a subgroup with higher mortality risk (1/3 of all patients) the 15 days' mortality rate in the placebo group was 8,5 per cent and in the metoprolol group 6,0 per cent, a difference of 29 per cent. In the low mortality risk group (2/3 of all) the mortality rate was 2,9 per cent in the placebo group and 3,3 per cent in the metoprolol group. Using a more complex LOGIT model for deaths it was found that in a high risk class (about 1/4 of all patients) a reduction in mortality by metoprolol was evident (39 per cent). It is thus possible that especially in patients with higher mortality risk, mortality might be reduced by very early betablocker institution already during the hospital stay (about 2 weeks). It should be stated that the subgroup analyses of the MIAMI trial has been done retrospectively and has to be interpreted with caution and in perspectives of other similar observations.

The MIAMI trial confirmed the positive findings of early metoprolol treatment what concerns the development of early and late mycardial infarction, enzyme estimated infarct size, incidence and severity of ischemic chest pain, supraventricular tachyarrhythmias and the need of antianginal and antiarrhythmic drugs. Somewhat unclear results were obtained on ventricular fibrillation. In contrast to the Swedish metoprolol study, a rather high proportion of the patients were given prophylactic antiarrhythmic treatment mainly with lidocaine despite the fact that the incidence of ventricular fibrillation was much lower than anticipated. The overall incidence of the adverse events was low and there were no unexpecting findings from the metoprolol treatment. Hypotension and bradycardia was reported more often as reasons for permanent withdrawal in the metoprolol group, whereas needs for betablockade was more common in the placebo group. The incidence of AV-block II and III, pacemaker inplantation, congestive heart failure and cardiogenic chock was not different between the two groups.

Based upon all studies reported on the use of betablockers in acute myocardial infarction in addition to the larger trials on metoprolol as being referred to early institution of betablockade results in a number of beneficial effects. Pooling studies on mortality [6, 24, 25] betablocker treatment seems to reduce mortality during the first 1–2 weeks by 10–15 per cent. In patients with high mortality risk this reduction might be much more marked [24]. The overall findings on infarct development, infarct size, supraventricular and ventricular arrhythmias, chest pain and use of other drugs are very positive when all available studies are considered. Most important, the tolerance seems also to be very good. It therefore seems reasonable to recommend start of treatment as early as possible after onset of symptoms in patients with suspected acute myocardial infarction. One ought to use drugs with proven efficacy and good tolerance for the dose regime given in the literature.

One important question in the postinfarction prophylaxis with a beta-locker is for how long this treatment should be continued. The majority of studies which have reported effects on mortality after myocardial infarction have a follow-up time of 1–2 years. The most convincing results were obtained from the Norwegian timolol study [5] and the American BHAT trial [7] in which the patients were followed for up to three years with an average of around two years. Both these studies as well as the pooled results from all long term studies have convincingly shown a reduction in mortality and reinfarction rate. Therefore beneficial effects have been demonstrated during a follow-up period of about two years. It can be recommended that the betablocker prophylaxis after myocardial infarction should be maintained for at least two years. Thereafter only patients with other indications for betablocker treatment such as angina pectoris, hypertension and tachyarrhythmias will be treated longer.

Conclusion

From a very large number of placebo-controlled postinfarction trials institution of a betablocker can reduce mortality and reinfarction rate by about 25 per cent. These results are very convincing and statistically highly significant. A number of studies and most convincing the Swedish metoprolol study and the multicenter international MIAMI trial have demonstrated that betablocker treatment can safely be started shortly after onset of symptoms in patients with suspected acute myocardial infarction. Based upon the results from the Swedish metoprolol study about 80 per cent of all patients with a definite infarction can be safely treated with metoprolol from the first few hours after onset of symptoms. Such treatment may influence early infarct development and reduce incidence and severity of chest pain and of arrhythmias. In view of available data from the literature, one might expect a reduction also in early mortality in the order of 10–15 per cent during the first two weeks. In patients with higher mortality risk a more marked reduction in mortality could be obtained. The value for long term prognosis is documented for a period of at least 2 years and it seems reasonable to recommend at least 2 years of postinfarction prophylaxis with a betablocker with proven effect. It is not year clear whether all betablockers have the same effects on postinfarction mortality and on morbidity.

References

1. Snow PDJ: Effect of propranolol in myocardial infarction. Lancet ii:551–553, 1965.
2. Wilhelmsson C, Vedin JA, Wilhelmsen L, Tibblin G & Werkö L: Reduction of sudden-deaths after myocardial infarction by treatment with alprenolol. Lancet ii:1157–1159, 1974.

3. A Multicenter International Study: Improvement in prognosis of myocardial infarction by long-term beta-adrenoreceptor blockade using practolol. Br Med J 3:735–740, 1975.

4. Andersen MP, Bechsgaard P, Fredriksen J, Hansen DA, Jürgensen HJ, Nielsen B, Pedersen F, Pedersen-Bjergaard O, Rasmussen SL: Effect of alprenolol on mortality among patients either definite or suspected acute myocardial infarction. Preliminary results. Lancet ii:865–872, 1979.

5. The Norwegian Multicenter Study Group: Timolol-induced reduction in mortality and reinfarction in patients surviving acute myocardial infarction. N Engl J Med 304:801–807, 1981.

6. Hjalmarson Å, Elmfeldt D, Herlitz J, Holmberg S, Målek I, Nyberg G, Rydén L, Swedberg K, Vedin A, Waagstein F, Waldenström A, Waldenström J, Wedel H, Wilhelmsen L, Wilhelmsson C: Effect on mortality of metoprolol in acute myocardial infarction. A double blind randomised trial. Lancet ii:823–827, 1981.

7. Beta-Blocker Heart Attack Trial Research Group: A randomized trial of propranolol in patients with acute myocardial infarction. I. Mortality results. JAMA 247:1707–1714, 1982.

8. The Göteborg Metoprolol Trial in Acute myocardial Infarction. Am J Cardiol 1984, 53/12:1D–50D.

9. Hansteen V, Moinichen E, Lorentsen E, Andersen A, Strom O, Soiland K, Dyrbekk D, Refsum A-M, Tromsdal A, Knudsen K, Eika C, Bakken J Jr, Smith P, Hoff PI: One year's treatment with propranolol after myocardial infarction: preliminary report of Norwegian multicentre trial. Br Med J 284:155–161, 1982.

10. Julian DG, Prescott RJ, Jackson FS, Szekely P: Controlled trial of sotalol for one year after myocardial infarction, Lancet ii:1142–1147, 1982.

11. Australian and Swedish Pindolol Study Group: The effect of pindolol on the two years mortality after complicated myocardial infarction. Eur Heart J 4:367–375, 1983.

12. European Infarction Study Group. A secondary prevention study with slow-release oxprenolol after myocardial infarction: Morbidity and mortality. European Heart Journal 5:189–202 (Mar 1984).

13. Olssen G, Rehnqvist N, Sjögren A et al. Long-term treatment with metoprolol after myocardial infarction. Report on 3 year mortality and morbidity. Am J Cardiology. In press.

14. Waagstein F, Hjalmarson Å: Effect of cardioselective beta-blockade on heart function and chest pain in acute myocardial infarction. Acta Med Scand, Suppl 587:193–200, 1976a.

15. Waagstein F, Hjalmarson Å: Double-blind study of the effect of cardioselective beta-blockade on chest pain in acute myocardial infarction. Acta Med Scand, Suppl 587:201–208, 1976b.

16. Hjalmarson Å, Herlitz J: Limitation of infarct size and its potential role for prognosis. Circulation 67, Suppl I:68–69, 1983.

17. Von der Lippe G, Lund-Johansen P: Effect of timolol on late ventricular arrhythmias after acute myocardial infarction. Acta Med Scand, Suppl 651:vol 210:253–258, 1981.

18. Lichstein E, Morganroth J, Harrist R, Hubble E for the BHAT Study Group: Effect of propranolol on ventricular arrhythmia. Circulation 67(suppl I):1-5–I-10, 1983.

19. Rydén L, Ariniego R, Arnman K, Herlitz J, Hjalmarson Å, Holmberg S, Reyes C, Smedgård P, Swedberg K, Vedin A, Waagstein F, Waldenström A, Wilhelmsson C, Wedel H, Yamamoto M: A doubleblind trial of metoprolol in acute myocardial infarction. Effects on ventricular tachyarrhythmias. N Engl J Med 308:614–618, 1983.

20. Singh BN, Collett JT, Chew CYC: New perspectives in the pharmacologic therapy of cardiac arrhythmias. Prog Cardiovasc Dis 22:243–301, 1980.

21. Norris RM, Barnaby PF, Brown MA et al.: Prevention of centricular fibrillation during acute myocardial infarction by intravenous propranolol. Lancet 1984, ii:883–886.

22. Yusuf S, Sleight P, Rossi P, Ramsdale D, Peto R, Furse L, Sterry H, pearson M, Motwani R, Parish S, Gray R, Bennett D, Bray C: Reduction in infarct size, arrhythmias and chest pain

by early intravenous beta blockade in suspected acute myocardial infarction. Circulation 67, Suppl I: 32–41, 1983.

23. International Collaborative Study Group: Reduction of infarct size with the early use of timolol in acute myocardial infarction. New England Journal of Medicine 310:310–315, 1984.

24. The MIAMI Trial: Rome, October 29–30, 1984. Drugs, Vol. 29, Suppl 1, 1985.

25. Yusuf S, Peto R, Lewis J, Collins R, Sleight P: Beta-blockade during and after myocardial infarction: an overview of the randomised trials. Prog Cardiovasc Dis 1985; in press.

10. Beta-blocking Agents in the Secondary Prevention after Acute Myocardial Infarction, with Special Reference to the European Infarct Study (EIS)

P.R. LICHTLEN

Abstract

The incidence of sudden coronary death is high in the first 6 months after myocardial infarction, amounting to 12–15% or more depending on the location and extent of infarction, the underlying coronary disease as well as the patient's age. Its mechanism, re-entry tachycardia in the area of scar tissue leading to ventricular tachycardia and fibrillation, provoked by PVCs, is well established today. Prevention was tried by various means, especially the administration of class I antiarrhythmic drugs and betablockers. Only some of the latter group proved to be successful, especially alprenolol, practolol, timolol, propranolol and metoprolol as shown in randomized studies. In Europe a multicenter double-blind, randomized, placebo-controlled study was performed with oxprenolol slow release 160 mg b.i.d. The study comprised 1,741 patients who were followed for 12 months. There were 57 deaths (6.6%) in the oxprenolol group (OX) and 45 (5.1%) in the placebo group (PL), the difference being insignificant. Some special features might explain some of the reasons for the 'negative' outcome of the study with regard to prevention of sudden coronary death. 275 patients in each group discontinued the trial medication; mortality in these patients was higher for OX (13.1%) than for PL (7.6%) even weeks and months after withdrawal. Mortality was also higher in patients 65–69 years, 16.7% for OX and 5.6% for PL. In the 1,472 patients less than 65 years mortality showed a tendency to be lower in the 478 patients at high risk, 6.9% under OX versus 10.2% under PL. Hence, the EIS failed to confirm previous positive results in this field. The reasons will be discussed as well as the rationale for betablocking treatment after acute myocardial infarction.

Introduction

During the last years several prevention studies for sudden coronary death using betablocking agents in the first year after myocardial infarction showed a positive outcome. A significant, approximately 25 to 30 % reduction of the incidence of sudden coronary death was shown especially with propranolol (the betablocker heart attack trial, BHAT, 1982), with timolol (the Norwegian Multi-Center Study Group, 1981), and alprenolol (Wilhelmsen, 1974). These few studies are contradicted by a large number of negative trials, some of them showing a trend for reduction of sudden death, especially of certain sub-groups, however, without significance (May, 1982). Hence, a cooperative study using slow release oxprenolol was started in Europe in July, 1979 (European Infarction Study, EIS) after extensive planning since 1977. As the main results of this trial are already published (see: European Heart Journal, 1984), this report will only give a short summary of the most important data and, in addition, try to analyse reasons for the negative outcome of this and any postinfarction betablocker trial.

Study design

EIS is a multicenter, double-blind, randomized study comparing the effects of oxprenolol slow release, 160 mg twice a day with placebo on survival, cardiac mortality and non-cardiac events in 1,041 patients aged 35 to 69 years, suffering from acute myocardial infarction. The patients were entering the study 14 to 36 days after onset of myocardial infarction and were followed over one year. Recruitment was stopped in July, 1981, before the scheduled 4,000 patients were included as at that time no trend towards

Table 1. Reasons for exclusion

Total number screened	8961 patients
Not eligible for randomization	5160
age out of range	3541
within age range but dead before possible entry	679
within age range and alive but no consent or expected non-cooperation	940
Considered for randomization	3801
Excluded	2060 (54.2 %)
Reasons:	
beta-blocker contraindicated	412 (10.8 %)
receiving beta-blockers, anti-arrhythmics, calcium antagonists or antiplatelet drugs	258 (6.8 %)
severe extracardiac conditions	131 (3.4 %)
post or scheduled cardiac surgery	115 (3.0 %)
other reasons	280 (7.4 %)
more than one exclusion criterion	832 (21.9 %)
no specified exclusion criteria	32 (0.8 %)
Randomized	1741 (45.8 %)

Table 2. Baseline comparison

Variable	Oxprenolol	Placebo
Male	83.7%	83.8%
Mean age (years)	54.7	54.9
1. Medical history		
Angina pectoris> 4 weeks *	28.4%	29.5%
Previous myocardial infarction	14.0%	16.9%
Hypertension	24.4%	25.3%
Congestive heart failure	6.9%	8.5%
Diabetes mellitus	9.2%	10.6%
Current smoker	56.3%	57.0%
2. Clinical data related to the acute myocardial infarction		
Anterior infarcion	37.1%	35.5%
Lateral infarction	3.4%	4.4%
Inferior infarction	47.7%	50.3%
Undefined infaction	11.2%	9.8%
Sinus tachyardia ($\geqslant$ 100/min)	21.8%	19.7%
Left heart failure	13.2%	13.1%
3.Treatment between qualifying M.I. and time of randomization		
Beta-blocker	10.2%	10.8%
Lidocaine	20.0%	24.7%
Other anti-arrhythmics	10.8%	9.3%
Inotropic substances	6.9%	5.9%
Digitalis	30.0%	28.0%
Diuretics	39.1%	37.5%
4. Conditions at time of randomization		
Mean heart rate/min	73.5	74.2
Systolic BP mmHg	127.1	128.1
Diastolic BP mmHg	80.4	82.0
Ventricular ectopic beats †	8.4%	9.1%
Persisting ST-elevation	22.5%	20.4%
Lung congestion (on x-ray)	18.5%	20.5%
Cardiomegaly ‡	42.4%	41.3%

reduction in mortality was observed in either group and no further changes were foreseen by the statisticians.

Reasons for exclusions are shown in table 1. The total number of patients screened amounted to 8,961 and 3,801 (42.4%) were considered for randomization, 1,741 (19.4% of all patients screened) were finally randomized.

The definition of myocardial infarction was based on the presence of at least two of the three following criteria: 1. typical chest pain, 2. develop-

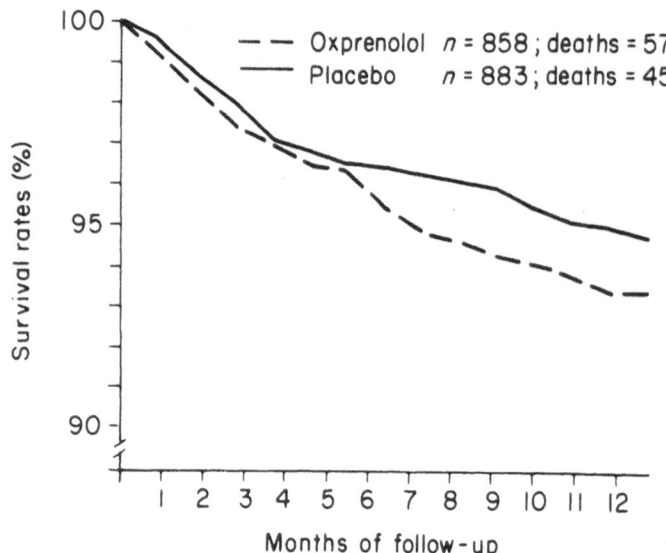

Figure 1. Life table cumulative mortality curves for groups allocated to oxprenolol and placebo, unadjusted for baseline differences. Note that after 6 months the survival rate for oxprenolol is lower than for placebo although the difference is not significant.

ment of typical Q-waves, 3. a twofold or higher increase in cardiac enzymes (CK, CK-MB, S-GOT, AST, alphaHBD or LDH). 1,725 patients (99%) fulfilled at least two of these criteria.

Baseline variables for the oxprenolol and the placebo treated group are shown in table 2. The majority were male patients, approximately 30% in both groups suffered from angina, approximately 15% showed old myocardial infarctions, 25% were hypertensive, and 7% presented with congestive heart failure. Patients with inferior myocardial infarctions prevailed in both groups with approximately 50%, approximately 36% suffered from anterior wall myocardial infarctions; approximately 30% of the patients were under digitalis, 40% under diuretics.

Figure 1 demonstrates the life table *cumulative mortality curves* for patients under oxprenolol or placebo. It is interesting to note that after 6 months mortality became slightly higher in the oxprenolol than in the placebo group. This was mainly due to an increased mortality in the group withdrawn from oxprenolol (see below). If only patients under active treatment were considered (Fig. 2), no difference in mortality could be observed between the two groups.

This is further illustrated on Figure 3, showing a more detailed analysis with regard to patients continuing and discontinuing treatment. Overall mortality amounted to 6.6% (57 deaths) in the oxprenolol and to 5.1% (45 deaths) in the placebo group, this small difference being insignificant. Furthermore, in patients still under treatment mortality was 3.6% in the oxprenolol and 3.9% in the placebo group, this difference also being insignificant.

actuarial rate (%)

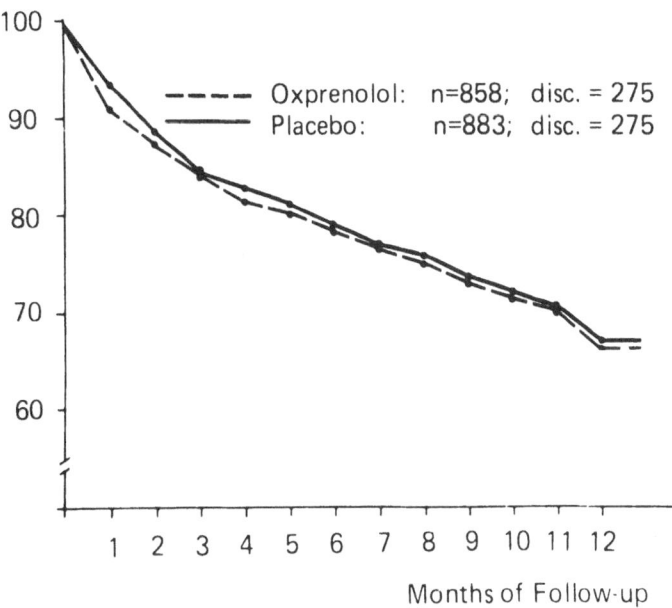

Figure 2. Survival rate of patients on trial medication in the two treatment group during the twelve months follow-up. Note that there is no difference whatsoever between the two groups.

Of special interest is the increased mortality of 13.1% in the group withdrawn from oxprenolol which is considerably higher than in the group withdrawn from placebo with 7.6%.

The analysis of the *cause specific mortality related to treatment* (Table 3) revealed 25 sudden death cases (mortality for sudden death 2.9%) in the oxprenolol and 24 cases in the placebo group (mortality of 2.7%); in contrast there were 26 non-sudden cardiac deaths in the oxprenolol (mortality 3%) in contrast to only 16 (mortality 1.8%) in the placebo group; most of these deaths were due to reinfarction (17 with oxprenolol against only 7 in the placebo group) or congestive heart failure (8 in the oxprenolol against 4 in the placebo group). Hence, patients under oxprenolol, especially when withdrawn from the drug had a higher risk to die from reinfarction or congestive heart failure than under placebo (see below).

Of special interest are the *mortality figures by selected baseline risk groups adjusted for age* (Table 4). Patients under age 65 at high risk (history of previous infarction or heart failure or pulmonary congestion at randomization) had a lower mortality under oxprenolol than placebo (6.9 versus 10.2%) whereas at age above 65 this was reversed (21.6% under oxprenolol against 9.5% under placebo). This increased mortality at high age (above 65 years) persisted also for the low risk group (none of the above mentioned

86

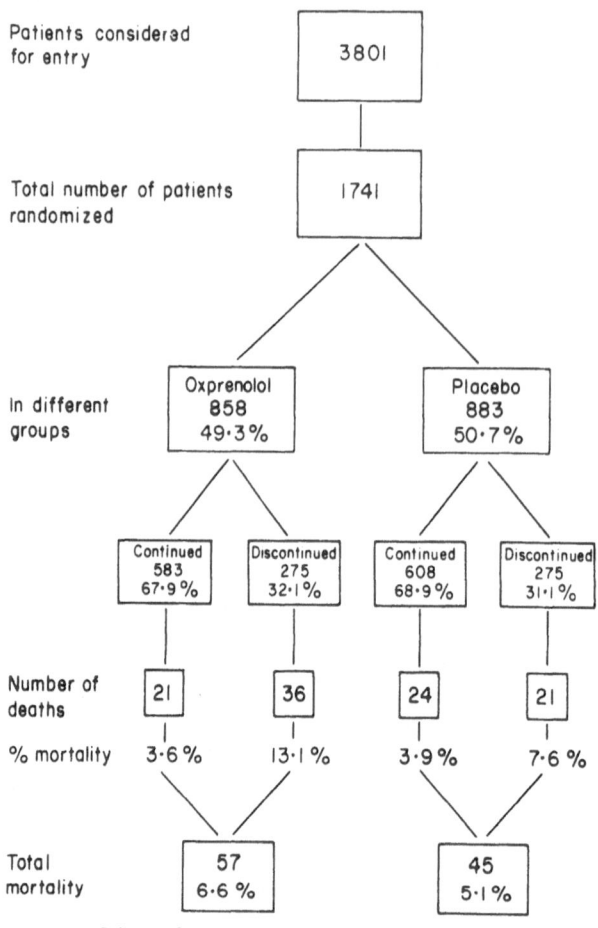

Scheme for data analysis of the E.I.S. trial

Figure 3. Data analysis of the EIS trial; the patients are grouped according to trial medication as well as to continuation or discontinuation of treatment (for details see text).

risks) with 13.3% in the oxprenolol and 1.5% in the placebo group. Treatment with digitalis did not really alter this pattern.

Hence, the course of patients in the high age group (above 65 years) was markedly more severe under the betablocker oxprenolol than under placebo, an observation which is in contrast to other studies (BHAT, Norwegian timolol trial). It is therefore of special interest to analyze separately the patients below 65 years (Fig. 4). Here again total mortality was equal in both groups with 4.9% and 5.0% for oxprenolol and placebo, respectively. It was slightly lower in the oxprenolol patients continuing treatment (3.0%) than in those under placebo (4.3%) and it was again markedly higher in patients withdrawn from medication.

If one compares the course of patients below and above aged 65 years (Fig. 5) several interesting points emerge:

Table 3. Cause-specific mortality by treatment group

	Oxprenolol	Placebo	Standardized deviate
Total deaths	57 (6.6%)	45 (5.1%)	1.37
Sudden death	25 (2.9%)	24 (2.7%)	0.25
Non-sudden cardiac death	26 (3.0%)	16 (1.8%)	1.66
Reinfarction	17	7	2.13
with rhythm disturbances	6	3	
with cardiac failure	6	2	
Congestive heart failure	8	4	1.21
Rhythm disturbances	2	3	
Death after cardiac surgery	0	2	
Death from non-cardiac reason	6 (0.7%)	5 (0.6%)	

Table 4. Mortality by selected baseline risk groups adjusted for age

	Age (years)	Oxprenolol		Placebo		Relative risk	Confidence interval (P = 99.5%)	Stan-dardized deviate
		n (pts)	% mor-tality	n (pts)	% mor-tality			
Clinical findings								
High risk [a]	<65	233	6.9	245	10.2	0.7	0.3 1.7	−1.30
	65–69	51	21.6	74	9.5	2.3	0.6 ⩾10.0	1.90
Low risk [b]	<65	499	4.0	495	2.4	1.7	0.6 4.8	1.41
	65–69	75	13.3	69	1.5	9.2	0.5 ⩾10.0	2.68
Treatment								
High risk [c]	<65	185	4.3	176	10.8	0.4	⩽0.1 1.3	−2.34
	65–69	50	14.0	61	8.1	1.7	0.3 ⩾10.0	0.98
Low risk [d]	<65	547	5.1	564	3.2	1.6	0.7 3.9	1.61
	65–69	76	18.4	82	3.7	5.0	0.9 ⩾ 10.0	2.99

[a] History of previous infarction or heart failure or pulmonary congestion at randomization.
[b] No history of previous infarction or heart failure or no pulmonary congestion at randomization.
[c] Treatment or [d] no treatment within last 4 weeks before infarction with digitalis or diuretics or nitrates.

88

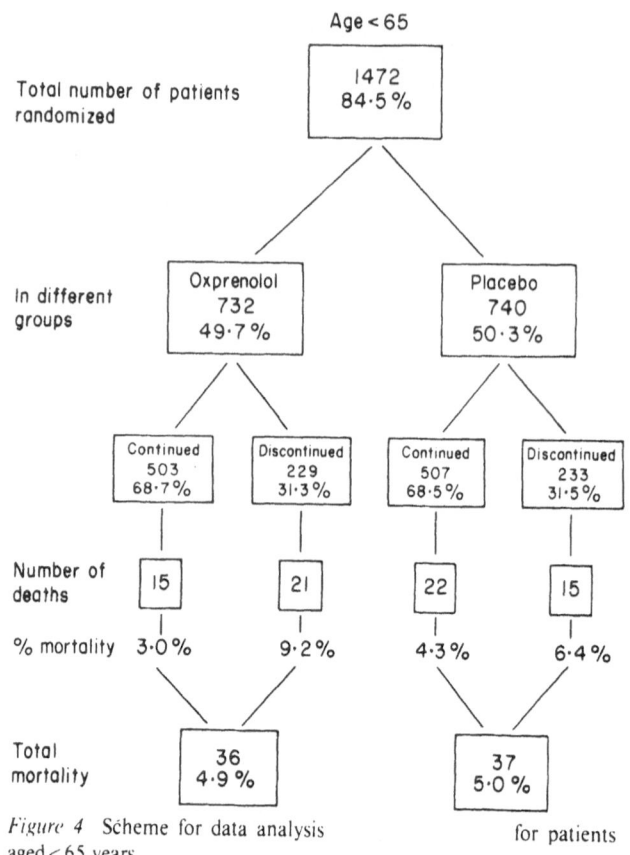

Age < 65

Total number of patients randomized

```
                    1472
                    84·5%
```

In different groups

```
   Oxprenolol              Placebo
      732                    740
     49·7%                  50·3%
```

Continued	Discontinued	Continued	Discontinued
503	229	507	233
68·7%	31·3%	68·5%	31·5%

Number of deaths

```
    15        21        22        15
```

% mortality 3·0%   9·2%   4·3%   6·4%

Total mortality

```
        36                  37
       4·9%                5·0%
```

Figure 4 Scheme for data analysis aged < 65 years.   for patients

Figure 4. Data analysis for patients aged below 65; again patients are grouped according to trial medication and continuation or discontinuation of treatment (for details see text).

EIS – DISTRIBUTION OF AGE

	< 65 YEARS				65 – 69 YEARS		
	OX		PL		OX		PL
	732		740		126		143
	cont.	discont.	cont.	discont.	cont.	discont.	cont.	discont.
	503	229	507	233	80	46	101	42
✝	15	21	22	15	6	15	2	6
	3.0%	9.2%	4.3%	6.4%	7.5%	32.6%	1.98%	14.3%
	4.9%		5.0%		16.7%		5.6%	

Figure 5. Comparison of survival in patients below and above 65 years under oxprenolol or placebo, according to continuation or discontinuation of treatment (vor details see text).

1. Total mortality in the oxprenolol group age above 65 is with 16.7% markedly higher than in the placebo patients above 65 years (5.6%) and, in addition, is also markedly higher than in the oxprenolol group below the age of 65 years (4.9%).
2. In contrast, total mortality under placebo is identical in patients below and above age 65 years with 5.0% and 5.6%, respectively.
3. Especially striking is the high mortality in patients above 65 years discontinuing oxprenolol; it amounted to 32.6% (!) against only 9.2% in the group below 65 discontinuing the betablocker. This figure is higher than in the discontinued placebo group age above 65 years where mortality amounted to 14.3%, a figure also markedly higher than in the discontinued placebo group below aged 65 years (6.4%). The low mortality of only 1.98% in the placebo patients treated age higher than 65 years remains unexplained and remarkable as it is the lowest mortality in all groups.

Hence, it seems that oxprenolol at higher age is not well tolerated, at least not in a high daily dose of 360 mg per day, and that this might have led to a certain 'rebound' effect in this group of patients which was finally reflected in the high mortality in the withdrawal group age above 65 years. This was the case both for reinfarction (12 in the oxprenolol and 2 in the placebo group), for heart failure (6 in the oxprenolol vs. 2 cases in the placebo group) as well as for sudden coronary death (16 in the oxprenolol and 9 in the placebo group) (Table 5). Interestingly enough, the reasons for discontinuation both of oxprenolol and placebo were obviously different from the com-

Table 5. Death and discontinuation of trial medication

Cause of death	Sudden death		M.I.		Heart failure		Other	
	Ox	Pl	Ox	Pl	Ox	Pl	Ox	Pl
Total	25	24	17	7	8	4	7	10
On study medication	9	15	5	5	2	2	5	2
Study medication discontinued	16	9	12	2	6	2	2	8
Reasons for discontinuation:								
Heart failure	3	4	3	0	2	2	0	0
reinfarction	2	1	7	2	2	0	0	0
Angina pectoris	3	1	0	0	1	0	0	2
non-compliance (phycician or patient)	2	3	2	0	0	0	2	0
other	6 [a]	0	0	0	1	0	0	5 [b]
treatment never commenced	0	0	0	0	0	0	0	1

[a] Reasons for discontinuation: 2 cardiac arrests, 1 syncope, 1 AV-block, 1 insomnia, 1 headache

[b] Cause of death: 2 strokes, 1 ventricular fibrillation, 1 sepsis, 1 bleeding.

90

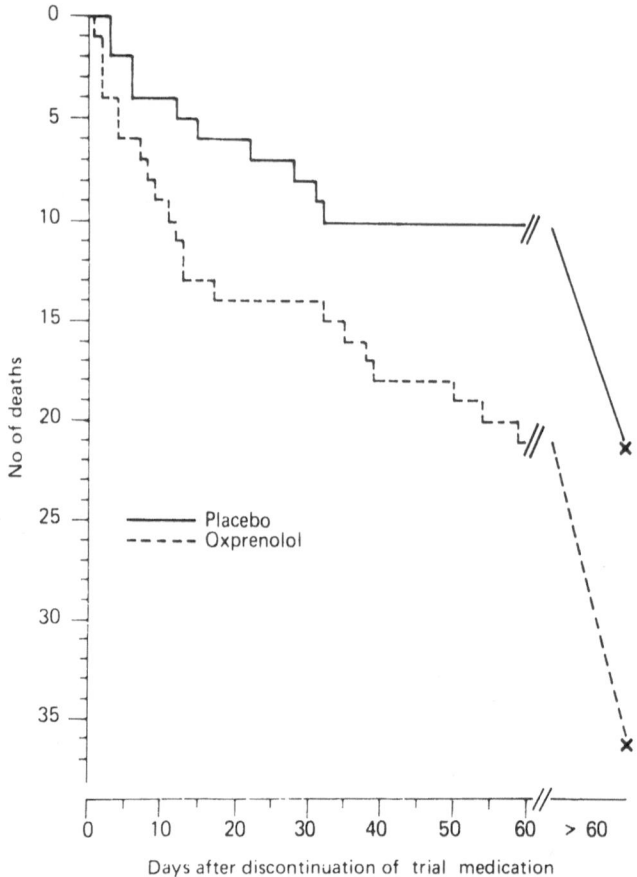

Figure 6. Number of deaths after discontinuation of trial medication in the placebo and oxpre-nolol group. Note the increasing difference in the number of deaths between the placebo and oxprenolol group, especially in the first 21 days, but also in the following days (for details see text).

plications occurring after withdrawal of trial medication. Hence, as Figure 6 demonstrates, the number of deaths after discontinuation increased more rapidly in the oxprenolol than in the placebo group, especially during the first 21 days, when 14 patients died in the oxprenolol group (7 suddenly, 6 due to reinfarction, 1 from heart failure) against only 6 patients the placebo group (2 suddenly, 1 due to reinfarction, 1 due to heart failure, 2 from non-cardiac causes). Also after 21 days up to 1 year mortality was still higher in the discontinued oxprenolol group (22 deaths) than in the placebo group (15 deaths); in the discontinued oxprenolol group 5 patients died due to heart failure against one in the placebo group.

Discussion

Although EIS had a 'negative' outcome with regard to the reduction of sudden death in the first year after myocardial infarction, especially if one follows 'intention of treatment', which includes by definition all discontinued cases, it shows some interesting features:

1. During trial medication the incidence of sudden death was lower under the betablocker, i.e. in the oxprenolol than in the placebo group (9 vs. 15 sudden death cases, mortality 1.54% vs. 2.46%). Although no significance was attributed to this figure, the reduction of 37.4% is close to the one observed in other studies (BHAT, Timolol Study).

2. In the high risk group below 65 years mortality was markedly lower in the oxprenolol than in the placebo group (6.9 vs. 10.2%), independent of trial discontinuation (−33%).

3. Of special concern is the mortality in the oxprenolol group above 65 years, both under trial medication (7.5%) and, especially after discontinuation (32.6%) in contrast to placebo (1.98 vs. 14.3%, respectively). This indicates an increased 'risk' for certain elderly patients when put under oxprenolol or eventually in general under betablocking agents. These results are in contrast to those demonstrated both in the timolol as well as in the BHAT trial where no undue increase in mortality was observed in this group. Nevertheless, it should be remembered that at high age sympathetic tone decreases and treatment with high doses of betablockers could easier lead to left heart failure and maybe to sudden death. This is supported by the fact that in this study, total mortality in the placebo group above 65 years was not increased in comparison to patients below 65 years, in contrast to the oxprenolol group. Hence, caution seems to be indicated in administering a betablocker in high doses at higher age, even if it contains intrinsic activity.

4. The increased death rate in the first three weeks after withdrawal in the oxprenolol group could be explained by a late 'rebound' effect, although such an effect on heart rate, blood pressure and contractility was not demonstrated beyond 4 to 6 days after discontinuation of a betablocker (Alderman, 1974; Rankno, 1982). In addition, the continuing higher death rate in the following months in this group in comparison to the placebo group is totally unexplained unless one accepts a difference in the severity of coronary disease and in the prognostic outcome between the two groups not evident from baseline variables. This cannot be excluded as in the majority of patients coronary and left ventricular angiography were not performed and also arrhythmia profiles were only established in approximately 1/3 of the cases using long-term ECGs; both anatomy as well as arrhythmia profile are, however, strong determinants of the prognosis in coronary artery disease.

5. EIS does not invalidate the results of other betablocker trials demonstrating a significant, approximately 25% reduction of sudden death in the first year after acute myocardial infarction. However, it emphasizes that obviously not all patients are candidates for such a treatment and that – even for betablocker trials with a positive outcome – a deterioration cannot be ruled out in some patients, especially in the elderly age group under betablockade. It should be remembered that betablocker treatment after myocardial infarction is not an all-or-nothing phenomenon; it might reduce the rate of sudden death but it does not suppress completely sudden coronary death.

Hence, indications have to be observed for this kind of treatment as for every treatment: patients with a combination of left ventricular failure and severe angina pectoris after myocardial infarction should undergo coronary angiography and if possible, revascularization, as this group profits from surgery as was shown both by CASS (Killip, 1983, 1984) and the European bypass-study (Varnauskas, 1984). Equally, patients with severe angina without cardiac failure should undergo angiography and possible revascularization. Patients with severe arrhythmias, especially clinically manifest tachyarrhythmias should undergo electrophysiological investigations (programmed stimulation, catheter mapping), and eventually intensive antiarrhythmic treatment or surgical or catheter ablation of the arrhythmogenic focus. This leaves the patient with an uncomplicated course of myocardial infarction for betablocker treatment. This group which has a mortality in the first year after myocardial infarction clearly below 10% (Bigger, 1984) is the target group of most of the betablocker trials. In patients with an extremely low risk course (small, first myocardial infarction, inferior myocardial infarction, no tachyarrhythmia, younger age etc.) betablocker treatment is a matter of discretion; here again the harm of betablockers might be greater than the profit. Furthermore, if treatment is installed, the dose should probably be kept at the lower level.

Finally, one should still recognize that the aim of all clinical trials is to proof a hypothesis by statistical means. Therefore, positive and negative outcome, if enough trials are performed, could represent a random phenomenon without any biological significance. Hence, it is still necessary to explain the large number of negative betablocker trials if one accepts that the positive ones represent a true biological event. Negative trials could be due to administration of an ineffective or less effective betablocker, one with not enough betablocking effect or class I antiarrhythmic properties. Also a too strong betablockade, too high a dose, could render a trial negative by provoking too many side effects and complications, especially also cardiac failure. Selection of patients could have been too strict, the risk of the included groups being too low. The baseline variables might be unbalanced with regard to criteria not evident in the patients history, such as anatomy only demonstrated by coronary angiography, i.e. the number of coronary arteries involved as well as the degree of obstructions or by different arrhythmia profiles not evident from long-term ECGs. Finally, in most of the trials the number of patients is too small for subgroup analysis and the trial is only positive for the entire group.

Nevertheless, as the situation stands today, the results of the large studies mentioned here suggest that betablocker treatment after myocardial infarction should be integrated into the management of patients in the first year after acute myocardial infarction. But only if the selection is done with great care will the patient really profit from this therapy which has its indications like other treatments.

References

1. The European Infarct Study Group: European infarct study (EIS). Eur Heart J 5:189–202, 1984.
2. Wilhelmsson C, Vedin JA, Wilhemsen L, Tibblin G, Werkö L: Reduction of sudden death after myocardial infarction by treatment with alprenolol. Lancet 1974; ii:1001, 57–60.
3. Multicentre International Study: Improvement in prognosis of myocardial infarction by long-term beta-adrenoreceptor blockade using practolol. Br Med J 3:735–740, 1975.
4. The Norwegian Multicenter Study Group: Timolol-induced reduction in mortality and re-infarction in patients surviving acute myocardial infarction. New Engl J Med 304:801–817, 1981.
5. Betablocker Heart Attack Trial Research Group: A randomized trial of propranolol in patients with acute myocardial infarction. I. Mortality results. JAMA 247:1707–1714, 1982.
6. Rose G: Prophylaxis with betablockers and the community. Br J Clin Pharm 14:455–485, 1982.
7. Alderman EL, Coltart DJ, Wettach GE, Harrison DC: Coronary artery syndromes after sudden propranolol withdrawal. Ann Internal Med 81:625–627, 1981
8. Rangno RE, Langloir S: Comparison of withdrawal phenomena after propranolol, metoprolol, and pindolol. Br J Clin Pharm 13:345S–351S, 1982.
9. Szecsi E, Kohlschütter S, Schiess W, Lang E: Abrupt withdrawal of pindolol or metoprolol after chronic therapy. Br J Clin Pharm 13:353S–357S, 1982.
10. May GS, Eberlein KA, Furberg CD, Passamani ER, DeMetz DL: Secondary prevention after myocardial infarction: A review of long-term trials. Progr Cardiovasc Dis 24:331–352, 1982.
11. Bigger TJ, Fleiss JL, Kleiger R, Miller JP, Rolnitzky LM, The Multicenter Postinfarction Research Group: The relationships among ventricular arrhythmias, left ventricular dysfunction, and mortality in the two years after myocardial infarction. Circ 69:250–258, 1984.
12. CASS: A randomized trial of coronary artery bypass surgery. Circ 68:939–950, 1983.
13. Varnauskas E: A multicenter randomized aorto-coronary bypass study; long-term survival. European Coronary Artery Study Group. In: Advances in Cardiology – Controversial views. Symposium Berlin 1984. Z f Kard: in preparation.

11. Platelet Aggregation Inhibitors

G. V. R. BORN

Abstract

In recent years there have been extensive and expensive clinical trials of drugs potentially effective against the most serious complications of atherosclerotic cardiovascular disease, namely cerebral thrombosis which causes stroke and coronary thrombosis which causes heart attacks. There is as yet no significant evidence to support the proposition that drugs designed to diminish thromboxane A_2 are effective against thrombogenesis. So far, the most effective antiplatelet drug has been acetyl salicylic acid, ie, aspirin. In seven large controlled trials of aspirin for the secondary prevention of myocardial infarction, involving a total of over 13,000 patients the drug produced no significant benefit although some showed a trend in that direction (May et al., 1982). However, in one recently published trial aspirin was very significantly effective in preventing myocardial infarction and death when the selection of patients was limited to those with unstable angina (Lewis et al., 1983). Controlled trials of aspirin for the prevention of stroke and of two clinical disorders which commonly precede stroke, namely transient ischaemic attacks and visual disturbances, have also demonstrated significant benefits (Fields, Lemak & Frankowski, 1977). This divergence suggests differences in the pathogenesis of these diseases. These differences may become understandable after considering thrombogenesis in atherosclerotic arteries, and how it may differ in carotid as against coronary arteries.

Recent evidence suggests that the antithrombotic effect of aspirin can be increased by dietary fish by a mechanism which, contrary to common claims, involves haemostatic factors other than platelets.

Introduction

Through an unusual and interesting development it has recently become possible to propose a pathogenetic mechanism for unstable angina as a result of a therapeutic success. Over several years there have been extensive and expensive clinical trials of drugs potentially effective against the most serious complications of atherosclerotic cardiovascular disease, namely cerebral thrombosis which causes stroke and coronary thrombosis which causes heart attacks. In several large controlled trials of aspirin for the secondary prevention of myocardial infarction involving a total of over 13,000 patients, the drug produced no significant benefit, although some of the trials showed a trend in that direction (May et al., 1982). However, in two recently reported trials, aspirin was very significantly effective in preventing myocardial infarction and death when the selection of patients was limited to those with unstable angina (Lewis et al., 1983; Cairns et al., 1984). Controlled trials of aspirin for the prevention of stroke and of two clinical disorders which commonly precede stroke, namely transient ischaemic attacks and visual disturbances, have also demonstrated significant benefit (Fields, Lemak & Frankowski, 1977). This divergence suggests differences in the pathogenesis of these diseases. These differences may become understandable after considering thrombogenesis in atherosclerotic arteries, and how it may differ in carotid as against coronary arteries.

The principal pathological facts of coronary thrombosis are as follows (Born, 1979): (1) Thrombi do not form in normal arteries, but in atherosclerotic arteries. (2) Atherosclerosis increases slowly, whereas thrombosis occurs rapidly and is individually unpredictable; therefore, atherosclerotic arteries must be subject to sudden, unpredictable events. (3) Most occlusive thrombi are associated with fissures in underlying atheromatous plaques. (4) The central portion of occlusive thrombi consists mainly of aggregated platelets.

Results and discussion

What is the mechanism responsible for initiating platelet aggregation in an atherosclerotic artery, as an apparently random event in time? Close serial sectioning (Friedman & Byers, 1965; Constantinides, 1966) and reconstruction of occluded segments of coronary arteries (Davies & Thomas, 1981, 1984) established that the central platelet-rich segment of an obstructive thrombus is usually, if not invariably, associated with recent haemorrhage into an underlying atherosclerotic plaque. Such haemorrhages occur through fissures or fractures in the plaque, and it is reasonable to assume that the sudden appearance of such a fissure or fracture is the random, individually unpredictable event affecting coronary arteries that has to be assumed to account for the clinical onset of acute myocardial infarction (Born, 1979). Why such a defect should develop at a particular moment is uncertain. Perhaps it is analogous to the sudden appearance of fine cracks in the wings of jet aircraft that is ascribed to the cumulative effects of variable stresses on metal known as fatigue failure (Born, 1979).

How does haemorrhage into a ruptured plaque trigger platelet thrombogenesis? This can be regarded as part of the general question of how platelets are caused to aggregate by haemorrhage. An explanation commonly put forward is that the process is initiated by platelets adhering to collagen that is exposed where damaged vessels walls are denuded of endothelium (Mustard et al., 1977). Adhering platelets then release other agents, including thromboxane A_2 and adenosine diphosphate, that in turn are responsible for the adhesion of more platelets as growing aggregates. This is unlikely, however, to be the complete explanation, for the following reasons. First, haemostatic and thrombotic aggregates of platelets grow very rapidly and without delay (Hugues, 1959; Born & Richardson, 1980). In contrast, platelet aggregation by collagen begins, even under optimal conditions for rapid reactivity, only after a delay or lag period of several seconds (Wilner, Nossell & LeRoy, 1968). Secondly, platelets tend to aggregate as mural thrombi when anticoagulated blood flows through plastic vessels (Didisheim, Panlovsky & Kobayashi, 1972) for example in artificial organs such as oxygenators or dialysers (Richardson, Galletti & Born, 1976) that contain neither collagen nor anything else capable of activating platelets similarly. This implies that there are conditions under which platelets are activated in the blood by something other than, or in addition to, the collagen in the walls of living vessels.

Recent *in vivo* experiments on three mammalian species, one of them man, indicate that the haemostatic aggregation of platelets is initiated by adenosine diphosphate (Zawilska, Born & Begent, 1982) which is released from injured cells in the blood vessels (Born, Görög & Kratzer, 1981; Born & Kratzer, 1984). It is reasonable to assume that cellular injury associated with the cracking of atheromatous plaques releases enough adenosine diphosphate locally to initiate thrombotic platelet aggregation in coronary arteries. The effect of this adenosine diphsophate, which is very rapid, is augmented first by thromboxane A_2 and later by much more adenosine diphosphate released from the platelets themselves. When a haemorrhage occurs through an atheromatous fissure into the arterial walls, the extravasated blood remains comparatively static; this condition can be presumed to favour the appearance of thrombin which initiates fibrin formation and contributes to platelet aggregation.

In this situation, therefore, platelets are apparently exposed simultaneously to several potent aggregating agents, only some of which are produced by the platelets themselves through their release reaction which is inhibited by aspirin. These considerations can therefore in principle account for the comparative ineffectiveness of aspirin in clinical trials of the secondary prevention of myocardial infarction; but they leave open the question why the drug is apparently effective when myocardial infarction is associated with unstable angina. Could it be that this type of angina points to a pathogenetic mechanism which differs from other antecedents of myocardial infarction and is more similar to the mechanism underlying cerebrovascular disturbances?

There is increasing evidence that in carotid as opposed to coronary arteries, haemodynamic disturbances alone can initiate the formation of embolising platelet thrombi. This conclusion is based mainly on non-invasive, ultrasound techniques that can be applied to carotid arteries but not to coronary arteries (Lusby et al., 1981, 1982; see also Born, 1985). In over 90% of patients affected by prestroke syndromes (characteristically transient ischaemic attacks and visual distrubances) two complementary imaging techniques demonstrate atherosclerotic lesions usually at the carotid bifurcation, that is, extracranially. In most of these cases the lesions constrict the arterial lumen severely, so that continuous vortices are established in the blood flow. At constant blood pressure the flow of blood is faster through the constriction than elsewhere in the artery. Therefore, high flow and wall shear rates are no hindrance to the aggregation of platelets as thrombi (Born, 1977). Indeed, the question arises of whether thrombogenic platelet aggregation can be brought about by abnormal haemodynamic conditions alone.

Evidence of increased platelet aggregation brought about by the operation of haemodynamic factors was provided by experiments in which blood was made to flow through branching channels in extra-corporeal shunts (Rowntree & Shionoya, 1927; Mustard et al., 1962). Deposits of platelets formed consistently on the shoulders of a bifurcation in the flow chamber, but nowhere else in the channels. When the chambers were perfused, not with blood, but with platelet-rich plasma, no deposit was formed, showing that red cells were also essential if deposition were to take place. The dependence that the deposition of platelets from flowing blood has on the red cells that surround and outnumber them could be caused by physical or chemical mechanisms; or by both acting together. A physical mechanism is contributed by the flow behaviour of the erythrocyte, which increases the diffusion of platelets in whole blood over that in plasma by up to two orders of magnitude (Turitto & Baumgartner, 1975). Thus, regions of flow separation and delays are evidently capable, as seen in similar flow in artificial vessels (Mustard et al., 1962), of causing platelet aggregates to form in the blood stream that are then carried as emboli into the cerebral circulation.

The exact mechanism that induces platelets to aggregate under these conditions is still uncertain. The established therapeutic effectiveness of aspirin in a high proportion of these cases would suggest that the platelets' release reaction is essential. Release of aggregating agents from platelets has long been assumed to subserve a 'chain reaction' or positive feedback mechanism (Born, 1965) that could, in principle, account for platelet aggregation in haemostasis and thrombosis. This assumption was based mainly on *in vitro* experiments that left considerable uncertainty about the contribution of the release reaction to the initiation of aggregation *in vivo*. The rapidity of the process, and the presence of other tissues, make it impossible to follow the release reaction quantitatively *in vivo* by the methods that permit its observation *in vitro*. Because it is the platelet reaction that is inhibited by aspirin, we adopted involving the postulated haemodynamic effects? Whatever the answer to this, recent evidence for the clinical effectiveness of at least one drug in the secondary prevention of myocardial infarction is very encouraging.

References

1. Born GVR: Platelets in thrombogenesis: mechanism inhibition of platelet aggregation. Ann R Coll Surg Engl 36:200–206, 1965.
2. Born GVR: Fluid-Mechanical and biochemical interactions in haemostasis. Br Med Bull 33:193–197, 1977.
3. Born GVR: Arterial thrombosis and its prevention. In: Hayase S, Murao S (eds) Proc VIII World Congress Cardiology. Excerpta Medica, Amsterdam, p 81–91, 1979.
4. Born GVR, Richardson PD: Activation time of blood platelets. J Membre Biol 57:87–90, 1980.
5. Born GVR, Görög P, Kratzer MAA: Aggregation of blood platelets in damaged vessels. Phil Trans R Soc Lond B 294:241–250, 1981.
6. Born GVR, Kratzer MAA: Source and concentration of extracellular adenosine tirphosphate during haemostasis in rats, rabbit and man. J Physiol Lond 354:419–429, 1984.
7. Born GVR: The carotid plaque. In: Robicsek F (ed) Extracranial cerebrovascular disease: diagnosis and management. Macmillan, New York (in press), 1985.
8. Cairns J, Gent M, Singer J, Finnie K, Froggatt G, Holder D, Jablonsky G, Kostuk W, Melendez L, Myers M, Sackett D, Sealey BQ, Tanser P: A study of aspirin (ASA) and sulfinpyrazone (S) in unstable angina. Circulation 70; suppl 2, Abstract 1659, 1984.
9. Constantinides P: Plaque fissures in human coronary thrombosis. J Atheroscler Res 6:1–17, 1966.
10. Davies MJ, Thomas T: The pathological basis and microanatomy of occlusive thrombus formation in human coronary arteries. Phil Trans R Soc Lond B 294:225–229, 1981.
11. Davies MJ, Thomas A: Thrombosis and acute coronary-artery lesions in sudden cardiac ischaemic death. New Engl J Med 310:1137–1140, 1984.
12. Didisheim P, Pavlovsky M, Kobayashi I: Factors that influence or modify platelet function. An Ann N Y Acad Sci 201:307–315, 1972.
13. Fields WS, Lemak RF, Frankowski RF: Controlled trials of aspirin in cerebral ischaemia. Stroke 8:301–328, 1977.
14. Friedman M, Byers SO: Induction of thrombi upon pre-existing parterial plaques. Amer J Path 46:567–575, 1965.
15. Hugues JC: Agglutination precoce des plaquettes au cours de la formation du clou hémostatique. Thromb Diathès haemorrh 3: 177–186, 1959.
16. Lewis HD Jr, Davies JW, Archibald DG, Steinke WE, Smitherman TC, Doherty JE III, Schnaper HW, LeWinter MM, Linares E, Maurice Pouget J, Sabharwal SC, Chesler E, DeMots: Protective effects of aspirin against acute myocardial infarction and death in men with unstable angina. New Engl J Med 309:396–403, 1983.

17. Lusby RJ, Machleder HI, Jeans W, Skidmore R, Woodcock JP, Clifford PC, Baird RN: Vessell wall and blood flow dynamics in arterial diseases. Phil Trans R Soc Lond B 294:231–239, 1981.

18. Lusby RJ, Ferrell LD, Ehrenfeld WK, Stoney RJ, Wylie EJ: Carotid Plaque hemorrhage: its role in production of cerebral ischemia. Arch Surg 117:1479–1488, 1982.

19. May GS, Eberlein KA, Furberg CD, Passamain ER, DeMets DS: Secondary prevention after myocardial infarction: a review of long-term trials. Prof Cardiovas Dis 24:331–352, 1982.

20. Mustard JF, Murphy EA, Rowsell HC, Downie HG: Factors influencing thrombus formation in vivo. Amer J Med 33:621–647, 1962.

21. Mustard JF, Moore S, Packham MA, Kinlough Rathbone RL: Platelets, thrombosis and atherosclerosis. Proc Biochem Phamracol 13:312–325, 1977.

22. Richardson PD, Galletti PMn Born GVR: Regional administration of drugs to control thrombosis in artificial organs. Trans Am Soc Artif Intern Organs 22:22–29, 1976.

23. Rowntree LG, Shionya T: Studies in experimental extracorporeal thrombosis. Part 1: Methods for the direct observation of extra-corporeal thrombus formation. J exp Med 46:7–12, 1927.

24. Turitto VT, Baumgartner HR: Platelet interaction with subendothelium in a perfusion system: physical role of red blood cells. Microvasc Res 5:167–179, 1975.

25. Wilner GD, Nossell HL, Le Roy EC: Agregation of platelets by collagen. J Clin Invest 47:2616–2621, 1968.

26. Zawilska KM, Born GVR, Begent NA: Effect of ADP-utilising enzymes on the arterial bleeding time in rats and rabbits. Br J Haematol 50:317–325, 1982.

12. Platelet Inhibitors or Anticoagulants for Prevention of Aorto-Coronary Bypass Graft Occlusion

M. E. ROTHLIN

Abstract

The effect of the anti-platelet drug Ticlopidine (T) on the thrombotic occlusion rate of coronary artery bypass (CABP) was studied by angiography 3 months postoperatively in 237 patients. A double blind trial with T 250 mg b.i.d. or Placebo (Pl) administered pre- and postoperatively with additional anticoagulation with Acenocoumarol postoperatively had to be interrupted prematurely when it became clear that T enhanced bleeding and the number of reoperations for hemostasis significantly. In the 87 patients included the number of perioperative infarctions was significantly reduced in patients receiving T (1/45) as compared to those receiving Pl (6/42) $P = 0,450$. After three months there was no significant difference in patency rate between the two treatment groups.

After a report on a significant reduction of graft occlusion by oral anticoagulation the question arose, whether simultaneous Acenocoumarol treatment concealed a beneficial effect of T in our patients. In a prospective randomized trial on 148 patients receiving T (250 mg b.i.d.) or anticoagulation by Acenocoumarol from the second or third postoperative day on it was examined, whether T is superior, equal or inferior to oral anticoagulants regarding CABP obstruction. Three months postoperatively angiography revealed an average patency rate of 84,2% after T as compared to 81.6% after Acenocoumarol (n.s.). Progression of stenosis in the native vessels was almost identical in both treatment groups. No side effects were observed which resulted in irreversible sequelae. Conclusions: In spite of the significant reduction of perioperative infarctions T can not be recommended preoperatively because of the significant increase of bleeding and reoperations for hemostasis. With postoperative administration T is easier to handle (standard dosage without determination of prothrombine time) and regarding CABP patency rate at least as effective as anticoagulation by Acenocoumarol.

Introduction

After aorto-coronary bypass graft surgery 10–30% of the bypasses get obstructed within the first few postoperative months (Bourassa et al., 1979; Bulkley and Hutchins, 1977, Chesebro et al., 1984; Lawrie et al., 1976; Sheldon et al., 1973; Vlodaver and Edwards, 1973). Apart from technical errors and vascular factors thrombosis plays an important role for early bypass obstruction. In an effort to reduce bypass occlusion we started a clinical trial in 1979 testing the effect of Ticlopidine, a platelet active drug, that had been proved to have a prophylactic effect on thrombosis of synthetic vascular grafts in the animal experiment (Walter et al., 1981).

Effect of pre- and postoperative ticlopidine on bypass occlusion

After informed consent male patients below age 65 were randomized. A treatment group received Ticlopidine, 250 mg twice daily, for 3 days before surgery and from the first to second postoperative day on, up to a postoperative angiography performed three months after surgery. A control group received a Placebo tablet in the same manner. All patients were anticoagulated by Acenocoumarol on the second postoperative day throughout the study period. When most severe bleeding occured in a patient, this trial had to be discontinued prematurely. It was found, that Ticlopidine significantly enhanced peri- and postoperative bloodloss and led to a six-fold increase of reoperation for bleeding (Rothlin et al., 1982). Therefore it was concluded, that preoperative administration of Ticlopidine is not justified.

Out of 100 patients included, when the study was discontinued, 87 completed the protocol. Patients compliance in the Ticlopidine group was 86% according to aggregation tests performed and 84% according to tablet counts.

Univariate comparison of the 45 Placebo patients and of 42 Ticlopidine patients showed, that patients in the Placebo group were older and had more severe symptoms, while there was no significant difference in stress test, ejection fraction, number of vessels involved or number of bypass implanted.

Graft patency is depicted on table 1. There was an overall patency of 80%, with 81% of patent grafts in the placebo group and 79% in the Ticlopidine group. Comparison of bypass to specific vessels or of single, double or multiple bypass did not reveal considerable differences.

On the other hand comparison of the incidence of perioperative infarction revealed one event in the Ticlopidine group but 6 in the Placebo group ($p = 0.045$). This significant difference in the incidence of perioperative infarctions is of interest, because postoperative angiography in patients with

Table 1. Patency rate of grafts after aorto – coronary bypass

	Placebo		Ticlopidine	
	no. of grafts	patent %	no. of grafts	patent %
All vessels	155	81 (74–87) [a]	136	79 (70–85)
LAD	69	84 (73–91)	67	85 (74–92)
RCA	42	81 (65–91)	40	82 (67–92)
RCX	44	77 (62–88)	29	59 (39–76)
Single bypass	56	84 (71–92)	40	78 (61–89)
Double bypass	72	90 (80–96)	68	84 (72–91)
Multiple bypass	27	52 (32–71)	28	68 (48–83)

[a]   95%confidence intervals

perioperative myocardial infarctions revealed obstruction of the corresponding aorto-coronary bypass and/or of the corresponding native vessel in almost all cases (Goebel et al., 1983).

The significant reduction of graft occlusion reported by Gohlke et al. (1981) raised the question, whether anticoagulants, administered after surgery to all patients in this trial, had concealed a possible effect of Ticlopidine on graft occlusion. A second study was therefore designed to compare the effect of postoperative treatment with Ticlopidine with that of oral anticoagulation by Acenocoumarol with respect to thrombotic occlusion of aorto-coronary bypass grafts.

Ticlopidine versus anticoagulants for prevention of bypass occlusion

A total of 166 patients consented to enter the trial. After the operation 83 patients each were assigned to Ticlopidine or Acenocoumarol treatment (Rothlin et al., 1985). Ticlopidine, 250 mg b.i.d. was administered orally starting the first postoperative day until angiography was performed three months postoperatively. Acenocoumarol was started after removal of the drainage tubes on the second or third postoperative day. Dosage was adjusted aiming at a prothrombine time of 20–25%.

Out of the 166 patients recruited, 17, namely 5 receiving Ticlopidine and 12 receiving anticoagulants could not submit to angiography. Numerous preoperative characteristics of the 78 patients in the Ticlopidine group and of the 71 patients in the anticoagulant group were compared by univariate methods without showing any significant difference at the 5% level. Logistic stepwise regression on a large number of preoperative findings of the two treatment groups did not reveal significant difference.

Cineangiographic examination of patency of the aorto-coronary bypass did not reveal any substantial difference between the two treatment groups.

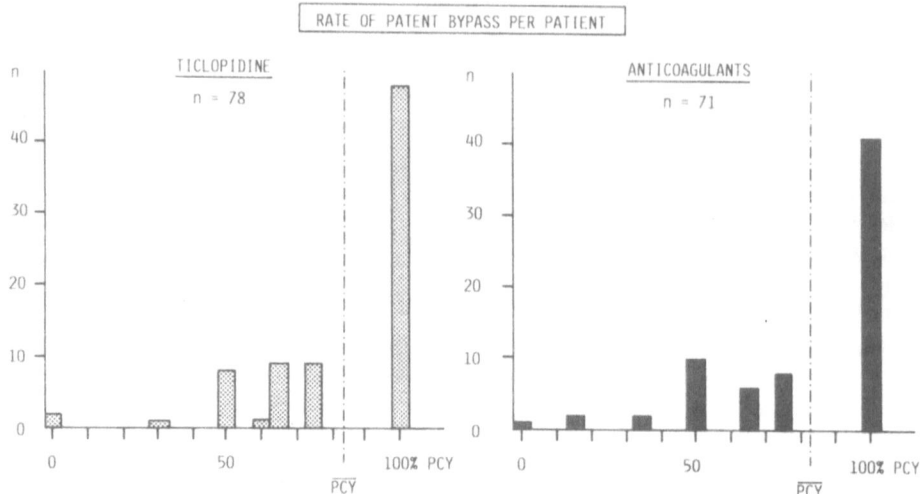

Figure 1. Histogram of individual patency rate (PCY) in patients treated with Ticlopidine (average PCY = 84.2%) or Acenocoumarol (average PCY = 81.6%).

There were 30 out of 78 patients with Ticlopidine and 30 out of 71 patients with anticoagulants, who had at least one occluded graft segment. Two patients out of 78 with Ticlopidine and one patient out of 71 with anticoagulants had all grafts occluded. The average patency rate per patient (PCY) was 84.2% for the Ticlopidine group and 81.6% for the Acenocoumarol group as can be seen from the histograms depicted on Figure 1. A regression characterizing patients before medication including the location of the bypass segment, the size of the anastomosed coronary artery, need for endarterectomy and type of bypass graft as possible risk factors for obstruction was done for PCY. Although a large number of possibly influencial variables was looked for, there was almost no influence on bypass patency. The presented findings indicate, that the regimens of Ticlopidine, an antiplatelet drug and Acenocoumarol, an oral anticoagulant, had virtually identical effects on aorto-coronary bypass graft patency studied three months after implantation.

Side effects of Ticlopidine were rare, only 3 patients discontinued the drug for nausea and anorexia. In the Acenocoumarol group there was cerebral hemorrhage, gastrointestinal hemorrhage and hematuria in one patient each. An indirect 'side effect' of Ticlopidine treatment may be seen in the occurance of pulmonary embolism in two patients and suspicion of this complication in an other two, all taking the platelet active drug instead of oral anticoagulants.

From our personal experience with Ticlopidine we may conclude that:
1. Although preoperative Ticlopidine treatment significantly reduces perioperative myocardial infarctions it is not justified because it enhances

perative and postoperative bleeding to a degree which may potentially be life threatening.

2. In the presented studies there is no direct evidence, that Ticlopidine has a beneficial influence on patency rate. The fact, that its effect is at least equal to that of anticoagulants, which were shown to improve patency rate significantly, is very much in favour of a beneficial effect of Ticlopidine. Moreover, in a very recent study Chevigné et al. (1984) found a beneficial effect of Ticlopidine on patency rate in a subgroup of patients studied in their randomized trial.

3. Postoperative administration of Ticlopidine for the first three months after bypass surgery is at least as effective as oral anticoagulation in regard to patency rate of bypass grafts. Antiplatelet drugs administered in a standard dose are easier to manage than oral anticoagulants. It appears, however, that anticoagulation during the first postoperative weeks is more effective in prevention of pulmonary embolism.

Other drug trials in prevention of bypass-occlusion

Since 1979 clinical trials aiming at the prevention of bypass-occlusion have been reported (Pantely et al., 1979; Gohlke et al., 1981; Mayer et al., 1981; McEnany et al., 1982; Chesebro et al., 1982 and 1984; Baur et al., 1982; Sharma et al., 1982; Lorenz et al., 1984; Chevigné et al., 1984; Brooks et al., 1984). Aspirin alone or in combination with Dipyridamole in different dosage, Sulfinpyrazone 4×200 mg and Ticlopidine 2×250 mg were tested as well as oral anticoagulants.

The result of the studies using Aspirin alone or in combination with Dipyridamole and Dicoumarol anticoagulants were conflicting. Mayer et al., 1981, Chesebro et al., 1982 and Lorenz et al., 1984 reported on a beneficial effect of these drugs. Pantely et al. (1979), McEnany et al. (1982), Sharma et al. (1982) and Brooks et al. (1984) were unable to show an effect.

The clinical trials with a beneficial effect had in common an early start of treatment on the first postoperative day or even preoperatively (Chesebro et al., 1982). On the other hand, in the clinical trials without positive effect treatment was withheld until the third to fourth postoperative day. Sulfinpyrazone and Ticlopidine were compared against placebo in one clinical trial each (Baur et al., 1982 and Chevigné et al., 1984). In both studies a beneficial effect was reported with starting the treatment on the first postoperative day.

A tentative conclusion from this review of clinical trials indicates that all platelet active drugs tested may exhibit an effect on early bypass obstruction. From the data available it cannot be said which drug is the most effective. On the other hand early start of treatment before the intervention

106

or at the latest on the first postoperative day, was the common factor in the protocols of all trials with a beneficial effect. Additional controlled clinical-studies are necessary to define the most effective drug, dosage and duration of treatment.

At our institution the present policy is Acetylsalicylate 0.5 g b.i.d. starting 6 hours postoperatively, after a tendency to hemorrhage has been ruled out. Acetylsalicylates are administered for 6 months. Moreover patients receive oral anticoagulation by Acenocoumarol starting on the second to third postoperative day, aiming at a prothrombin time of 30–40%. This treatment is directed to the prevention of venous thrombosis and pulmonary embolism and it is maintained for about two weeks.

References

Baur HR, van Tassel AR, Pierach CA, Gobel FL: Effects of sulfinpyrazone on early graft closure rate after myocardial revascularization. Am J Cardiol 49:420–424, 1982.

Bourassa MC, Lespérence J, Campeau L, Simard P: Factors influencing patency of aortocoronary vein grafts. Circulation 45(Suppl I):179–185, 1972.

Brooks N, Wright JEC, Sturridge MF, Balcon R: Randomized trial of the effect of aspirin and dipyridamole on coronary vein graft patency. Personal comunication. Eur. Heart J. 5(Suppl 1), 1984.

Bulkley BH, Hutchins GM: Accelerated 'atherosclerosis' a morphologic study of 97 saphenous vein coronary artery bypass grafts. Circulation 55:163–169, 1977.

Chesebro JH, Clements IP, Fuster V, Elveback LR et al.: A platelet inhibitor drug trial in coronary artery bypass operations. N Engl J Med 307:73–78, 1982.

Chesebro JH, Fuster V, Elveback lr, Clements JP et al.: Effect of Dipyridamole and Aspirin on late vein-graft patency after coronary bypass operations. N Engl J Med 310:209–214, 1984.

Chevigné M, David JL, Rigo P, Limet R: Effect of Ticlopidine, on saphenous vein bypass patency rates: A double blind study. Ann Thorac Surg 37:371–378, 1984.

Gohlke H, Gohlke-Bärwolf CH, Stürzenhofecker P, Görnandt L et al.: Improved graft patency with anticoagulant therapy after aorto-coronary bypass surgery: A prospective randomized study. Circulation 64(Suppl II):22–27, 1981.

Lawrie GM, Lie JT, Morris GC, Beazley HL: Vein Graft patency and intimal proliferation after aortocoronary bypass: early and longterm angiographic correlations. Am J Cardiol 38:856–862, 1976.

Lorenz RL, Weber M, Kotzur J et al.: Improved aortocoronary bypass patency by low dose Aspirin. Lancet 8:969–971, 1984.

Mayer JE, Lindsay WJ, Castaneda W, Nicoloff DM: Influence of aspirin and dipyridamole on patency of coronary artery bypass grafts. Ann Thorac Surg 31:204–210, 1981.

McEnany MT, Salzman EW, Mundt ED, De Sanctis RW et al.: The effect of antithrombotic therapy on patency rates of saphenous vein coronary artery bypass grafts. J Thorac Cardiovasc Surg 83:81–89, 1982.

Pantely GA, Goodnight SH, Rahimtoola SH, Harlan BJ et al: Failure of antiplatelet and anticoagulant therapy to improve patency of grafts after coronary artery bypass. N Engl J Med 301:962–966, 1979.

Rothlin ME, Pfluger N, Speiser K, Geroulanos S et al.: Clinical experience with antiplatelet drugs in aorto-coronary bypass surgery. In: Coronary artery surgery today. Ed.: Bruschke AVG, van Herpen G, Vermeulen FEE. Excerpta Medica, International Congress Series 557:413–419, 1982.

Rothlin ME, PFluger N, Speiser K, Goebel N et al.: Platelet inhibitors versus anticoagulants for prevention of aorto-coronary bypass graft occlusion. In press.

Sharma GVRK, Khuri SF, Folland ED, Josa M et al.: Lack of benefit from aspirin-dipyridomale therapy in aorto-coronary vein graft patency. Circulation 66(Suppl II9; II-94 abstract, 1982.

Sheldon WC, Rincon G, Effler DB, Proudfitt WL, Sones FM: Vein graft surgery for coronary artery disease. Circulation 48(Suppl III): 184–189, 1973.

Vlodaver Z, Edwards JE: Pathologic changes in aortocoronary and saphenous vein grafts. Circulation 44: 719–728, 1971.

Walter P, Geroulanos S, Rothlin ME, Turina M et al.: Die rasterelektronenoptischen Oberflächenränderungen der Gefässinnenfläche gewobener Dacron-Gefässprothesen nach Verabreichung von Ticlopidine. Folia Angiol 29: 20–32, 1981.

13. Cardiovascular Protection by Calcium Antagonists

A. FLECKENSTEIN, M. FREY and G. FLECKENSTEIN-GRÜN

Abstract

As shown in animal experiments, one of the most important effects of the new pharmacological family of Ca antagonists is to prevent deleterious myocardial Ca overload which is the decisive etiological factor in the production of cardiac necroses by overdoses of β-adrenergic catecholamines, vitamin D3, dihydrotachysterol, or following alimentary K^+ or Mg^{++} deficiency as well as genetic defects (hereditary cardiomyopathy of Syrian hamsters). Furthermore in our experiments on rats, a pathogenic myocardial and arterial Ca accumulation producible by chronic oral administration of nicotine did no longer appear if nicotine was given together with suitable oral doses of verapamil, diltiazem or nifedipine. On the other hand, nicotine-induced myocardial and arterial Ca uptake as well as tissue damage are greatly enhanced by measures which increase the extracellular Ca supply. For instance vitamin D3 or dihydrotachysterol elevate the plasma Ca level, and can thereby potentiate within a few days, the calcifying potency of nicotine to a dramatic extent. Again with the help of suitable Ca antagonists, tremendous cardiovascular toxicity of the incompatible drug combination (vitamin D3 plus nicotine) could be neutralized.

However even in simple anoxia or ischemia, Ca overload seems to play an additional pathogenic role in that the inevitable structural decay is precipitated. Thus also in humans, certain Ca antagonists have proved to be useful additives to cardioplegic solutions for providing better myocardial preservation.

Physiological Control of Myocardial Contractile Performance

Excitation occurs at the sarcolemma membrane whereas contraction is an intracellular phenomenon. Therefore, there is a need for some kind of information transfer from the fibre surface to the intracellular contractile elements, if the internal mechanical reactions should be linked with the superficial excitation process. Nature has solved this difficult problem of 'excitation-contraction coupling' with the help of Ca-ions, serving as messengers. During the past decade evidence has been obtained of the existence of a dual membrane carrier system in atrial and ventricular myocardium: a fast channel for Na-ions that initiate the cardiac fibre action potentials and a separate slow channel for Ca-ions that activate the contractile machinery. Thus a sudden transmembrane Ca-influx takes place during cardiac excitation together with a liberation of Ca-from certain endoplasmic stores. The resulting increase in the intracellular concentration of free Ca-ions initiates the splitting of ATP by the Ca-dependent myofibrillar ATPase. In this way, phosphate-bond energy is transformed into mechanical work. Positive inotropic agents such as β-receptor stimulating catecholamines or histamine, acting on H_2-receptors, potentiate the transmembrane Ca influx during cardiac excitation, thus augmenting splitting of ATP, contractile force and, finally, oxygen requirement. The catecholamines and histamine probably enhance Ca-binding at superficially located sarcolemmal storage sites by phosphorylation of membrane proteins (via formation of cyclic AMP and activation of a phosphokinase) so that more Ca is made available to the slow channels. Butyryl-cyclic-AMP promotes Ca-influx more directly.

Table 1. Classification of calcium antagonists into the groups A and B according to the degree of specificity

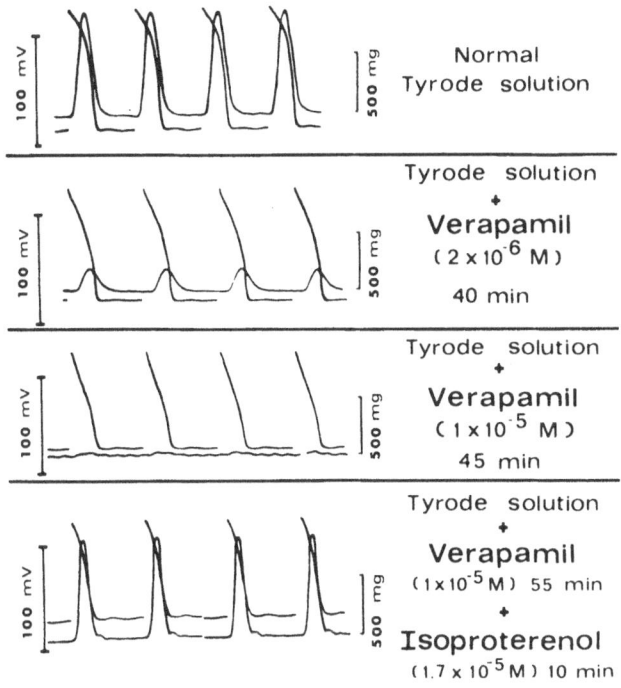

Figure 1. Selective loss of cardiac contractility under the influence of a high overdose of verapamil, and the reversal of this effect by isoproterenol. Experiments on an electrically driven (2 shocks/sec) isolated papillary muscle of a guinea-pig in Tyrode solution with 2 mM Ca^{2+}. Reproduced from Fleckenstein (1968), Verh Deutsch Ges Kreisl-Forsch 34:15–34.

Reduction of Cardiac Contractile Energy Expenditure by Calcium Antagonists

The most powerful opponents of the positive-inotropic promoters of Ca influx are the Ca antagonists verapamil, D 600 (methoxy-verapamil), nifedipine, niludipine, nimodipine, and diltiazem (see the review articles 1–7). According to our studies, these drugs are capable of blocking the Ca-conductivity of the slow channels by 90 to 100% before a concomitant reduction of the fast Na-current becomes also discernible. The transmembrane Mg-influx is not affected [8]. Fleckenstein has proposed to designate these compounds as Ca-antagonists of group A (see Table 1). Diltiazem was introduced as a Ca-antagonist by Japanese authors [9], and identified as a member of group A in our laboratory. In an elevated concentration range, all Ca-antagonists of group A can totally suppress contractile performance of isolated mammalian myocardium without an appreciable inhibition of the Na-dependent action potential parameters (upstroke velocity, height of overshoot (Fig. 1)).

The Ca-antagonists prenylamine, fendiline and perhexiline are somewhat less potent and specific. Nevertheless these drugs too, designated by Fleckenstein as Ca-antagonists of group B, can produce a preferential suppression of the slow Ca-current by 50 to 70% without major impairment of the Na-dependent excitatory processes. All Ca-antagonists probably act by competing with Ca-ions at superficial Ca-binding sites in the sarcolemma membrane or in the slow channels. There is in all cases a rigid correlation between the inhibition of transsarcolemmal Ca-influx, contractile energy expenditure and respiration rate. No other drugs are known that restrict Ca-dependent ATP consumption, tension development, and oxygen requirement of the active myocardial fibres so effectively with no or only minor concomitant influences on atrial or ventricular excitability and impulse propagation. Moreover the degree of contractile inhibition is strictly dose-related and readily reversible by all measures that restore transmembrane Ca-influx as for instance, administration of extra-calcium or β-adrenergic catecholamines. Thus, the Ca-antagonists can be considered as safe drugs with particular value also for clinical purposes in the therapy of hyperkinetic cardiac dysfunctions.

Slowdown by Ca-Antagonists of Cardiac Pacemaker Activity

However the situation is different with respect to the action of Ca-antagonists on spontaneous cardiac pacemaker excitation in the SA or AV node and, particularly, in case of ectopic atrial or ventricular automaticity which can be suppressed by inhibition of the Ca inward current. In fact, the electrogenesis of nomotopic and ectopic pacemaker action potentials requires Ca-ions as transmembrane electric charge carriers because in SA and AV nodal cells as well as in ectopic foci, the fast carrier mechanism for Na is absent or inactivated [2-4, 6]. Thus automaticity is as Ca-dependent as contractility is (Fig. 2). This explains why β-adrenergic agents, by promoting the transfer of Ca through the slow channels not only cause an increase in contractile force, but also produce an analogous rise in heart rate and AV conduction velocity. Conversely, organic Ca-antagonists exert negative inotropic, chronotropic and dromotropic influences mostly in combination, and also suppress ectopic atrial or ventricular foci.

Arterial Smooth Muscle Relaxation by Ca-Antagonists

Interestingly enough, excitation and, particularly, excitation-contraction coupling of vascular smooth muscle cells is also highly susceptible to the action of Ca-antagonistic substances. Here again, as in cardiac fibres, the transmembrane Ca conductivity is inhibited so that all Ca-dependent con-

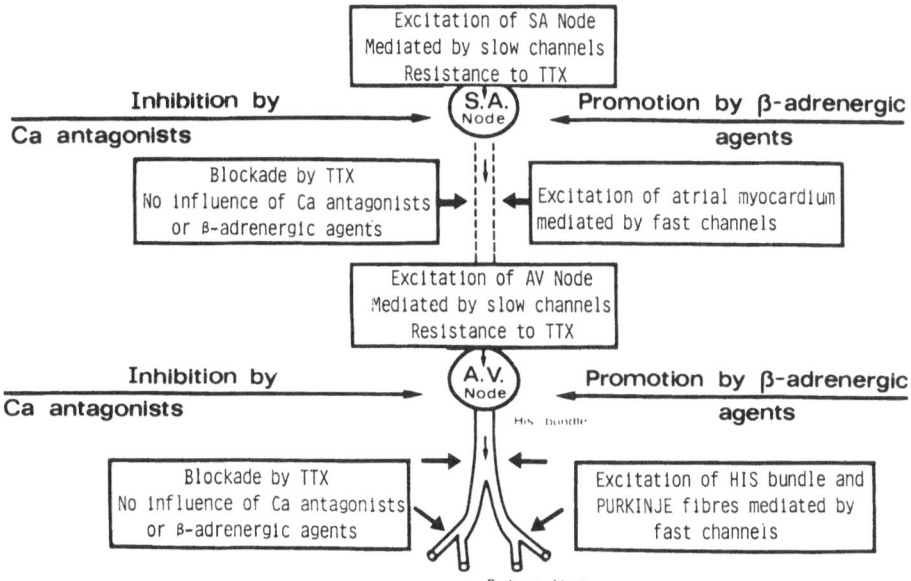

Figure 2. Opposite effects of calcium antagonists and calcium promoters (beta-adrenergic agents) on slow-channel-mediated, tetrodotoxin (TTX)-insensitive sinoatrial (S.A.) node automaticity and atrioventricular (A.V.) node conductivity. Refractoriness to calcium antagonists and beta-adrenergic catecholamines of normal TTX-sensitive impulse propagation in atrial, His bundle, Purkinje and ventricular fibres. Reproduced from Fleckenstein (1980), Proc Symposium on Calcium Antagonism in Cardiovascular Therapy, Florence 2-4 October 1980, (Zanchetti A, Krikler DM (eds)), pp 10–29, Excerpta Medica, Amsterdam-Oxford-Princeton.

tractile phenomena such as vascular tone and spastic vasoconstriction can be suppressed even with very small doses (Fig. 3). This explains the coronary and peripheral vasodilator effects of Ca-antagonistic compounds. As to the influence on diseased coronary vessels, it is commonly known that more than 95% of the obstructive intima lesions are located in large extramural stem arteries, and that blood flow through these vessels is often additionally jeopardized by superimposed spasms. Therefore, it is important to note that nifedipine and related Ca-antagonistic compounds are the most powerful smooth muscle relaxants of the extramural coronary vessels, including extramural anastomoses and collaterals [6, 10, 11]. Accordingly, all forms of vasospastic angina (particularly Prinz-metal's 'Variant Angina') are outstandingly responsive to these drugs. Moreover, Ca antagonists exert antihypertensive effects by inducing systemic arteriolar vasodilation.

Cardioprotection by Ca-Antagonists

Another important finding is that Ca-antagonists provide direct cardioprotection against Ca-induced functional and structural damage [1, 3, 5–7]. In

114

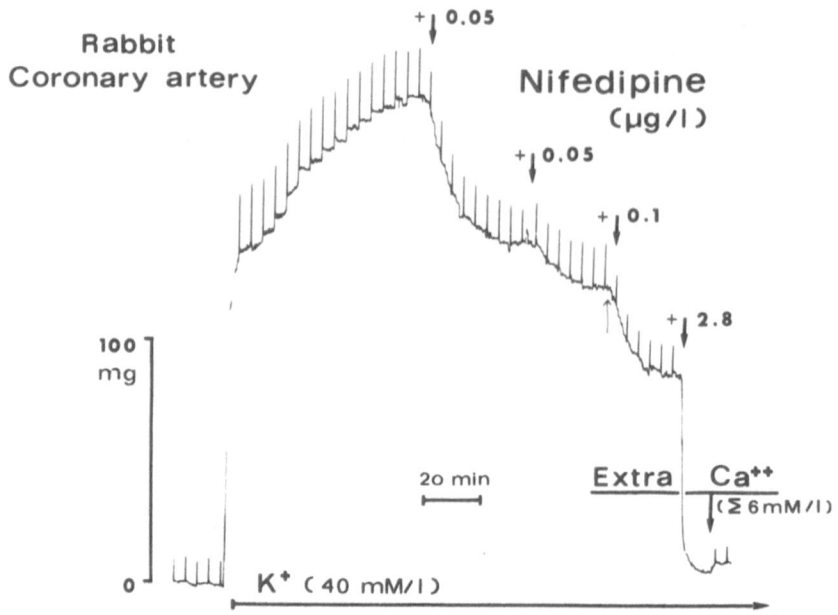

Figure 3. Suppression by nifedipine of a spastic in vitro contraction of a rabbit coronary strip depolarized with high K$^+$ (40 mM) in Tyrode solution. In addition to the high K concentration, alternating electric square wave stimuli were applied to test excitability. Minute amounts of nifedipine, successively administered to the bath after the climax of shortening had been reached, produced gradual relaxation. With a total dose of 3 μg nifedipine/l (1×10^{-8} M) relaxation was completed, and electric excitability abolished. Nifedipine blocks Ca entry across the K$^+$-depolarized coronary smooth muscle cell membrane and thereby produces excitation-contraction uncoupling. Extra calcium, given at the end of the experiment, restored excitability. (Experiment of Nakayama and Fleckenstein, see Fleckenstein [6].)

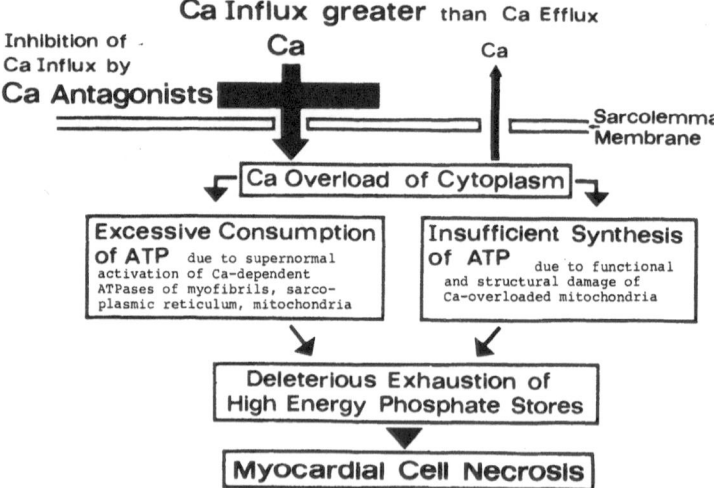

Figure 4. Scheme of myocardial necrotization, produced by intracellular calcium overload, and of cardioprotection, provided by Ca-antagonists. Reproduced from Fleckenstein (1980), reference see figure 2.

fact, heart muscle fibres undergo severe alterations, finally resulting in necrotization, as soon as free extracellular Ca-ions penetrate excessively through the sarcolemma membrane into the myoplasm, so that the capacities of the Ca-binding or extrusion processes become insufficient (Fig. 4). The crucial event in the development of such lesions is high-energy phosphate deficiency which results (a) from excessive activation of Ca-dependent intracellular ATPases, and (b) from Ca-induced impairment of the mitochondria (swelling, vacuolization, cristolysis, loss of respiratory control and phosphorylation capacity). Intracellular Ca overload proved to be the decisive pathogenic factor in the etiology of myocardial fibre necroses produced under the following circumstances: Overdoses of β-adrenergic catecholamines, dihydrotachysterol [AT10], vitamin D3 or cardiac glycosides; extreme physical or emotional stress; alimentary potassium or magnesium deficiency; hereditary cardiomyopathy of Syrian hamsters. Moreover, intracellular Ca-overload develops in the course of myocardial hypoxia or ischemia thus causing additional deterioration of the mitochondria. In rat hearts, the number and size of catecholamine-induced cardiac lesions are obviously determined by the extent and, particularly, by the duration of the Ca-mediated high-energy phosphate penury. Conversely, Ca-antagonistic compounds are capable of partially or totally protecting the structural integrity of the heart muscle fibres in that they restrict transmembrane Ca-influx and, consequently, prevent ATP and creatine-phosphate exhaustion. Thus, also the tolerance of heart muscle to anoxia or ischemia is considerably increased following prophylactic administration of verapamil [12], nifedipine [13] or diltiazem [14].

Prophylactic Effects of Calcium Antagonists against Experimental Vascular Calcinosis

Our studies have provided experimental evidence that, in vascular smooth muscle too, Ca-overload is a highly pathogenic event, finally leading to necrotization and calcinosis of the arterial media, similar to Mönckeberg's type of arteriosclerosis. In humans, arterial Ca-overload progressively develops with age (Fig. 5), but it can also be observed in hypertensive or alloxan-diabetic rats, and in animals treated with overdoses of vitamin D_3 or dihydrotachysterol (AT 10), particularly if combined with administration of nicotine [15–18]. Our observations have revealed that in accordance with our original findings on heart muscle, Ca-antagonists are also capable of interfering with deleterious Ca accumulation in the arterial wall. Thus in our experiments, verapamil and diltiazem provided excellent protection against vascular calcinosis in aging, vitamin D3-treated, nicotine-treated, and alloxan-diabetic rats, whereas in other experiments, nifedipine was most effective

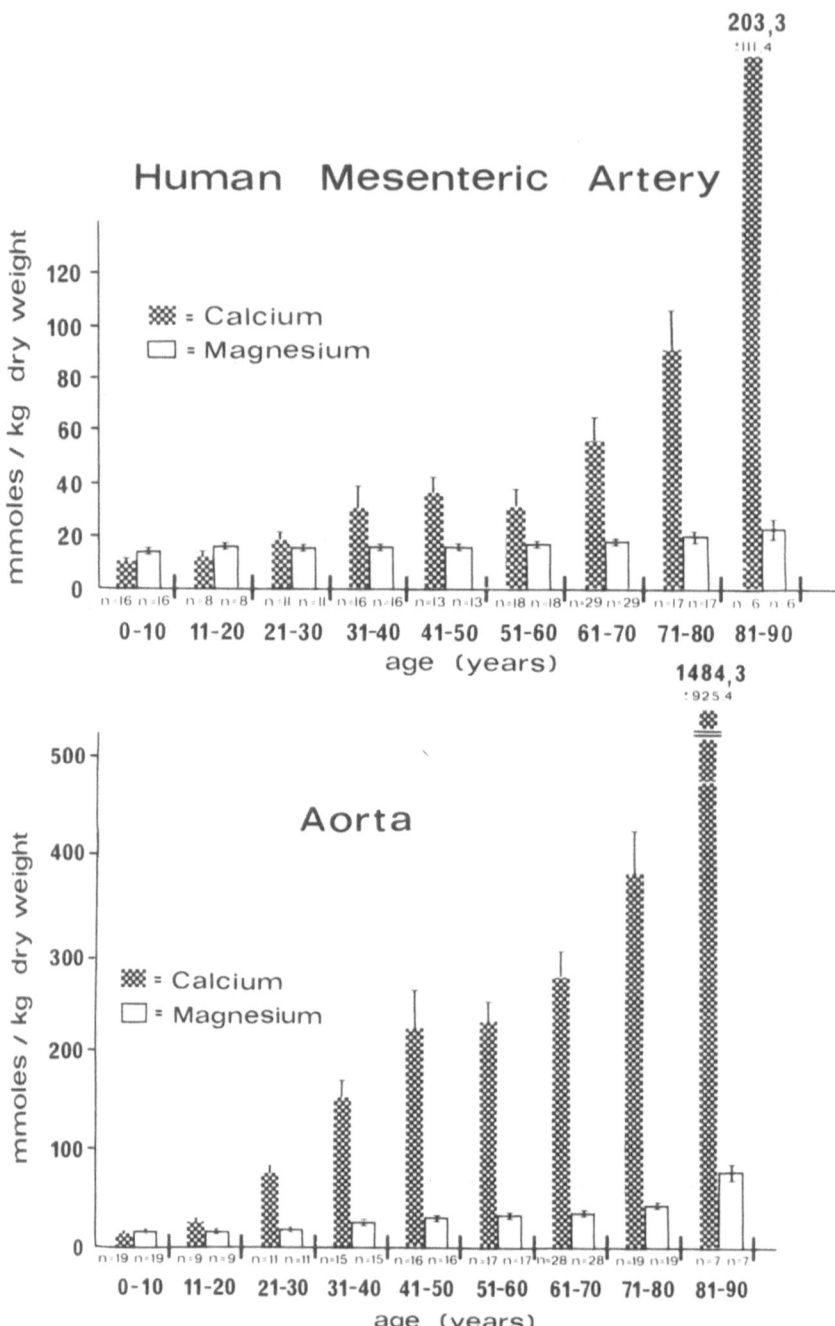

Figure 5. Progressive arterial Ca overload and increase in the ratio Ca:Mg with advanced age. Tissue samples were taken from the superior mesenteric artery (N = 134) and the aorta (N = 141). The arteries mostly originated from autopsies of traffic victims. Only artery segments without visible plaques were analyzed using atom absorption spectrometry.

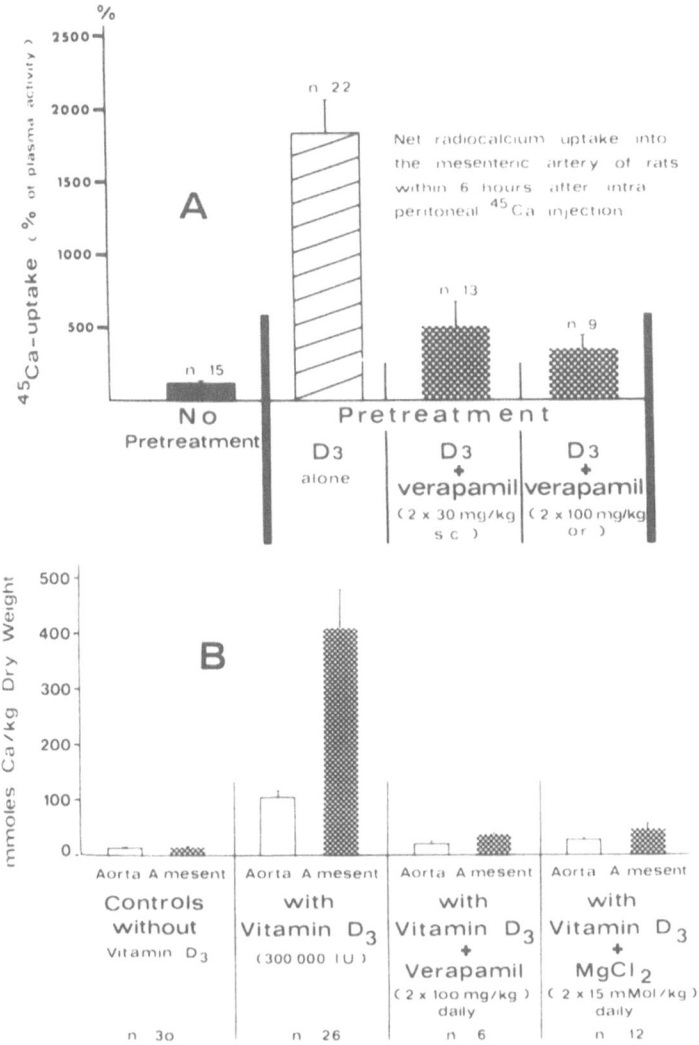

Figure 6. A. Inhibition of vitamin-D$_3$-stimulated (300,000 I.U./kg) net radiocalcium uptake into the wall of the mesenteric artery of rats by verapamil, administered subcutaneously or orally during 4 days. B. Prevention of vitamin-D$_3$-induced (300,000 I.U./kg) rise in absolute Ca content of the aortic and mesenteric walls by oral treatment with verapamil or MgCl$_2$ for 4 days (see Fleckenstein et al. [17, 18]).

against excessive vascular Ca-uptake in hypertensive rats (Fig. 6–8). Thus our experimental data suggest that the natural age-dependent increase in arterial Ca-content, and particularly the enhancement of this process by risk factors such as diabetes, hypertension nicotine, as well as uncontrolled vitamin D intake, plays an important etiological role also in the development of arteriosclerosis of humans. Ca-overload represents perhaps the

118

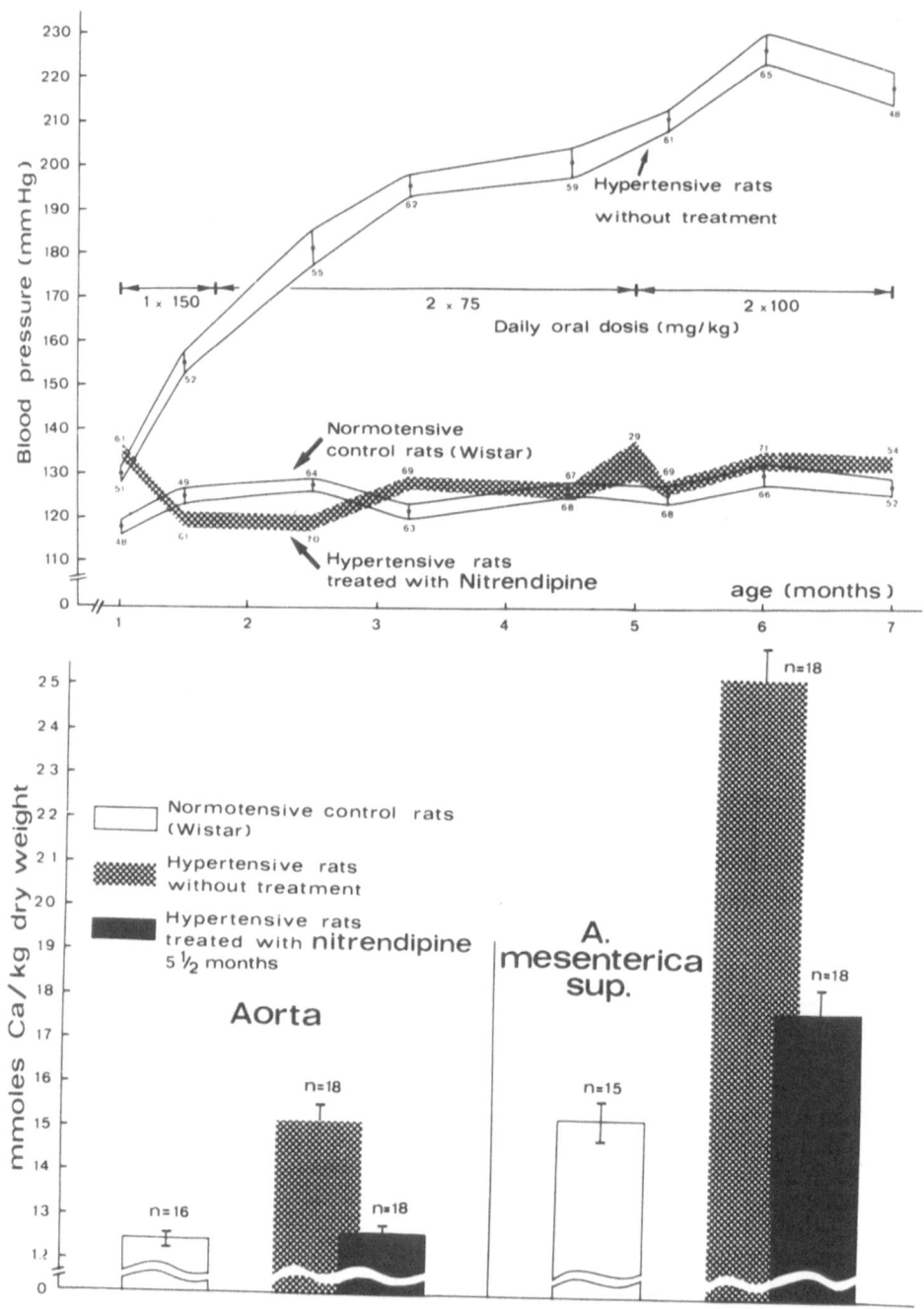

Figure 7. A. Normalization of mean arterial blood pressure of rats suffering from spontaneous hypertension by chronic oral administration of nitrendipine during 6 months. Treatment with nitrendipine lasted from the end of the first to the end of the seventh month of age. B. Restriction of Ca overload of the arterial walls of spontaneously hypertensive rats by the treatment with oral nitrendipine over 5½ months (same rat population as in [A]).

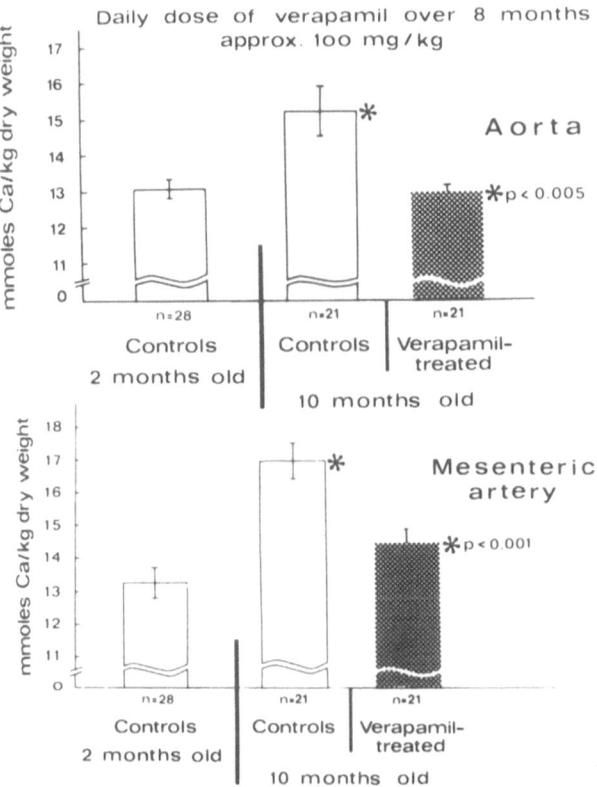

Figure 8. Graphical illustration of the inhibitory influence of verapamil on Ca accumulation in the arterial walls of aging rat aortae and mesenteric arteries (see Fleckenstein et al. [17]).

common denominator that underlies the predisposition to arteriosclerosis by these different risk factors. There is no doubt that at an age of more than 60 years, the steady increase in Ca content of the arterial walls reaches a cytotoxic concentration range which is otherwise only attainable in animal experiments with overdoses of dihydrotachysterol or vitamin D (alone) or in combination with nicotine (Figs. 5 and 6).

Admittedly there is still a missing link between the calcium and the lipid accumulation in arteriosclerotic vessels. Hopefully, future studies about the interaction of calcium with phospholipids and phosphoproteins will help to fill up this gap in present knowledge. However, notwithstanding these pending problems, all our results point to the possibility of an eventual retardation of age-dependent arterial calcinosis (and of the effects of complicating risk factors) by a suitable long-term Ca-antagonist therapy. Hence a definite clarification of the possible significance of Ca-antagonists as anticalcinotic or antiarteriosclerotic drugs is certainly one of the most intriguing prospects in future clinical research. Interestingly in our experiments, both myocardial and arterial Ca overload, although highly responsive to Ca antagonists, were refractory to nitrate compounds (nitroglycerin, isosorbide dinitrate).

Summary

In conclusion it is to be stated that the application of Ca-antagonists as antianginal, antiarrhythmic, antihypertensive, cardioprotective or antisclerotic drugs makes use of the different manifestations of the same fundamental inhibitory action on cardiac and vascular transmembrane Ca-conductivity. The beneficial influence of Ca-antagonists in coronary disease is probably complex because several therapeutically important factors seem to work together:
(a) direct reduction of myocardial energy expenditure and, therefore, of oxygen demand,
(b) indirect decrease in cardiac oxygen requirement by facilitation of heart work at a reduced level of arterial blood pressure,
(c) improvement of oxygen supply to the myocardium due to vasodilator or spasmolytic effects particularly on extramural coronary vessels, i.e. stem arteries, collaterals, anastomoses,
(d) cardioprotection and increase in ischemic tolerance by prevention of myocardial Ca-overload, and lastly,
(e) suppression of ectopic dysrhythmias (and re-entry tachycardias).
Moreover, many experimental observations indicate that Ca-antagonists also interfere with vascular calcinosis thus antagonizing the promoter effects of coronary risk factors (i.e. hypertension, diabetes, nicotine, advanced age) on arterial Ca accumulation.

References

1. Fleckenstein A: Specific inhibitors and promoters of calcium action in the excitation-contractioncoupling of heart muscle and their role in the prevention or production of myocardial lesions. In: Calcium and the Heart, (Harris P, Opie L eds.), PP 135–188, Academic Press, London-New York, 1971.
2. Fleckenstein A: Specific pharmacology of calcium in myocardium, cardiac pacemakers, and vascular smooth muscle. Ann Rev Pharmacol Toxicol 17:149–166, 1977.
3. Fleckenstein A: Steuerung der myocardialen Kontraktilität, ATP-Spaltung, Atmungsintensität und Schrittmacher-Funktion durch Calcium-Ionen – Wirkungsmechanismus der Calcium-Antagonisten. In: Calcium-Antagonismus, Proceed. of an Internat. Symposium 1978 in Frankfurt, (Fleckenstein A, Roskamm H, eds.), pp 1–28, Springer-Verlag, Berlin-Heidelberg-New York, 1980.
4. Fleckenstein A: Fundamental actions of calcium antagonists on myocardial and cardiac pacemaker cell membranes. In: New Perspectives on Calcium Antagonists, Weiss GB (ed), Clin Physiol Series, Amer Physiol Society, 59–81, 1981.

5. Fleckenstein A: History of calcium antagonists. In: Calcium Channel Blocking Drugs: A Novel Intervention for the Treatment of Cardiac Disease. Schwartz A, Taira, N (eds), pp 3–16, Monograph Nr. 95 of the American Heart Association, Circulation Research, Part II, Vol 52, Nr. 2, 1983.

6. Fleckenstein A: Calcium Antagonism in Heart and Smooth Muscle – Experimental Facts and Therapeutic Prospects. Monograph published by John Wiley & Sons, New York-Chichester-Brisbane-Toronto-Singapore, 1983.

7. Fleckenstein A, Döring HJ, Janke J, Byon YK: Basic actions of ions and drugs on myocardial high-energy phosphate metabolism and contractility. In: Handbook of Experimental Pharmacology, Vol. XVI/3, pp 345–405, Springer Verlag, Berlin-Heidelberg-New York, 1975.

8. Späh F, Fleckenstein A: Evidence of a new, preferentially Mg-carrying, transport system besides the fast Na and the slow Ca channels in the excited myocardial sarcolemma membrane. J of Mol and Cell Cardiology 11:1109–1127, 1979.

9. Nakajima H, Hoshiyama M, Yamashita K, Kiyomoto A: Effect of diltiazem on electrical and mechanical activity of isolated cardiac vantricular muscle of guinea pig. Japan J Pharmacol 25:383–392, 1975.

10. Grün G, Fleckenstein A: Die elektromechanische Entkoppelung der glatten Gefäß-Muskulatur als Grundprinzip der Coronardilatation durch 4-(2′-Nitrophenyl)-2,6-dimethyl-1,4-dihydropyridin-3,5-dicarbonsäure-dimethylester (Bay a 1040, Nifedipin). Arzneim.-Forsch. (Drug Res) 22:334–344, 1972.

11. Fleckenstein-Grün G, Fleckenstein A: Calcium-Antagonismus, ein Grundprinzip der Vasodilatation. In: Calcium-Antagonismus, Proceed. of an Internat. Symposium 1978 in Frankfurt, (Fleckenstein A, Roskamm H (eds)), pp 191–207, Springer Verlag, Berlin-Heidelberg-New York, 1980.

12. Nayler WG, Grau A, Slade A: A protective effect of verapamil on hypoxic heart muscle. Cardiovasc Res 10:650–662, 1976.

13. Henry PD, Shuchleib R, Borda LJ, Roberts R, Williamson JR, Sobel BE: Effects of nifedipine on myocardial perfusion and ischemic injury in dogs. Circ Res 43:372–380, 1978.

14. Weishaar R, Ashikawa K, Bing RJ: Effect of diltiazem, a calcium-antagonist, on myocardial ischemia. Am J Cardiol 43:1136–1143, 1979.

15. Janke J, Hein B, Pachinger O, Leder O, Fleckenstein A: Hemmung arteriosklerotischer Gefässprozesse durch prophylaktische behandlung mit $MgCl_2$, KCl und organischen Ca^{++}-Antagonisten (quantitative Studien mit Ca^{45} bei Ratten). In: Vascular Smooth Muscle, Proceed. of a Satel. Symp. 25th Congress Internat. Union Physiol. Sciences. Tübingen Juli 1971, E Betz ed, pp 71–72, Springer-Verlag, Berlin-Heidelberg-New York, 1972.

16. Frey M, Keidel J, Fleckenstein A: Verhütung experimenteller Gefäss-Verkalkungen (Mönckeberg's Typ der Arteriosklerose) durch Calcium-Antagonisten. In: Calcium-Antagonismus, Proceed. Internat. Symp. on Calcium-Antagonism, Frankfort, December 1978, A Fleckenstein a. H Roskamm eds, pp 258–264, Springer-Verlag, Berlin-Heidelberg-New York, 1980.

17. Fleckenstein A, Frey M, Leder O: Prevention by calcium antagonists of arterial calcinosis. In: Drug Development and Evaluation 'New Calcium Antagonists – Recent Developments and Prospects', diltiazem Workshop, Freiburg, May 1982, Fleckenstein A, Hashimoto K, Herrmann M, Schwartz A, Seipel L (eds), pp 15–31, Gustav Fischer Verlag, Stuttgart – New York, 1983.

18. Fleckenstein A, Frey M, Fleckenstein-Grün G: Protection by calcium antagonists against experimental arterial calcinosis. In: Secondary Prevention of Coronary Heart Disease, Workshop of the Internat. Soc. and Federation of Cardiology, Titisee, Oct. 1983, PyöräläK, Rapaport E, König K, Schettler G, Diehm C (eds), pp 109–122, G. Thieme Verlag, Stuttgart-New York, 1983.

14. The Influence of Nitrates on Prognosis in Patients with Coronary Heart Disease

W.-D. BUSSMANN

Abstract

No hard data are available today to prove that nitrates may influence prognosis in patients with coronary heart disease. The very few available studies are incomplete and can serve at best as pilot studies to stimulate new trials in larger patient population.

There are some authors who reported mortality data in patients with *acute myocardial infarction* who received intravenous nitroglycerin during the acute phase. However, the number of patients studied were too small to reach definite conclusions. Chiche et al. found two deaths in nitroglycerin treated patients ($n = 35$) compared to seven deaths in the control group ($n = 35$). Bennet found according to a personal communication an early mortality rate of 7.8% in 70 patients treated with nitrogyclerin compared to 13% in the control group ($n = 70$, n.s.). Flaherty et al. registered a reduced incidence of left ventricular failure and mortality rate in a group of 52 treated patients compared to an equal number of untreated patients. In our own randomized controlled study ($n = 60$) which showed a 30% decrease of CK and CKMB indices of infarct size, no early death was observed in the nitroglycerin group ($n = 29$) compared to five deaths in the control group ($n = 31$).

The influence of *chronic use of nitrates* in patients with coronary heart disease has not been analysed for prognosis. We were able to study mortality rates in patients who initially were randomized for nitroglycerin treatment or control 1 ½ year following the acute event. 3/28 patients died compared to 7/23 in the control group. Sudden death and reinfarction occurred in three compared to eleven of the control group. The grade of angina pectoris and the dose of nitrates were strikingly higher in patients initially treated with nitroglycerin during follow up.

The phenomenon stimulated us to conduct a retrospective study on the influence of small and large doses of nitrates in the treatment of patients with angiographically proven coronary disease. In 168 patients followed over a period of 7 years 98 were on low (< 40 mg/die) and 70 patients on a high dose of nitrates (> 40 mg/die). Despite the same severity of ventricular damage and the same amount of coronary lesions in both groups the survival rate in patients treated with large doses of isosorbide dinitrate was improved by 30–40%. This interesting result, however, should be viewed with scepticism and prospective studies are warranted.

Introduction

The question whether nitrates influence prognosis in patients with coronary heart disease cannot be answered with today's knowledge.

There are only few tentative data available from a small group of investigators [1, 6, 7, 14–18, 20]. These studies can serve at best as pilot studies to stimulate new trials in larger patient populations.

The first part is concerned with the use of nitrates during acute myocardial infarction [1–4, 7–10, 12, 20]. Can intravenous nitroglycerin influence morbidity and mortality in these patients?

In the second part the effect on prognosis will be discussed when patients with coronary artery disease are treated with nitrates on a long term basis. Here, only two studies are available [6, 11, 13–15].

Acute myocardial infarction

What do we know about the early phase following acute myocardial infarction when nitroglycerin is used by the intravenous route? In a prospective randomized trial, we evaluated 60 patients [12]. 31 patients received nitroglycerin for 2 to 4 days. 29 patients served as controls. Both groups were comparable as to age, site of myocardial infarction and baseline hemodynamics. Note, that diastolic pulmonary artery pressure was around 20 mm Hg in both groups.

Morbidity was favorably influenced in nitroglycerin treated patients.

The patients had less pain, less dyspnea and fewer ventricular arrhythmias. Bradycardia was less frequent. There was evidence for less ischemia and reduced infarct size [10].

Ventricular ectopic beats and ventricular fibrillation were less frequent in patients treated with nitroglycerin compared to the control group [9].

Frequent ventricular ectopic beats were present in 20% of nitroglycerin treated compared to 50% of the control group. The need for lidocaine was reduced as well.

The effect on ventricular arrhythmias may have prognostic significance for patients with reinfarction or recurrent myocardial ischemia.

There was less ischemia as evidenced by the reduction of ST-segment elevation during acute intervention and infarct size was smaller. CK and CK-MB was used as an index for infarct size. A 30% reduction was found compared to untreated control patients [5, 12].

The development of Q-waves was much smaller in patients treated with nitroglycerin. Compared to day 1, smaller Q-waves were present on day 5 and day 30 [19]. Chiche and coworkers reported similar results: R-wave reduction following treatment was half of that in the control group [17, 18].

When morbidity is apparently lower in treated patients should this imply reduced mortality?

In our study five control patients died. None of the nitroglycerin patients expired except 1 during emergency bypass surgery due to severe angina pectoris (Fig. 1) [8, 15].

In Chiche's randomized study 7 of 35 controls and 2 of 35 nitroglycerin treated patients died [17]. David Bennett from St. George's Hospital, London, conducted a doubleblind study on the effect of intravenous nitroglycerin in 140 patients with acute myocardial infarction. 9 died in the control group compared to 5 during nitroglycerin treatment [1]. Bennett found a 30% reduction in cumulative CK-MB values as well. Flaherty and coworkers had results pointing in the same direction: less mortality and less congestive failure were present in the group treated with nitroglycerin [20].

It is interesting to note that one cause of death in our cohort was a higher incidence of reinfarction during the first days. The current patient population, however – and this is important – is too small to draw any definite conclusions. These preliminary data must be confirmed by future studies in larger patient populations.

Post infarction period

Obtaining conclusive data for the *post-infarction period* in respect to the possible influence of nitrates during this time span appears to be even more difficult. We evaluated our own patients 2 years later following the acute myocardial event (Fig. 1).

The mortality was 11% in patients initially treated with nitroglycerin and 27% in untreated patients [8, 15].

One important aspect is the difference in the severity of angina pectoris between the groups. The nitroglycerin treated patients had less necrosis as mentioned before and consequently more angina during follow-up. Patients with complete extension of their infarction had less severe angina pectoris during follow-up. The dose of nitrates used in these patients correlated with the severity of angina. Daily dose was 38 mg of isosorbide dinitrate compared to 21 mg/day in the control group [8, 15].

126

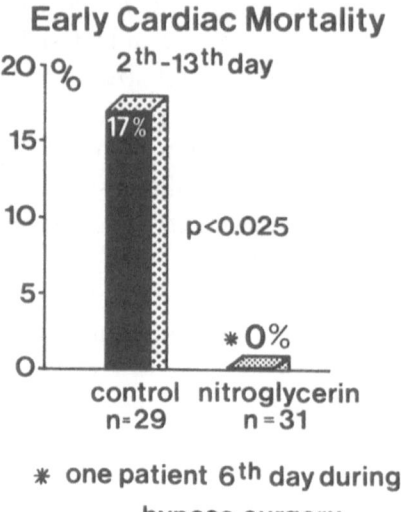

Early Cardiac Mortality

Figure 1. Early and late cardiac mortality in patients whose myocardial infarctions were treated or untreated with nitroglycerin during the acute phase. None of the nitroglycerin treated patients died except one during emergency bypass surgery. In the control group 5 patients died.

On the other hand, reduced late mortality may be primarily due to the higher dose of nitrates. The only paradox, however, is that patients with severe angina pectoris seem to have a better prognosis than those with a less severe type of angina.

Reduced infarct size due to nitroglycerin treatment may also play a role for the better outcome in this group, since some fatalities were related to heart failure.

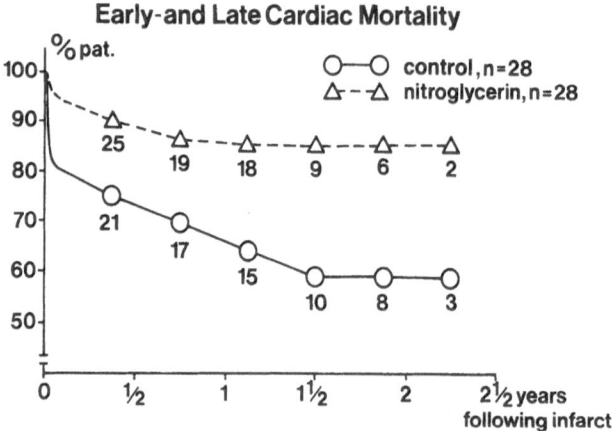

Figure 2. Cardiac mortality was 11 % in the nitroglycerin treated group, in the controls 39 %. In addition to the reduced infarct size of the nitroglycerin-treated patients the higher daily dose of nitrates possibly causes these findings. Angina pectoris was more frequent in the nitroglycerin group.

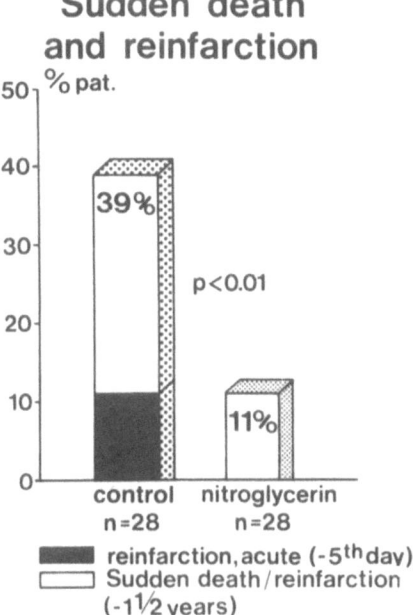

Figure 3. Incidence of sudden death and reinfarction with or without death in the treated and untreated group. Nitroglycerin treated patients had 3 events compared to 11 events in the control group.

In our study we found a large difference between the groups due to less early and less late cardiac mortality in patients initially treated with nitroglycerin and on sustained high dose of nitrates during follow-up (Fig. 2) [8, 15].

Again, however, this result should be viewed with scepticism since the number of patients randomized is not large enough to be convinced on statistical grounds.

We then evaluated the causes for death acutely and during follow-up.

The incidence of sudden death and reinfarction with or without death was 39% of the control patients but only 11% in the nitroglycerin treated group (Fig. 3).

Thus, sudden death and reinfarction seemed to be reduced when nitroglycerin is given during the acute phase and an effective dose of isosorbide dinitrate is used during follow-up.

Patients with coronary heart disease: longterm effects

The study just reviewed was related to patients undergoing nitrate therapy during the acute *and* chronic phase. Another study was carried out exclu-

128

sively in patients with coronary heart disease receiving nitrates during the *chronic phase* [11, 14]. At least, some similarities between the two can be shown.

In 293 patients who had undergone coronary angiography and ventriculography 7 years before, a questionnaire was filled out by those still living. Medical records and information provided by the family physician were used for those who had died during the intervening period.

The daily dose of nitrates (isosorbide dinitrate, Pharma Schwarz Monheim) could be ascertained in a total of 168 patients: 112 were survivors and 56 were non-survivors. The patients were divided into two groups: group 1 was on a daily dose of isosorbide dinitrate of less than 40 mg (mean dose 16 mg/day) and group 2 on a dose of more than 40 mg (mean dose 55 mg/day).

2/3 of the case fatalities occurred in patients taking the low dose – less than 40 mg of isosorbide dinitrate and only 1/3 following intake of the higher dose. Assessing the dose of nitrates in the survivors' group half of the patients were on low and half of the patients were on a high dose of nitrates (Fig. 4).

Left ventricular function was assessed by scoring hypo-, a- and dyskinesis in 6 different wall segments. The same mean value 6.2 and 6.3 was present in the groups on high and low dose of nitrates.

Since this important prognostic parameter is identical in both groups the difference in mortality may be related to the dose of nitrates. Again, this

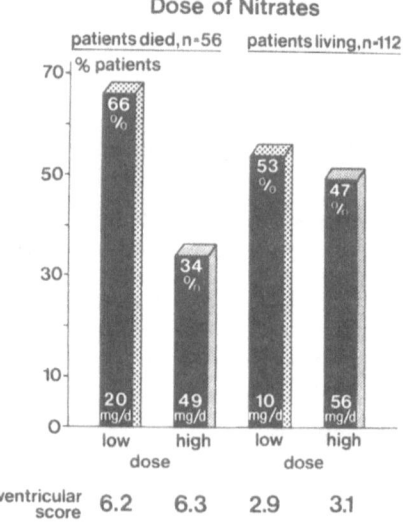

Figure 4. 2/3 of the case fatalities occurred in patients taking the low dose but only 1/3 in patients taking the high dose of nitroglycerin. Left ventricular damage was equal in both groups (6.2 versus 6.3). The percentage of the patients who survived, was equally distributed between low and high dose of nitrates.

result seems to say that less patients die when they are on a high dose regimen.

With time there was an increasing separation between the high and low dose survival curves. The mean dose of isosorbide dinitrate was 55 mg/day in the upper and 16 mg/day in the lower curve (Fig. 5).

Patients on a high dose have a better outcome. Mortality was reduced by 30% compared to the low dose group.

Comparison of both groups were assessed according to the extent of coronary lesions and of ventricular dysfunction using a score. Ventricular and coronary score were the same in both groups. The heart volume determined by x-ray did not differ significantly.

Thus, based on these parameters comparison can be assessed on a satisfactory basis.

However, angina pectoris was more severe in these patients and ST-segment depression in the exercise ECG was significantly more extensive in the group on the large dose of nitrates. There was no major difference in the use of beta-blockers, calcium-antagonists or patients with aggregation inhibitors.

Despite the fact that this is the first study evaluating this important item, the design of the study in itself has several important limitations:

1. The study was carried out retrospectively in a limited number of patients. Prospective studies are warranted. However, the first study showing the beneficial effect of beta-blockers on prognosis was a retrospective one [22].

2. The type of information we got from survivors and non-survivors was different. Survivors had to fill out a questionnaire for non-survivors charts or the family physicians were interviewed.

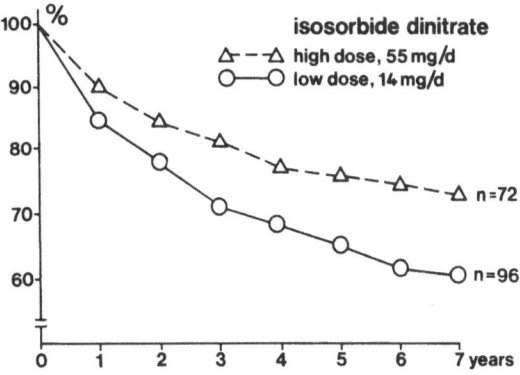

Figure 5. Mortality in patients on a high dose of isosorbide dinitrate was reduced by 30–40% compared to the low dose group. The probability of surviving was significantly higher in the high dose group (2p< 0,06, Gehan-test).

3. The dose of nitrates is the dose taken at the end of the seven year observation period in survivors and the last dose in non-survivors. We don't
know if these patients took the dose regularly over the entire period.

4. The structure in both groups is comparable in respect to the ventricular
and coronary score and to heart volume which were nearly identical in
both groups. However, the severity of angina pectoris and the ST-segment depression during exercise differed: patients on a high dose had
more angina and a more pronounced ischemia during exercise than those
on a low dose.

5. Patients with more angina pectoris may develop better collaterals which
in turn relates to a better prognosis. Thus, the higher dose of nitrates may
be not more than an indicator for the group but not a clear causal factor [21].

Due to these limiting circumstances a conclusion should be drawn with
caution: the result of this retrospective study seems to give some evidence
for a favorable influence of a higher dose of nitrates on the prognosis in
patients with coronary heart disease. In February 1980 we initiated a doubleblind multicenter study in the Frankfurt area. 1000 patients will be randomized in a low and high dose group. The high dose group receives 200 mg
isosorbide dinitrate per day and will be compared to 12.5 mg in the low
dose group. Our objective is to determine ultimate mortality and morbidity
in the two collectives. This will take 3 to 5 years.

In conclusion, there seems to be at least some evidence that nitrates
favorably influence early and late mortality in patients following acute myocardial infarction or in those with coronary heart disease. Preliminary findings are encouraging enough to warrant additional investigation of this
aspect of nitrate therapy in the future.

References

1. Bennett D: Double blind study of the effects of intravenous infusion of nitroglycerin in
   patients with acute myocardial infarction, Personal communication 1982
2. Bussmann W-D, Vachalowa J, Kaltenbach M: Wirkung von Nitroglycerin beim frischen
   Herzinfarkt Z Kardiol, Suppl I, 25, 1974, Abstract)
3. Bussmann W-D, Schöfer H, Kaltenbach M: Wirkung von Nitroglycerin beim akuten Myokardinfarkt. II. Intravenöse Dauerinfusion von Nitroglycerin bei Patienten mit und ohne
   Linksinsuffizienz und Auswirkung auf die Infarktgröße. Dtsch med Wschr 101:642–648,
   1976.
4. Bussmann W-D, Barthe G, Klepzig Hjr, Kaltenbach M: VII Nitroglycerindauertherapie
   beim frischen Herzinfarkt im Vergleich zu einer nicht behandelten Kontrollgruppe. Med
   Klin 74:191–198, 1979.

5. Bussmann W-D, Schöfer H, Kurita H, Ganz W: Nitroglycerin in acute myocardial infarction. X. Effect of small and large doses of i.v. nitroglycerin on ST-segment deviation, experimental and clinical results. Clin Cardiol 2:106–112, 1979.

6. Bussmann W-D: Do nitrates influence prognosis? European Congress of Cardiology, Paris, 1980.

7. Bussmann W-D: Nitroglycerin bei Herzinfarkt – Von der Kontraindikation zur Indikation –. Dtsch med Wschr 105:1551–1554, 1980.

8. Bussmann W-D, Haller M, Kalkenbach M: Nitroglycerin bei frischem Herzinfarkt. Einfluß auf spätere Angina pectoris. Beeinflussung der Prognose? Z Kardiol 69:201, 1980.

9. Bussmann W-D, Neumann K, Kaltenbach M: Die Wirkung von Nitroglycerin auf die ventrikuläre Extra-systolie beim frischen Herzinfarkt. Dtsch med Wschr 105:369–373, 1980.

10. Bussmann W-D: Nitroglycerin in the treatment of acute myocardial infarction Acta Med Scand 210:Suppl 651, 165–175, 1981.

11. Bussmann W-D, Giebeler B, Kaltenbach M: Beeinflussen hochdosierte Nitrate die Prognose bei koronarer Herzkrankheit? Z Kardiol 69:201, 1981, Abstract.

12. Bussmann W-D, Passek D, Seidel W, Kaltenbach M: Reduction of CK and CK-MB Indexes of Infarct Size by intravenous Nitroglycerin. Circulation 63:615–622, 1981.

13. Bussmann W-D, Schneider W, Kaltenbach M: Anfalls- und Langzeittherapie der Koronaren Herzkrankheit mit Nitraten. Z Kardiol 71:583, 1982, Abstrakt.

14. Bussmann W-D, Giebeler B: Beeinflußt eine Dauertherapie mit hochdosierten Nitraten die Prognose bei koronarer Herzkrankheit? Klin Wschr (in press).

15. Bussmann W-D, Haller M: Hinweis auf eine Abnahme der Früh- und Spätmortalität beim frischen Herzinfarkt unter Nitroglycerintherapie Klin Wschr. (in press).

16. Chatterjee K Swan HJC, Kaushik VS, Jobin DMG, Magnusson P, Forrester JS: Effects of vasodilator therapy for severe pump failure in acute myocardial infarction on short-term and late prognosis. Circulation 53:797–802, 1976.

17. Chiche P, Bahgadoo SJ, Dørrida JP: A randomized trial of prolonged nitroglycerin infusion in acute myocardial infarction. Circulation 57+60:Suppl II, 693, 1929, Abstract.

18. Derrida JP, Sal R, Chiche P: Favorable effects of prolonged nitroglycerin infusion in patients with acute myocardial infarction. Am Heart J 96:833, 1978, Annotation.

19. Dowinsky S, Rose D-M, Bussmann W-D: Abnahme von QRS-Nekrosezeichen unter Nitroglycerintherapie beim frischen Herzinfarkt. Jahrestagung Dtsch, Ges. Herz- und Kreislaufforschung, Bad Nauheim 1982. Z Kardiol 71:252, 1982, Abstrakt.

20. Flaherty JT, Becker lc, Weisfeldt ML, Weiss JL, Gerstenblith G, Kallmann CH, Bulkley BH: Results of prospective randomizes clinical trial of intravenous nitroglycerin in acute myocardial infarction. Circulation 62:Suppl III, 299, 1980, Abstract.

21. Schneider W, Stahl B, Kaltenbach M, Bussmann W-D: Dosis-Wirkungs-Beziehungen bei der Behandlung der Angina pectoris mit Isocorbiddinitrat. Dtsch med Wschr 107:771–776, 1982.

22. Snow PJD: Effect of propranolol in myocardial infarction. Lancet 551–553, 1965.

15. Metabolic Aspects of Preventive Drug Administration

H. KAMMERMEIER

Abstract

The dependence of cardiac energy metabolism and tissue integrity on oxygen supply is a well established fact. Whether substrate supply, which is equally important for cardiac energy metabolism, can also be a limiting factor for cardiac energy metabolism and integrity is scarcely considered. There are, however, clear indications at least from animal experiments, that under severe work load substrates supplied from blood are not sufficiently available. This is indicated first by the marked utilization of endogenous myocardial glycogen under severe work load, second by the fact that according to numerous investigations on capillary permeability glucose cannot serve as the sole substrate of cardiac energy metabolism, and third by the observations that in isolated hearts interstitial glucose concentration can reach hypoglycemic values under the condition of high oxygen consumption. Accordingly, as well established the myocardium utilizes free fatty acids and under severe work load mainly lactic acid for substrate supply. Plasma levels of both substrates are markedly increased during work load, due to catecholamine-mediated glycolysis in liver and lactate release from skeletal muscle, which is also dependent partly on sympathetic activity. All three mechanisms involved in additional cardiac substrate supply i.e. myocardial glycogen utilization, UFA mobilization from fat stores and glycogen mobilization from skeletal muscle are at least partly dependent on β-agonistic mechanisms. However, one main preventive intervention concerns administration of β-blocking drugs or drugs which reduce plasma lipids. Thus the possibility of insufficient substrate supply has to be considered at least when exercise programs and β-blockade are used in combination.

Introduction

The energy metabolism of the myocardium depends on adequate supply of substrate and oxygen. Due to its high lipid solubility and the high permeability of the capillary wall resulting therefrom the oxygen supply depends almost exclusively on blood flow. In contrast, the exchange of substrates is mainly determined by the diffusional resistance of the capillary wall, which follows from the absence of lipid solubility as for instance is the case for lactate and glucose. The transcapillary exchange of free fatty acids is not yet well understood but seems complicated and restricted as well. Due to these facts and also based on some observations of our group, it does not seem evident that substrate supply of the myocardium is sufficient under all physiological and pathophysiological conditions. This is valid in particular, when substrate utilization is limited by administration of drugs as for instance β-blocking agents. This should be relevant especially for the condition of increased cardiac work during exercise, which is increasingly applied also in secondary prevention.

In exercising man β-blocking agents exhibit various effects on levels of substrates and other blood constituents. According to table 1 a marked decrease in levels of blood glucose, lactate and free fatty acids can be observed, whereas levels of cortisol, STH, noradrenaline, adrenaline and potassium can be markedly increased [7, 9]. The changes in plasma potassium levels are only loosely linked to the subject of this paper. However, due to its clinical interest it should be described briefly.

Direct recording of potassium in working man reveals an increase in arterial plasma potassium levels by about 50% and a decrease within about 2 min after the cessation of exercise [9]. Following acute administration of propranolol the increase in plasma potassium is more pronounced. The plasma potassium response to exercise after acute-on-chronic blockade does not seem to level off during 5 min and reaches almost 8 mM [9], which seems of clinical relevance.

The main subject of this paper concerns myocardial energy metabolism and in particular the possible role of diffusion limitation of substrate supply. The diffusional resistance of the capillary wall should be reflected among others by a decreased interstitial concentration of substances which are taken up by the heart. The concentration differences between plasma and interstitial fluid can be calculated from data of capillary permeability using

Table 1. Effects of β-receptor blocking agents on blood/plasma levels of various substances in man during exercise

— Decrease in glucose (< 50%) [7]
— Decrease in lactate (< 25%) [7]
— Decrease in UFA (< 50%) [7]
— Increase in cortisol (< 50%) [7]
— Increase in STH, nor-adrenaline, adrenaline [7]
— Increase in K^+ (< 50%) [9]

Table 2. Maximum transcapillary concentration differences calculated from maximum uptake rate and capillary permeability

	O_2-Consumption [ml/min·100 gl			
	8	20	40	
	Concentration differences [mM/l]			
Glucose				
$P \cdot S^a$ = 0.45 (13 [b], 15 [b])	1.2	3.0	6.0	Saturable
= 0.9 (2 [b])	0.6	1.5	3.0	K_m 7 mM (3)
Lactate				
$P \cdot S$ = 0.6 (2 [b])	1.7	4.3	9.1	Saturable
= 1.0 (13 [b], 15 [b])	1.0	2.6	5.5	k_m 8 mM (6)
= 2.6 (8)	0.4	1.0	2.1	
Palmitate				
$P \cdot S$ = 1.8 (5, 10 [b])	0.07	0.2	0.4	linearily concentration dependent 8, 9

[a] Permeability × surface area [ml/min·g_{ww}]
[b] Calculated from the respective reference

Fick's law: $J = P \cdot S \cdot \Delta C$ (J = uptake rate, P = Permeability coefficient, S = Surface area, ΔC = Concentration difference). Capillary permeability can be expressed best by the so called permeability × surface area product, which is the reciprocal of the diffusional resistance and comparable to a conductance. Permeability data shown in Table 2 obtained by various investigators and various methods were used to calculate transcapillary concentration differences for 3 cardiac oxygen consumption levels (8, 20, 40 ml · 100 g^{-1} · min^{-1}) considering the theoretical borderline condition that the respective substrate is the only one consumed. This, however, is only the case approximately for lactate at maximum work load conditions.

Transcapillary concentration differences of glucose according to these calculations (Tab. 2) could range between 1.4 and 3.0 mM for intermediate cardiac oxygen consumption and between 3 and 6 mM at high cardiac oxygen consumption. Taking into account physiological blood glucose levels of about 5 mM this indicates already that glucose because of the diffusion limitation of the capillary wall cannot serve as the sole substrate at intermediate and high cardiac oxygen consumption, particularly facing the high K_m-value of about 7 mM.

The transcapillary concentration gradients of lactate calculated range between 1 and 4 ml · min^{-1} for intermediate cardiac oxygen consumption and between 2 and 9 ml · min^{-1} for high cardiac oxygen consumption (Tab. 2).

Respecting the high lactate levels which occur at severe work load, limitation of substrate supply by diffusion might only be inferred from the data obtained with the lower PS-values. In the case of endurance exercise where lactate levels are below 4 mM a certain limitation can be expected taking in account the half saturation value of 8 mM. The transcapillary concentration differences for palmitate resulting from the calculation are between 0.2 and 0.4 mM for intermediate and high cardiac oxygen consumption respectively. Similar data were obtained by Rose and Gorsky [10] who calculated an interstitial concentration of UFA of 30 to 50% of that of plasma. The resulting values indicate a marked reduction of UFA availability from the interstitial fluid. Therefore unesterified fatty acids presumably cannot serve as the sole substrate at high cardiac oxygen consumption as well. Considering the situation of high cardiac oxygen consumption without increased plasma lactate levels the data even cast doubt whether glucose and unesterified fatty acids together are capable of coping with the substrate demand of the myocardium.

The date of Tab. 2 might only be of theoretical interest if no real data on interstitial substrate concentration were available. However, we investigated interstitial substrate concentrations also directly in isolated perfused hearts. Transcapillary concentration differences between the interstitial fluid and the perfusate reached values in fact which were similar to those calculated in Tab. 2. In an isoprenaline treated isolated rat heart with an oxygen consumption of about $25 \, ml \cdot min^{-1} \cdot 100 \, g^{-1}$ the transcapillary concentration difference of glucose amounted to about 2.5 and that of lactate to about 1.0 mM (Fig. 1).

The subsequent question is now, whether this transcapillary concentration differences and reduced interstitial availabilities of substrates have any impact on cardiac energy metabolism. This question appears to be answered

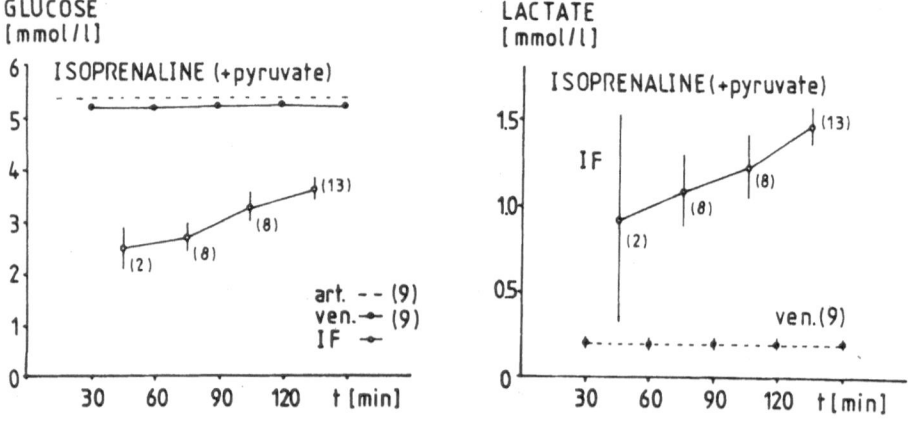

Figure 1. Interstitial (IF), arterial, and venous concentration of glucose and lactate in isolated rat hearts under the influence of isoprenaline (14) ($\bar{x}\pm$, SEM, N).

FASTED ANIMALS

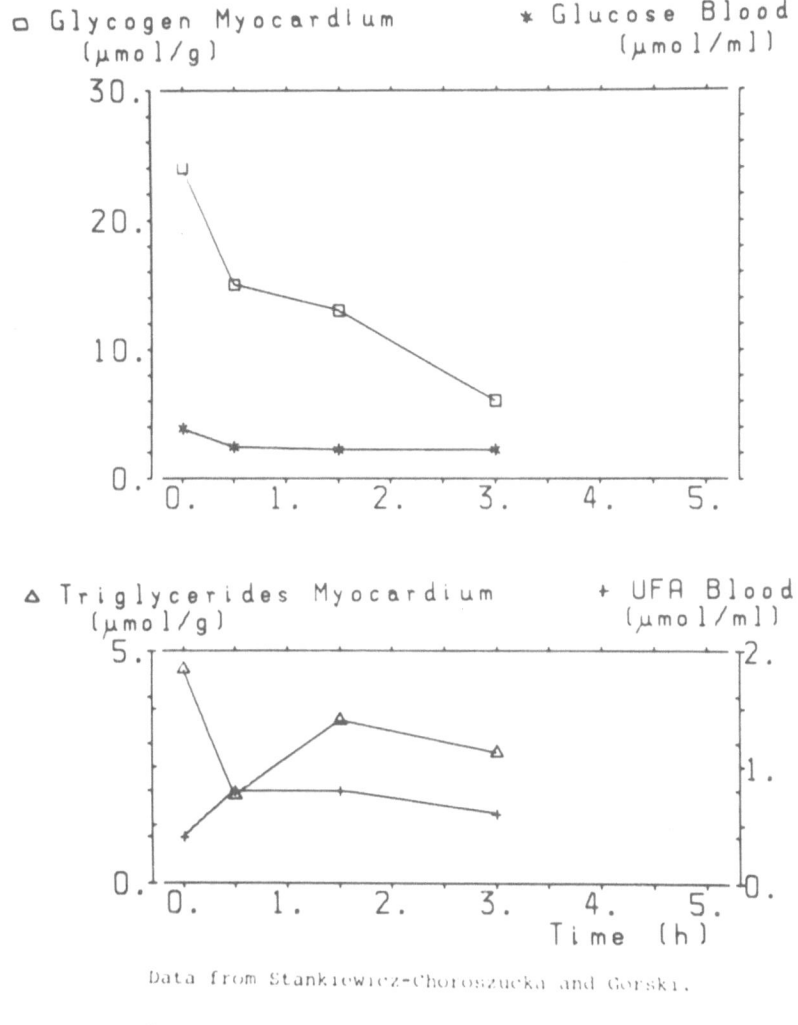

Data from Stankiewicz-Choroszucka and Gorski.

Eur. J. Appl. Physiol 43:11-17 (1980)

Figure 2. Levels of glucogen (glucose units), glucose, triglycerides and unesterifies fatty acids in myocardium and blood of fasted rats during 3 h swimming, Graph according to data of (12).

to a major part by an experimental study published a few years ago [12].

In heart of rats swimming for several hours, where cardiac oxygen consumption certainly is not at maximum, the myocardial glycogen stores and to a smaller extent the myocardial stores of triglycerides exhibited a transient and marked decrease during the first hour of exercise which presumably is a consequence of increased glycogenolysis and lipolysis due to sympathetic overdrive. During the subsequent 4 hours of the experiments both return to normal values indicating no substrate limitation under these circumstances.

In contrast, reduction of substrate availability by fasting or administration of nicotinic acid with the same experimental protocol induced a pronounced decrease in cardiac glycogen stores by about 75% and a premature exhaustion after 3 hours of swimming (Fig. 2). This marked reduction of glycogen and in addition of triglycerides appears in spite of the fact that the glucose concentration was still about 50% of that of controls and about that observed in the interstitial fluid of isoprenaline treated hearts (Fig. 1). Free fatty acid concentration of blood was even increased relative to controls. Thus, moderate reduction of availability of substrate from blood seems to require additional substrate mobilization from myocardial substrate stores.

In propranolol treated animals neither a reduction of cardiac glycogen nor of cardiac triglycerides stores was observed. This missing reduction of cardiac substrate stores in propranolol treated animals, however, is no evidence of sufficient substrate supply. Mobilisation of both substrate stores depend to a major part of β-adrenoceptor mediated glycogenolysis and lipolysis. These mechanisms are depressed under β-blockade. In all these experiments on swimming rats in addition one has to take into account that increased plasma lactate levels though not measured in this study, contribute markedly to cardiac substrate supply during exercise.

Taking all these observations together, there are rather strong indications that an already moderately reduced plasma concentration of substrates makes additional mobilisation of intracardiac substrate stores necessary. This seems to be already the case in long lasting exercise, where cardiac metabolism presumably is not the limiting factor and lactate is available as additional substrate. More pronounced limitation of substrate supply from blood can be expected if either in exercise of intermediate duration cardiac performance is at a maximum or if lactate is not available as an additional substrate. The latter can be the case if high cardiac oxygen and substrate consumption occurs without exercise. The shortage of substrate supply appears to be buffered under physiological conditions for a limited period of time of the intramyocardial substrate stores. If the substrate availability is reduced in addition by administration of β-receptor blocking agents or nicotinic acid there might in fact occur a critical reduction of substrate availability with certain exercise conditions, which finally should have similar consequences as reduced oxygen supply. With respect to the clinical relevance of these considerations and the controversy on secondary prevention with β-receptor blocking agents it seems of interest to look for incidents in exercise during selective and non-selective β-blockade.

Summary

Data on capillary permeability indicate reduced substrate concentrations in the interstitial fluid. These were observed in fact in isolated hearts. With reduced concentrations of glucose and fatty acids in blood limited substrate supply apparently causes consumption of intramyocardial substrate stores in exercise which might reach a critical extent during treatment with β-receptor blocking agents and nicotinic acid.

References

1. De Grella RF, Light RJ: Uptake and metabolism of fatty acids by dispersed adult rat heart myocytes. J Biol Chem 255:9739–9745, 1980.
2. Duran WN, Yudilevich DL: Estimate of capillary permeability coefficients of canine heart to sodium and glucose. Microvasc REs 15:195–205, 1978.
3. Gerards P, Graf W, Kammermeier H: Glucose transfer studies in Isolated cardiocytes of adults rats. J Mol Cell Cardiol 14:141–149, 1982.
4. Hütter JF, Piper HM, Spieckermann PG: Myocardial fatty acid oxidation: Evidence for an albumin-receptor – mediated membrane transfer of fatty acid. Basic Res Cardiol 79:274–282, 1984.
5. Kammermeier H: Endothelial diffusion limitation of cardiac substrate supply and transport mechanisms supporting substrate exchange. In: Microcirculation of the heart. Kübler W, Tillmanns H, Zebe H (ed) Springer, Berlin, Heidelberg, 1982.
6. Kammermeier H, Wein B, Graf W: Characteristics of lactate transfer in isolated cardiac myocytes. Basic Res Cardiol (in press).
7. Kindermann W, Scheerer W, Salas-Fraire O, Biro G, Wölfing A: Verhalten der köperlichen Leistungsfähigkeit und des Metabolismus unter akuter Beta$_1$ und Beta$_{1/2}$-Blockade. Z Kardiol 73:380–387, 1984.
8. Lang U, Wendtland B, Kammermeier H: Direct measurement of unidirectional capillary transfer of small hydrophilic substances in isolated perfused rat hearts. J Mol Cell Cardiol 16:S2, 55, 1984.
9. Linton RAF, Lim M, Wolff CB, Wilmshurst P, Band DM: Arterial plasma potassium measured continuously during exercise in man. Clinical Science 67:427–432, 1984.
10. Rose CP, Goresky CA: Constraints on the uptake of labeled palmitate by the heart. Circ Res 41:534–545, 1977.
11. Schmitz D, Kammermeier H: Apparent transfer coefficients of substrates across the capillary wall of isolated perfused rat hearts calculated from concentration differences between the interstitial fluid (IF) and venous effluent (VE). Pflügers Arch 402:R21, 1984.
12. Stankiewicz-Choroszucha B, Gorski J: Effect of substrate supply and beta-adrenergic blockade on heart glycogen and triglyceride utilization during exercise in the rat. Eur J Appl Physiol 43:11–17, 1980.
13. Trap-Jensen J, Lassen NA: Capillary permeability for smaller hydrophilic tracers in exercising skeletal muscle in normal man and in patients with long-term diabetes mellitus. In:
14. Capillary permeability; Crone C, Lassen NA (ed). Munksgaard, Copenhagen pp 135–152, 1970.
15. Wendtland B, Jüngling E, Kammermeier H: Interstitial concentration of metabolites in isolated perfused rat hearts as function of myocardial metabolism and capillary permeability. Pflügers Arch 294:R11, 1982.
16. Yipintsoi T, Tancredi R, Richmond D, Bassingthwaighte JB: Myocardial extraction of sucrose, glucose, and potassium. In: Capillary Permeability; Crone C, Lassen NA (ed). Munksgaard, Copenhagen pp 153–156, 1970.

IV. The Role of Physical Exercise in Secondary Prevention

16. The Role of Physical Exercise in Secondary Prevention 'Evidence to Date'

G.T. GAU

Abstract

The evidence that physical activity plays a direct role in the prevention of coronary artery disease is difficult to ascertain. Epidemiologic studies in occupations relating activity versus inactivity, different levels of leisure activity, athlete versus nonathlete, and continued active aerobic exercise of various levels have indicated protective effects related to increased physical activity in both morbidity and mortality.

The beneficial effect of exercise on risk factor reduction, (body weight and percentage fat, blood lipids, smoking, blood pressure, stress, and diabetes) has been established. This positive role relationship may explain much of the gain that exercise plays in secondary prevention of coronary disease.

Direct beneficial effects of exercise on cardiac function, coronary collateral formation, and reduction in the development of atherosclerosis has been shown in animal studies, but only limited potential benefit has been shown in humans. Improved cardiovascular functional capacity and reduced myocardial oxygen demand result from exercise training with reduced symptomatology.

As illustrated by Jim Fixx's death while running, exercise is not the cure for coronary disease, but may still have an ameliorating influence on this multifactorial disease.

Introduction

The recent tragic death of Jim Fixx, internationally known author of *'The Complete Book of Running'* and *'Jim Fixx's Second Book of Running'* has refocused interest on the role of exercise in primary and secondary prevention of coronary atherosclerosis. Jim Fixx was 52 years of age when he died while running on July 20, 1984 in rural Vermont. He had started his exercise program at age 35, the age his father had his first heart attack. Up to that date Jim Fixx was a two pack per day smoker and was overweight. With running he decreased his weight to 159 pounds, quit smoking, wrote four books, and became famous as an author, speaker, and proponent of cardiovascular fitness. His autopsy showed severe three vessel disease, two nearly completely obstructed vessels, and one 50% occluded. Despite many years of running at high performance levels (marathon), Jim Fixx did not obtain immunity to coronary artery disease.

The concept that exercise would give immunity to coronary artery disease was postulated by Bassler T.J. in 1975 in his statement that marathon runners are immune to coronary heart disease as long as they maintain fitness, train at distances over six miles, and do not smoke. Currens J.H. in 1961 had stimulated interest in the role of exercise when he published the autopsy data on Clarence De Mar, a long distance runner who continued to run up until the time of his death from cancer at age 70 years. His coronary vessels were shown to be two to three times normal size with only mild atherosclerosis. This concept of immunity was not true for Jim Fixx and has been shown to not be true for many other published deaths in runners.

Despite the fallibility of the Bassler hypothesis and the tragic deaths of men like Jim Fixx, there is a ray of hope for the role of exercise in limiting progression of coronary atherosclerosis.

Pollock et al., 1984 and Froelicher V., 1977 and 1980, have summarized the studies relating to exercise in primary prevention and this background is important to understand the scope and hope for secondary prevention. The ideal study is yet to be completed and probably can never be carried out. There is much data on the prevalence of coronary artery disease in relation to exercise which supplies indirect support for the beneficial effect of exercise. This data takes the form of epidemiologic studies of occupations and leisure time activity, active versus nonactive, studies of athletes versus non-athletes, studies of risk factor reduction and improved cardiovascular endurance with exercise, studies in animals, and finally, morbidity and mortality studies in secondary prevention.

Previous studies

Morris, 1953 pointed out that bus drivers on London double decker buses had 1.5 times age adjusted incidence of coronary artery disease over conductors who were more physically active with their job. In Morris' study, drivers also had a 2 times higher sudden death and 3 month post myocardial infarction mortality rate. These findings were assumed to be related to the exercise differences with their individual jobs. Morris, 1956 and in 1966 pointed out that drivers had larger gerths when hired (bigger uniforms) and also had more hypertension and higher cholesterol values. Oliver, 1967 later pointed out that the recruits to these jobs differed in weight and lipid values. These later observations pointed out the difficulty of trying to assess a single factor (exercise) in coronary artery disease which has multiple factors.

Other authors Zukel, 1959 in studies with North Dakota farmers, Taylor, 1962 with U.S. railroad workers, Kahn, 1963 with U.S. postal clerks versus mail carriers, and Frank, 1960 in the health insurance plan of New York all showed the trend that Morris had published with exercise resulting in decreased coronary artery disease incidence and a reduced mortality.

Morris later in 1973 and 1980 evaluated the role of leisure activity in executive grade civil servants and noticed that those who were involved in vigorous sports and kept fit over 8½ years had less than 50% the incidence of coronary disease than those less active colleagues.

Paffenbarger, 1977 published his data on 3,686 long-shoremen, age 35 to 74 years, followed up for 22 years. They found that younger workers who are more active had three times less incidence of fatal heart attacks and sudden deaths. Their data suggested that sedentary work, smoking, and hypertension increased the risk of sudden death twenty times.

Kannel, 1967 in reporting the Frammingham data described the inverse relationship of exercise to incidence of coronary artery disease as well as coronary artery disease mortality.

All of these studies are inconclusive because the data are not standardized, complete, or known. Many assumptions are made and multiple variables are not controlled. There is no good way of documenting exercise carried out over many years and questionnaire data is subject to considerable bias. Despite these problems, a definite trend is evident indicating the beneficial effect of exercise on decreasing coronary artery disease prevalence and mortality.

Williams, 1982; Wood and Haskel, 1979; Cooper, 1976; Zuti, 1976; Carleton, 1981 and Pollock et al., 1984 have published that data showing the direct assocation of endurance exercise training and lowering cardiovascular risk factors (lipids, blood pressure, cigarette smoking incidence, obesity, and stress). Williams, 1982 pointed out that exercise reduces cholesterol, triglycerides, very low density lipoproteins, low density lipoproteins, cholesterol/high density lipoprotein cholesterol (HDLc) ratio, and raises HDLc. He also pointed out that for HDLc to increase it was necessary to exercise 10 miles per week. The beneficial association of exercise with reduction in multiple risk factors may be the major way that exercise exerts a limiting effect on atherosclerotic progression, however, a primary role for exercise may still exist.

Froelicher, 1981 summarized the beneficial cardiovascular changes in animals subjected to chronic exercise. These benefits include cardiac hypertrophy in younger animals, increased myocardial blood flow, improved myocardial function, increased coronary artery diameter, increased ratio of capillary to muscle fiber, faster cardiac relaxation making possible more complete filling at higher heart rates, improved left ventricular performance during ischemia, decreased infarct size, changes in sympathetic innervation and responses to catecholamines, more effective coronary dilatation and improved coronary collateral development.

Two particular animal studies are worthy of further expansion. Eckstein, 1957 demonstrated that animals with coronary stenosis subjected to chronic exercise developed increased collateral flow to the involved area. This has not been reproduced by other authors and is yet to be demonstrated in man. Kramsch, 1981 studied monkeys on an atherogenic diet at rest and subjected to chronic exercise compared to a sedentary control normal diet group. Ischemic ECG changes, positive coronary angiograms and sudden death was limited to the sedentary atherogenic group. The exercising group, despite the atherogenic diet, had reduced overall atherosclerosis, larger hearts, and wider coronary arteries. They concluded that moderate exercise may prevent or retard coronary heart disease in primates.

Perhaps the best epidemiological data, both primary and secondary, comes from Paffenbarger's Harvard Alumni Study 1984. In following the 16,936 Harvard alumni he had shown that the benefit in reduced coronary artery disease incidence and reduced mortality derived by habitual exercise greater than 2,000 Kcal/wk is independent of smoking, obesity, weight gain, hypertension, and family history of coronary artery disease or hypertension. Paffenbarger also published the data on the 782 men who developed coronary artery disease during the follow-up. 607 alumni had survived a myocardial infarction and 175 had angina alone. Over 12 to 15 years of follow-up there were 197 coronary heart disease deaths (25%) and 82 deaths from other causes (10%). Men who maintained exercise greater than 2,000 Kcal/wk experienced 71% of the coronary artery disease mortality of nonactive subjects. They concluded that men who exercise appropriately after recovery from a myocardial infarction have a lower risk of death from a subsequent myocardial infarction.

Shaw, 1981 in the National Exercise and Heart Disease Project reported on 651 men ages 30 to 64 years followed for three years in five different centers. 23% of the exercise group stopped exercise and 31% of the nonexercise group began regular exercise during the follow-up period. The exercise group had a myocardial infarction rate of 5.3% ($N = 17$) and coronary artery disease mortality of 4.6% ($N = 15$) compared to the nonexercise group myocardial infarction rate of 7% ($N = 23$) and coronary artery disease mortality rate of 7.3% ($N = 24$). These figures tend to indicate a trend but are too small to be of significance. Rechnitzer, 1983 in the Ontario study of high versus low intensity exercise showed no difference in the two groups and the study was inconclusive.

Kallio, 1979 in a multifactorial intervention study after myocardial infarction reported on 375 patients, 301 males, 74 females, less than 65 years of age who were randomized into an intervention and control group and followed for three years. Total coronary heart disease deaths were lower in the intervention group, 18.6% versus the control group 29.4% and this was particularly prominent with sudden deaths in the first six months, intervention 5.8%, control 14.4%. Both groups had similar exercise capacity and smoking incidence but other risk factors, blood pressure, cholesterol, triglycerides, and body weight were reduced in the intervention group. These data suggested that mortality particularly in the first six months post myocardial infarction can be reduced by comprehensive rehabilitation. A similar study from Sweden (Veden, 1976) showed different results with only a trend toward reduced mortality. Both the Veden and Kallio studies showed better survival with reinfarction in the intervention group.

Cody, 1983 reviewed 32 patients with poor LV function as manifested by ejection fractions of 10–22% (mean 18%) followed in a rehabilitation program over one year. The observed mortality was 3/32 or 9% versus the expected mortality of 35–40%. It should be noted that careful electrophysiologic studies were performed in 17 out of 32 patients and treatment of ventricular dysrhythmias may have contributed to the good result reported. There were no deaths during training and the MET exercise workload increased from 3.7 METs at 4 weeks post myocardial infarction to 7 METs at 12 months.

Jensen et al., 1980 using radionuclide ventriculography in patients with coronary artery disease active in a rehabilitation program demonstrated improved left ventricular performance with increased submaximal left ventricular ejection fraction at the same workload in selected patients. Williams et al., 1984 showed similar changes at submaximal pretraining workload but not at peak effort. These findings are consistent with the decreased oxygen demand at the same workload due possibly to bradycardia induced by training which could explain the improved left ventricular ejection fraction data.

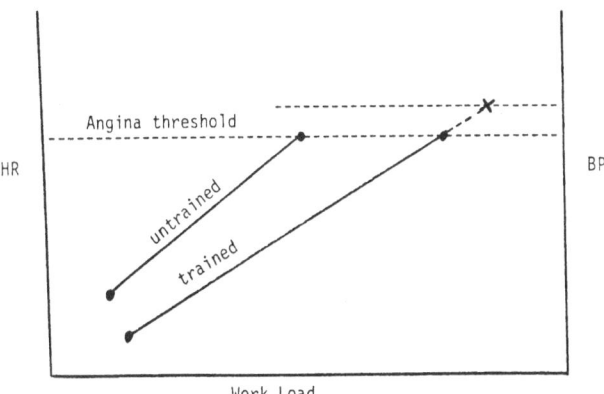

Figure 1. Exercise and Secondary Prevention.

They reported no definite evidence of improved myocardial contractility.

Figure one shows the main cardiovascular benefits to be derived from exercise training. In the trained state heart rate and blood pressure are lower at all work levels and a higher peak workload can be achieved before angina threshold is reached. In selected patients, a higher double product may be achieved. Ehsani, 1982 using echo measurements of the left ventricle at rest and with handgrip exercise in 8 men with coronary artery disease demonstrated for the first time cardiac adaptations to intense exercise training. All 8 patients after training exhibited improvement in left ventricular function as evidenced by lack of decline in fractional shortening or mean velocity of circumferential fiber shortening at similar levels of blood pressure attained during isometric exercise. These data indicate that prolonged exercise training not only results in peripheral adaptations but also in cardiac changes with left ventricular enlargement and probable improvement in left ventricular performance in selected patients with coronary disease.

Figure two presents the possible role of exercise in secondary prevention of atherosclerosis. In the patient with coronary artery disease who has a regular exercise program and a healthful lifestyle, all the major risk factors are reduced and even the effect of a positive family history of coronary artery disease or hypertension can be overcome as demonstrated by the Harvard Alumni study. This combined multifactorial effect could alter the atherosclerotic progress and could delay the onset of symptomatic ischemic heart disease. More important, the mortality from recurrent myocardial infarction is less in the exercising individual.

In summary, the evidence to date would indicate that exercise has several beneficial effects. Risk factors are reduced and there is a reduction in total and sudden death mortality resulting from recurrent myocardial infarction. Exercise improves physical work capacity by peripheral adaptations and may improve left ventricular performance in selected patients. Life may be

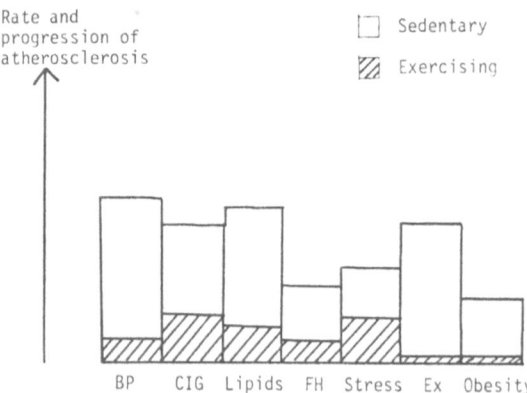

Figure 2. Exercise and Secondary Prevention (BP = blood pressure, CIG = cigarettes, FH = family history, EX = exercise).

prolonged as a result of the reduction in myocardial infarction mortality and with the reduced multiple risk factors progression of atherosclerosis may be delayed. Jim Fixx lived to age 52 years, 9 years longer than this father, suggesting that he may have been successful in his rehabilitation goal and might well be alive yet if he had sought medical assistance. Patients with poor left ventricular function may have reduced mortality and have improved clinical status.

Exercise does not give immunity to coronary artery disease and warning signs of ischemia are meant to be heeded and investigated. The high risk patient should exercise with others or under supervision. Jim Fixx was running from the truth.

References

1. Bassler TJ: Marathon running and immunity to heart disease. Physician Sportsmedicine 3:77–80, 1975.
2. Carleton RA, Blomqvist CG, Mitchell JH, Hartley LH, James F, McHenry PL, Oliverio M, Pollock ML, Selvester RH, Yanowitz FG, Sterling, Brinkley B: American Heart Association: Statement on Exercise. Circulation 64:(6) 1327A–1329A, 1981.
3. Cody DV, Denniss AR, Ross DA, Russell PA, Young AA, Uther JB: Early exercise testing, physical training, and mortality in patients with severe left ventricular dysfunction. Journal of American College Cardiology 1:(2) 718, 1983.
4. Cooper KH, Pollock ML, Martin RP, White SR, Linnerud AC, Jackson A: Physical fitness levels versus selected coronary risk factors. Journal of the American Medical Association 236:(2) 166–169, 1976.
5. Currens JH, White PD: Half a century of running. New England Journal of Medicine 265:988, 1961.
6. Eckstein RW: Effect of exercise and coronary artery narrowing on collateral circulation. Circulation Research 5:230–235, 1957.
7. Ehsani AA, Martin WH, Heath GW, Coyle EF: Cardiac effects of prolonged and intense exercise training in patients with coronary artery disease. The American Journal of Cardiology 50:246–254, 1982.
8. Frank CW, Weinblatt E, Shapiro S, Sager RV: Physical inactivity as a lethal factor in myocardial infarction among men. Circulation 34:1022–1033, 1966.
9. Froelicher VF: Does exercise conditioning delay progression of myocardial ischemia in coronary atherosclerotic heart disease? In: Corday E, Brest A (ed): Controversy in Cardiology (Cardiovascular Clinics series, vol 8, no 1). Philadelphia, e.a. Davis p 11–31, 1977.
10. Froelicher V, Battler A, McKirnan MD: Physical activity and coronary heart disease. Cardiology 65:153–190, 1980.
11. Froelicher VF, Brown P: Exercise and coronary heart disease. Journal of Cardiac Rehabilitation 1:(4) 277–288, 1981.
12. Jensen D, Atwood JE, Froelicher V, McKirnan D, Battler A, Ashburn W, Ross J: Improvement in ventricular function during exercise studies with radionuclide ventriculography after cardiac rehabilitation. The American Journal of Cardiology 46:770–777, 1980.
13. Kahn HA: The relationship of reported coronary heart disease mortality to physical activity of work. American Journal of Public Health 53:(7) 1058–1067, 1963.
14. Kallio V, Hämäläinen H, Hakkila J, Luurila OJ: Reduction in sudden deaths by a multifactorial intervention programme after acute myocardial infarction. The Lancet 2:1091–1094, 1979.

15. Kannel WB: Habitual level of physical activity and risk of coronary heart disease. The Frammingham Study. Canadian Medical Association Journal 96:811, 1967.
16. Kramsch DM, Aspen AJ, Abramowitz BM, Kreimendahl T, Hood WB: Reduction of coronary atherosclerosis by moderate conditioning exercise in monkeys on an atherogenic diet. The New England Journal of Medicine 305:(25) 1483–1489, 1981.
17. Morris JN, Heady JA, Glasg MA, Oxfd MA: Coronary heart disease and physical activity of work. The Lancet 2:1053–1057,. 1111–1120, 1953.
18. Morris JN, Heady JA, Glasg MA, Oxfd MA: Physique of London busmen epidemiology of uniforms. The Lancet 2:569–570, 1956.
19. Marris JN, Kagan A, Pattison DC, Gardner MJ: Incidence and prediction of ischemic heart disease in London busman. The Lancet 2:553–559, 1966.
20. Marris JN, Adam C, Chave SPW, Sirey C, Epstein L: Vigorous exercise in leisure-time and the incidence of coronary heart disease. The Lancet 1:333–339, 1973.
21. Morris JN, Pollard R, Everitt MG, Chave SPW, Semmence AM: Vigorous exercise in leisure-time: Protection against coronary heart disease. The Lancet 2:1027–1210, 1980.
22. Oliver RM: Physique and serum lipids of young London busmen in relation to ischemic heart disease. British Journal Industrial Medicine 24:181, 1967.
23. Paffenbarger RS, Hale WE, Brand RJ, Hyde RT: Work energy level, personal characteristics, and fatal heart attack: A birth-cohort effect. American Journal of Epidemiology 105:200–213, 1977.
24. Paffenbarger RS, Hyde RT, Wing AL, Steinmetz CH: A natural history of athleticism and cardiovascular health. Journal of the Americal Medical Association 252:(4) 491–495, 1984.
25. Paffenbarger RS, Hyde RT: Exercise in the prevention of coronary heart disease. Preventive Medicine 13:3–22, 1984.
26. Pollock ML, Wilmore JG, Fox SM: Exercise in Health and Disease, W.B. Saunders Company P 3–28, 1984.
27. Rechnitzer PA, Cunningham DA, Andrew GM, Buck CW, Jones NL, Kavanaugh T, Oldridge NB, Parker JO, Shephard RJ, Sutton JR, Donner AP: Relation of exercise to the recurrence rate of myocardial infarction in men. Ontario exercise-heart collaborative study. American Journal of Cardiology 51:65–69, 1983.
28. Shaw LW: Effects of a prescribed supervised exercise program on mortality and cardiovascular morbidity in patients after a myocardial infarction. The American Journal of Cardiology 48:39–46, 1981.
29. Taylor HL, Klepetar E, Keys A et al.: Death rates among physically active and sedentary employees of the railroad industry. American Journal of Public Health 52:1697, 1962.
30. Vedin A, Wilhelmsson C, Tibblin G, Wilhelmsen L: The post infarction clinic in Goteborg, Sweden. A controlled trial of a therapeutic organization Acta Medica Scandinavian 200:453–456, 1976.
31. Williams PT, Wood PD, Haskell WL, Vranizan K: The effects of running mileage and duration on plasma lipoprotein levels. The Journal of the American Medical Association 247:(19) 2674–2679, 1982.
32. Williams RS, McKinnis RA, Cobb FR, Higginbotham MB, Wallace AG, Coleman RD, Califf RM: Effects of physical conditioning on left ventricular ejection fraction in patients with coronary artery disease. Circulation 70:(1) 69–75, 1984.
33. Wood PD, Haskell WL: The effect of exercise on plasma high density lipoproteins. Lipids 14:(4) 417–427, 1979.
34. zuti WB, Golding LA: Comparing diet and exercise as weight reduction tools. The Physician and Sportsmedicine 4:49–53, 1976.
35. Zukel WJ, Lewis RH, Enterline PE, Painter RC, Ralston LS, Fawcett RM, Meredith AP, Peterson B: A short-term community study of the epidemiology of coronary heart disease. The American Journal of public Health 49:(12) 1630–1639, 1959.

17. The Behavior of the Ejection Fraction at Rest and Exercise in Myocardial Infarction Before and After a 4-week Training Period. Comparison to a Control Group

E. GRODZINSKI, W. SCHOOP, G. BLÜMCHEN and
J.S. BORER*

Abstract

99 myocardial infarction patients were divided randomly an average of 6.5 weeks after M.I. into a training group and a control group. The training group performed 2×30 minutes of physical training at 80% of their maximal performance level 5 days a week. Before and after the 4 week observation period, the ejection fraction at rest and during exercise was determined with the help of radionuclide ventriculography. Differences between the training group and the control group were, as a whole, negligible. The control group demonstrated a significant rise in the resting ejection fraction ($p < 0.05$) compared to the resting ejection fractions of the training group. The ejection fraction during sub-maximal exercise showed a distinct rise in the training group ($p < 0.005$). As the control group also showed a tendency for improvement of the ejection fraction during exercise, the overall behaviour of the exercise ejection fraction between the two groups was not significantly different. The increase in ejection fraction from rest to exercise (ΔEF) in the training group was significantly lower compared with the control group. The training group had first shown a decline of ejection fraction from rest to exercise, whereas the control group demonstrated a negligibel rise. After four weeks, this relationship reversed. The total change in ejection fraction from rest to exercise between the training group and control group was, after four weeks, highly significant ($p < 0.005$). This improvement can be explained by the already existing, significant difference in the behavior of the ejection fraction from rest to exercise before training. The remainder is explained by the lack of improvement in ejection fraction at rest in the training group. This would make a peripheral target of the effect of the training more likely than a cardiac one.

---

* Dr. Borer is an Established Investigator of the American Heart Association.

Introduction

Exercise is considered beneficial to patients with myocardial infarction (MI) in a chronical stage [5, 11, 12, 15–17, 19, 20, 22]. Above all, numerous works attribute the beneficial training effect to the training condition of the peripheral system. Other authors presume it to be a direct training influence on the heart muscle. Using the non-invasive method of radionuclide ventriculography (RNVA), ejection fraction (EF) at rest and during exercise was examined with a training group (T-group), and a control group (C-group), 5–8 weeks after MI. The question should be persued as to whether or not training has a conceivable effect on the ejection fraction.

Methods

99 patients (93 male, 6 female), with an average age of 48 years (from 33–62 years), were examined. The myocardial infarction had occurred on an average of 6,5 weeks prior to this study (from 5–8 weeks) and was documented through anamnesis, ECG and increases in enzymes. The 99 MI-patients were randomly divided into a T-group (53 patients: of which 25 had an anterior MI and 28 had an inferior MI and in a C-group (46 patients: of which 22 had an anterior and 24 a inferior MI).

10 of the 99 patients had an intramural MI and 8 had suffered a re-infarction. The T-and C-groups were comparable according to the following criteria: distribution in anterior and inferior, intramural and reinfarctions, age, time after infarction, duration of the history of coronary heart disease (CHD), sex, heart volumes, size of the infarct (R-reduction in ECG at rest), work tolerance during ergometry, aneurysm (found by RNVA), PCP and cardiac index at rest and during exercise by using the floating catheter (Swan-Ganz-procedure).

In the 4 weeks between the 1st and 2nd RNVA, 8 patients had to undergo a change of medication because of arrhythmias or hypertension. 4 patients were placed in the C-group and 4 in the T-group. However, the medication (digitalis, isosorbiddinitrate, calciumantagonist, betablocker) remained the same in all other patients.

Training Program

The training program was supervised by an experienced calisthenics director. The T-group underwent training 5 times per week in the following manner: During the first week (examination), light ergometry exercise was performed at 40 watts for 15 minutes in a sitting position, as well as taking walks and performing calisthenics with the goal of improving coordination. Afterwards, the actual 4 week training program began: dynamic endurance training 2 times daily at 80% of the maximum performance capability. Calisthenics and ergometry training took place in the morning. In the afternoon, running or walking training took place [18], and afterwards the group played ball. According to a determined exercise level which depended on the body weight, the running or walking training was calculated in watts.

The heart rate of every patient was recorded during the running training with the help of Holter-ECG, to determine if 80% of the achieved maximum heart rate was reached. Those patients who could perform at an 80 watt level, without signs of ischemia and without arrhythmias, were involved in a 30 minute swimming exercise period in the afternoon.

No physical efforts were demanded from the C-group during the in-patient stay. The patients were informed about the examination program and its set objectives. They participated in light recreational activities. The exercises were chosen so that a training-heart-rate would not be reached. In addition, ergometry exercise was performed in a supine position for 15 minutes at a 25 to 30 watt level. In the afternoon, the patients walked for 30 minute walks on level terrain.

Examination Methods

The examination program during the 6 week in-patient stay was as follows:

1st week:
Anamnesis and clinical examination, ECG at rest, X-ray of the thorax with determination of the heart volume, a symptom limited exercise-ECG (or the achievement of a heart rate of 180/min minus the age), radionuclide ventriculography (RNVA), floating catheter method (in 72 patients).

2nd-5th week:
Dynamic endurance training of the T-group and exercise program of the C-group 5 times per week with a Holter-ECG recording at least once.

6th week:
ECG at rest, X-ray of the thorax, exercise-ECG (stopping criteria as above) and radionuclide ventriculography. Coronary angiography and left ventricular angiography was performed in 19 patients.

a) *Radionuclide ventriculography*

The examination was done in a supine position at rest and during submaximal exercise using Borer's et al. method [1, 2, 6–9] to measure the ejection fraction (EF). A conventional gamma camera and the data processing system VP 450 (Siemens) was used for the recording, storage, processing, and depiction of the heart, which had been triggered by the ECG [1].

A dosage of 15–20 mCi 99^m-technetiumpertechnetate was injected into the cubital vein 30 minutes after the injection of 5 mg pyrophosphate. After 10 minutes, that is, following equal distribution of the indicator, the first images were done at rest in 2 planes [27] (RAO at approximately 35° and LAO between 30°–35°). The LAO projected image was chosen in such a manner that the superficial detector was placed perpendicular to the interventricular septum, so that an optimal separation of the left ventricle from the right one was reached. The demarcation of the left ventricle from the left atrium was due to additional angling of about 15° in a caudal direction. The projected image of the maximum achieved exercise level resulted from an identical LAO-view.

The 2nd RNVA after the 4 week training (observation program) was done again at comparable submaximal exercise levels. However, the improved exercise capacity, with decreasing risk of myocardial infarction (after the training program), allowed a higher work load in the follow-up examination. The average exercise level in the initial study was 99 watts for the T-group and 106 watts for the C-group. The average level in the follow-up study was 103 watts for the T-group and 104 watts for the C-group.

After the data were collected, the wall motion of the left ventricle in RAO and LAO projected images was well described by one and the same author (E.G.) and was judged as possibly being hypokinetic, akinetic, or dyskinetic. The quantitative automatic determination of the left ventricular ejection fraction (EF) in the LAO-plane under resting conditions, as well as during exercise, resulted in the following formula:

$$EF = \frac{ED \: cts - ES \: cts}{ED \: cets} \times 100,$$

whereby:

ED cts = maximal enddiastolic counts.
ES cts = maximal endsystolic counts.

A comparison between 2 observers was made in 18 patients (E.G. and J.S.B.). The value of the RNVA at rest agreed with a correlation coefficient of $r = 0.89$, the exercise RNVA with a value of $r = 0.82$.

Statistical Procedure

The exercise EF values were respectively adjusted with the equivalent value at rest. These differences were shown with the ΔEF:

$$\Delta EF_1 = EF_{E1} - EF_{R1}$$
$$\Delta EF_2 = EF_{E2} - EF_{R2}$$

Therefore, index 1 indicates the values before training and index 2 shows the values after training.

The increase of this difference between the 1st and 2nd RNVA was determined to be the main objective for measuring the training results:

$$\Delta\Delta EF = \Delta EF_2 - \Delta EF_1$$

The increases of the EF values at rest (EF_R) were examined, as well as the EF values during exercise (EF_E), between the 2 points of time:

$$\Delta EF_R = EF_{R2} - EF_{R1}$$
$$\Delta EF_2 = EF_{E2} + EF_{E1}$$

Not only the influence of the training, which is assumed to be the standard distributed main objective, but also the localization of the infarct was taken into account.

Furthermore, the possibility of error should be smaller than 0.05.

Results

The individual results are given in Figures 1 through 8 and in Tables 1 and 2.

Table 1 shows the mean, maximal, and minimal values of the ejection fraction in 25 anterior and in 28 inferior MI-patients before and after a 4 week training program (T-group). It also shows the ejection fraction at rest and during submaximal exercise in 22 anterior and 24 inferior MI-patients, after a 4 week observation period without training (C-group). A large distribution of the single value of EF at rest and ΔEF during exercise can be detected. It extended from 21 up to 81%. In Table 1, the significances between anterior and inferior infarctions are also given. The study of the

Table 1.

		T-group		C-group		Significance between AMI and IMI
		AMI n = 25	IMI n = 28	AMI n = 22	IMI n = 24	
EF_{R1}	$\bar{x}$	46,76	54,61	45,91	51,83	p<0,004
	s	±13,68	±10,80	±12,36	±8,72	
	max	74	81	67	75	
	min	21	36	18	40	
EF_{R2}	$\bar{x}$	47,12	53,00	49,00	54,79	p<0,025
	s	±14,64	±10,55	±13,48	±10,63	
	qsmax	77	76	74	76	
	min	25	28	19	36	
Significance (EF_{R1} and EF_{R2})		p<0,45	p<0,15	p<0,05	p<0,1	
EF_{E1}	$\bar{x}$	43,20	49,54	47,05	52,42	p<0,03
	s	±16,03	±10,88	±14,27	±10,40	
	max	75	77	70	71	
	min	18	31	18	25	
EF_{E2}	$\bar{x}$	46,24	53,96	47,14	54,29	p<0,005
	s	±16,26	±10,58	±13,60	±9,86	
	max	80	70	67	74	
	min	25	22	21	37	
Significance (EF_{E1} and EF_{E2})		p<0,1	p<0,003	p<0,5	p<0,2	
ΔEF_1	$\bar{x}$	−3,56	−5,07	+1,14	+0,58	p<0,55
	s	±9,33	±6,51	±8,55	±8,31	
	max	+13	+11	+22	+20	
	min	−23	−16	−15	−15	
ΔEF_2	$\bar{x}$	−0,88	+0,96	−1,86	−0,50	p<0,55
	s	±10,56	−8,70	±8,06	±9,93	
	max	+25	+15	+13	+14	
	min	−19	−21	−16	−15	
$\Delta\Delta EF$	$\bar{x}$	+2,68	+6,04	−3,00	−1,08	p<0,55
	s	±13,48	±9,02	±9,20	±11,00	
	max	+43	+25	+23	+21	
	min	−22	−8	−17	−23	
ΔEF_R	$\bar{x}$	+0,36	−1,61	+3,09	+2,96	p<0,055
	s	±8,08	±6,56	±7,03	±9,77	
	max	+20	+11	+15	+20	
	min	−14	−14	−10	−14	
ΔEF_E	$\bar{x}$	+3,04	+4,43	+0,09	+1,88	p<0,55
	s	±9,09	±6,37	±7,32	±8,96	
	max	+29	+14	+14	+17	
	min	−12	−3	−17	−14	

		T-group		C-group		
		AMI n = 25	IMI n = 28	AMI n = 22	IMI n = 24	Significance
$\Delta\Delta EF$	$\bar{x}$	+2,68	+6,04	−3,00	−1,08	p<0,005
	s	±13,48	±9,02	±9,20	±11,00	
	max	+32 +25	+25	+23	+21	
	min	−22	−8	−17	−23	
ΔEF_R	$\bar{x}$	+0,36	−1,61	+3,09	+2,96	p<0,025
	s	±8,08	±6,56	±7,03	±9,77	
	max	+20	+11	+15	+20	
	min	−14	−10	−10	−14	
ΔEF_E	$\bar{x}$	+3,04	+4,43	+0,09	+1,88	p<0,1
	s	±9,08	±6,37	±7,32	±8,96	
	max	+29	+14	+14	+17	
	min	−12	−13	−17	−14	

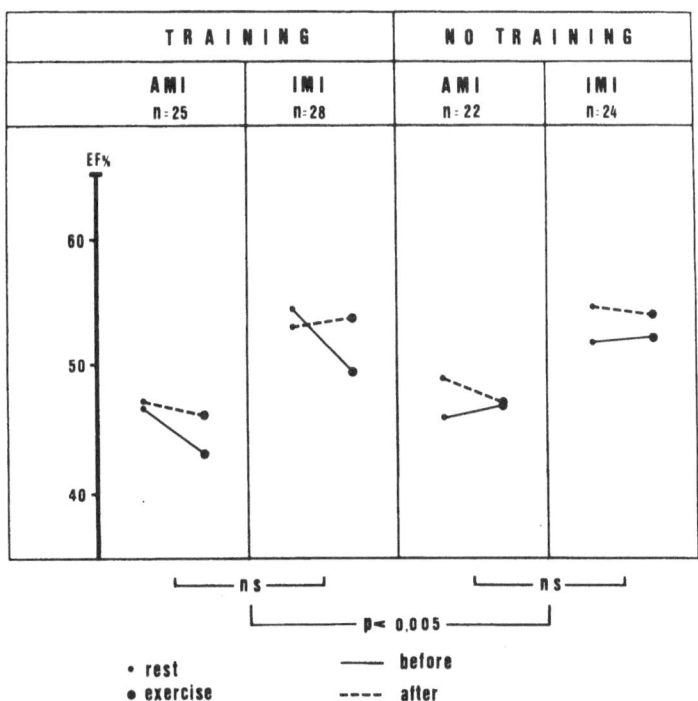

Figure 1. Mean values of EF at rest and during exercise before and after the 4 week program in T-group (Training) and C-group (no Training), divided in anterior (AMI) and inferior (IMI) MI.

158

individual values showed, that patients with a very low EF at rest could show an increase during exercise and that patients with a pronounced higher EF at rest could display a decrease during exercise. That holds true for the T-, as well as the C-group.

Table 2 shows the comparison between the training and the control group.

Figure 1 shows the behaviour of the EF at rest and during submaximal exercise before and after a 4 week training program (left side of the figure) and also the control group (right side of the figure). The anterior and inferior infarction groups are depicted. It can be recognized that the EF of the inferior MI are higher than those of the anterior infarctions which holds true not only for the values at rest but also during exercise. The difference between the T- and C-groups from rest to exercise is significant before and after the 4 week program ($p < 0.005$). It can also be recognized, that the exercise

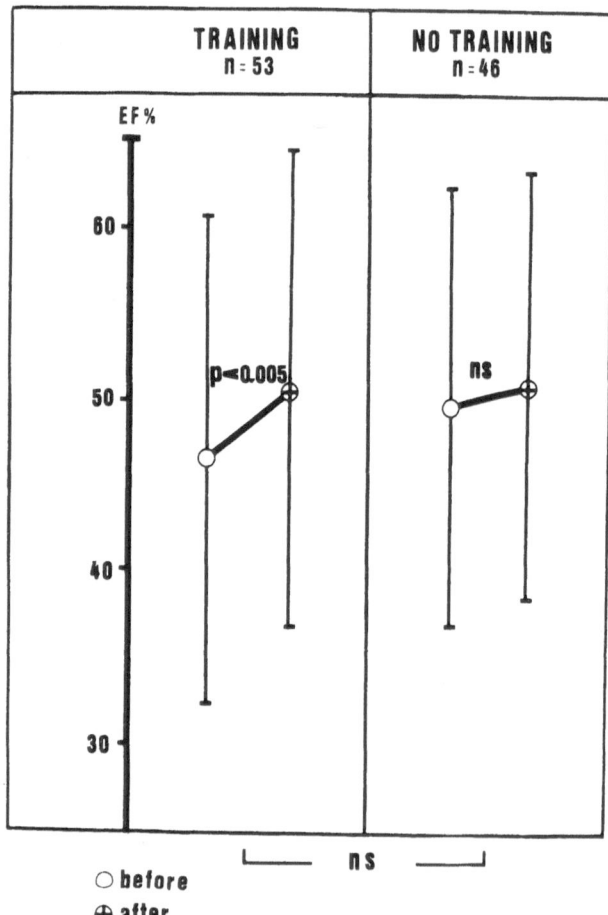

Figure 2. EF during exercise (EF$_E$) before and after the 4 week program in T-group (training) and in C-group (no training)

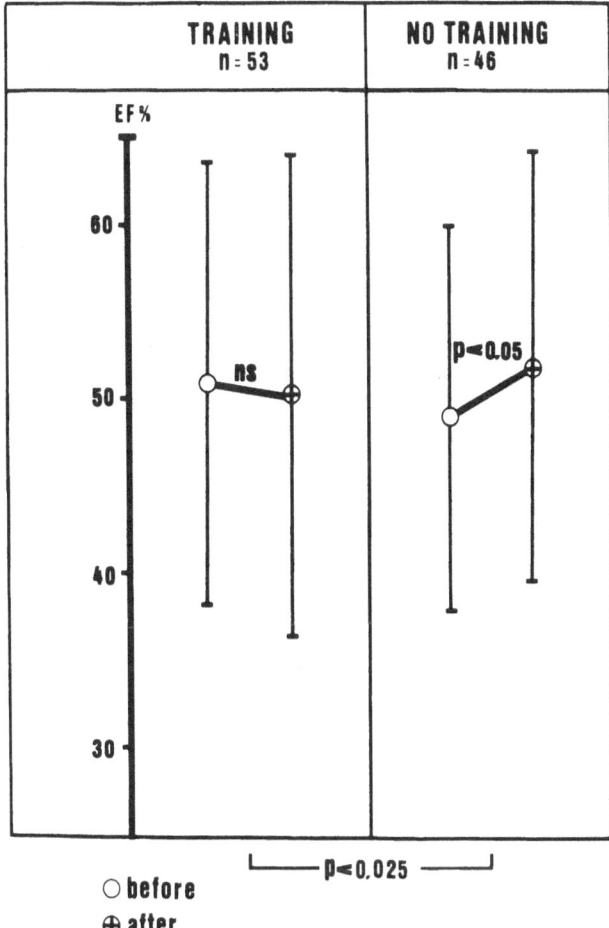

Figure 3. EF at rest (EF_r) before and after the 4-week program in T-group (training) and in C-group (no training)

values in the training group are clearly better ($p < 0.005$) than those in the control group (Fig. 2). Furthermore, a slight improvement of the values at rest in the control group was noted, however not in the T-group ($p < 0.05$). This is significantly different between the 2 groups ($p < 0.03$) (Fig. 3).

Figure 4 shows the ΔEF ($\Delta EF = \Delta EF_E - EF_R$) before and after a 4 week training program (left side of figure) and in the control group (right side). It is recognized that the training group (in patients with anterior as well as those with inferior MI) has an increase in the ΔEF after training, however this did not occur in the control group. The difference between the T-and C-groups is significant at the time of the initial study ($p < 0.0025$), but not in the 2nd study.

Figure 5 shows the behaviour of the $\Delta\Delta EF$ ($\Delta\Delta EF = \Delta EF_2 - \Delta EF_1$) in the training group (left side of figure) and the control group (right side). It is

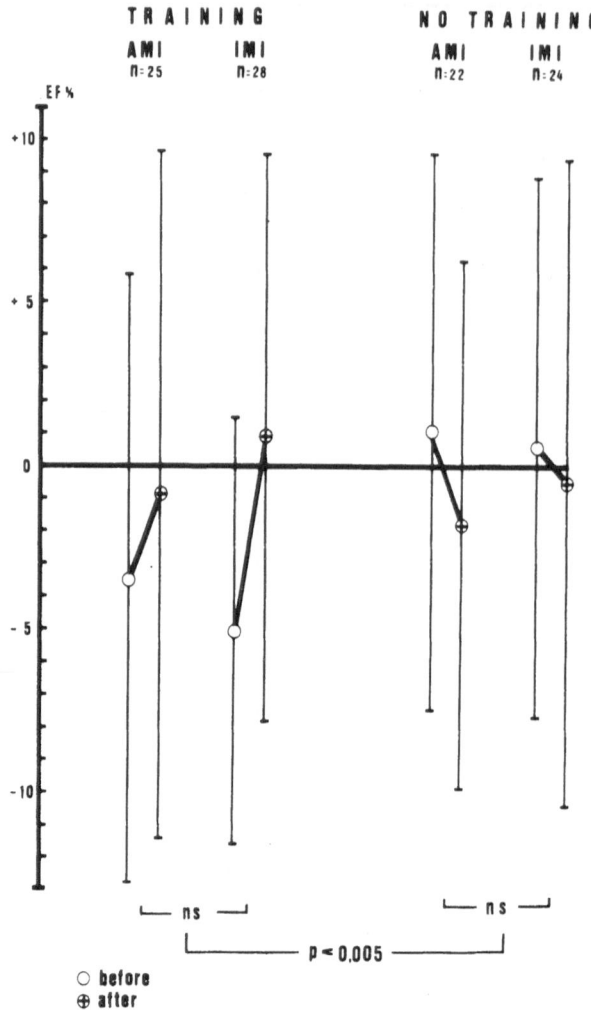

Figure 4. Behaviour of ΔEF (ΔEF = $EF_E - EF_R$) before and after the 4 week program in T-group (training) and C-group (no training), divided in anterior (AMI) and inferior (IMI) MI

recognized that the ΔEF of anterior and inferior infarct paients in the training groups increased, and decreased in the control groups. The difference between the T- and C-groups is significant.

Figure 6 shows the behaviour of the so-called double product (heart rate × systolic blood pressure) at rest and during comparable exercise with RNVA. That is, in the training group and in the control group at rest (left side) and during comparable exercise levels (right side). The behaviour of the double product of the T- and C-groups was not significantly different at rest, nor during exercise.

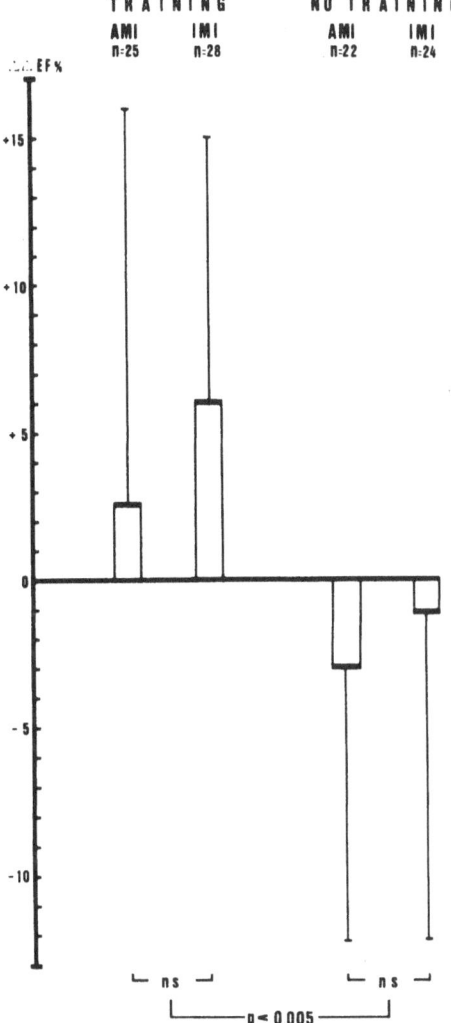

Figure 5. Mean values of $\Delta\Delta EF$ ($\Delta\Delta EF = \Delta EF_2 - \Delta EF_1$) in T-group (training) and C-group (no training), devided in AMI and IMI

Discussion

The EF, in comparison to a randomized control group without training, shows the following results:

1. In comparison to the non-trained control group, a distinct increase in the EF from rest to exercise can be found in the training group. It is more pronounced in inferior rather than in anterior MI-patients.
2. The control group shows an improvement of the EF at rest, 5 to 8 weeks after MI, within a 4 week period. This is a spontaneous improvement in the left ventricular function.

162

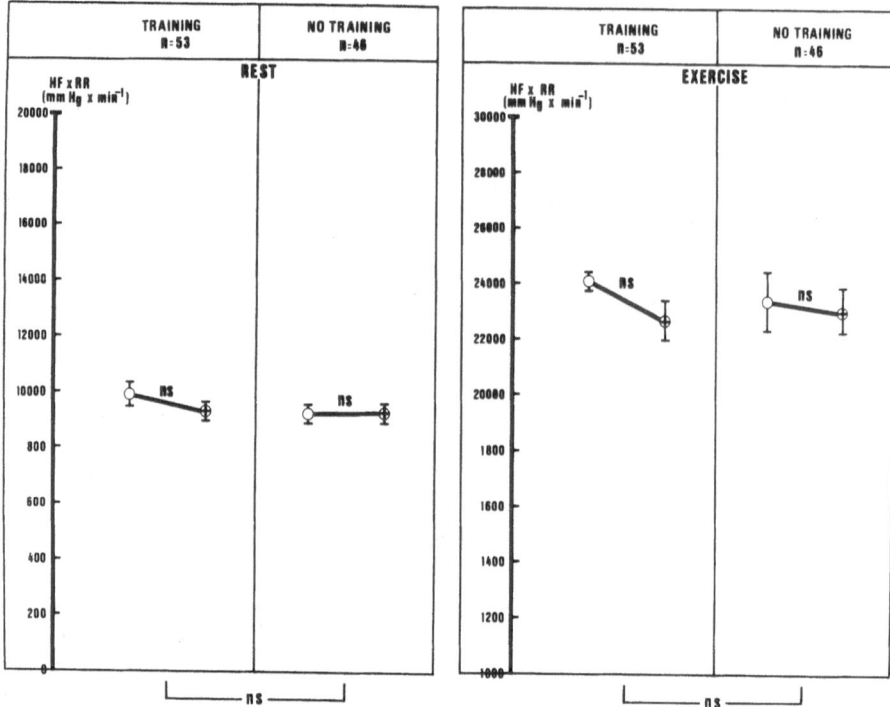

Figure 6. Double product (heart rate x systolic blood pressure) before and after the 4-week program in T-group (TRAINING) and C-group (NO TRAINING)

3. A more distinct increase of the EF during exercise can be noted in the training group than in the control group.

Comparison of the behaviour of the ejection fractions between the T- and C-groups

In coronary disease, we view the reaction of the EF from rest to exercise as an essential parameter. We followed the given criteria of Borer et al. [9]: An increase of the EF, of at least 5%, is the normal reaction during submaximal exercise. This 5% increase does not show in patients with coronary heart disease during submaximal exercise, therefore the behaviour of the EF is pathological.

The anterior MI-patients of the T-group show a clear decrease of the EF during exercise, before the 4 week training treatment. After 4 weeks of training, a decrease of the EF during exercise did persist. However, it is not as marked as before the training. The control group of anterior infarct patients shows a slight increase in the exercise EF at the time of the initial study and a slight decrease after 4 weeks. It may also be discussed that the improvement of the EF of the anterior infarct patients in the T-group comes about because the EF-value to begin with is lower than in the C-group.

Coincidentally, at the time of the initial study, a decrease of the EF during exercise in inferior infarctions in the T-group is found, however, not in the C-group. In comparison to the C-group, the improvement of the EF behaviour in inferior infarct patients in the T-group can also predominantly come about via the low EF-value to begin with. The difference in the behaviour of the EF from rest to exercise is significant between the T- and C-groups ($p < 0.005$) and is independant of the infarct localization.

Like Jensen et al. [17], we found no significant changes of the double product during submaximal exercise. The decrease of the double product is indeed more pronounced in the T-group, but in comparison to the C-group, the difference is insignificant. At the time of the initial study and after 4 weeks, the behaviour of the double product between the T-group and the C-group is not statistically different. Because of statistically significant differences in the behaviour of the ejection fractions from rest to exercise (ΔEF), between the T- and C-groups at the time of the initial and second RNVA, it could be argued that the training treatment had a direct cardiac effect. The effect is, especially in comparison to the control group, certainly not very distinct. The differing EF-values at the begin of the study of both groups, from rest to exercise, could by itself, explain the significantly differing behaviour. Because the inferior infarct patients benefit more through training than the anterior infarct patients, the extent of the myocardial damage probably plays a role in the achieved adaptation procedures on the left ventricle through training. This direct training effect on the heart muscle was also assumed by Jensen et al. According to our results, the improvement of the EF through physical training was found between the 5th and 8th week after a MI. These results were still obtainable in the following six months, according to the results of Jensen et al.

We did not succeed in finding out if sub-groups had especially benefited from the training treatment. It can only be said that the reaction of the ejection fraction during exercise was more improved in inferior MI in contrast to anterior MI. It could also not be forseen in which patients the reaction of the ejection fraction would worsen during training. The group consisted of patients which all showed a myocardial scar, but only 16 complained about angina pectoris discomfort during the first RNVA. In these 16 patients, it must also be assumed that, in addition to the existing scar, exercise coronary insufficiency plays a role in the reaction of the ejection fraction during exercise. The size of the infarct, the location of the infarct and, in addition, the possible appearance of silent ischemia during exercise will have influenced the behaviour of the ejection fraction differently in the T- and C-groups.

Angiocardiography was performed in 19 patients. Besides the infarct vessel, an additional 50% of stenosis was found in other vessels in 8 out of 9 patients from the T-group and in 6 out of 10 from the C-group. In both groups, at the time of the initial study, a decrease of the EF from rest to exercise (ΔEF) was recognized. This decrease was more distinct in the patients of the T-group. After 4 weeks, both groups had an average decrease of the ΔEF, which was more distinct in the control group. Increases in the EF from rest to exercise were found in patients who had undergone angiocardiography and who did not have additional higher degrees of stenosis (1 from the T-group and 4 from the C-group). Statistically significant differences were not found between those trained and those untrained in this sub-group of paients who underwent coronary angiography. The number of patients who underwent coronary angiography is too small in order to be able to draw conclusions from both groups (with and without additional stenosis). The trend though, reveals that patients with apparent training induced ischemia show no improvement in the EF reaction after 4 weeks.

Spontaneous course in the control group

There is no report in the literature about the spontaneous course of the EF at rest and during exercise, 5 to 8 weeks after a myocardial infarction. For that reason, our control group can be used as an observation for the spontaneous course of the EF at this time.

The RNVA at rest and during exercise was done in the control group in the course of 4 weeks, without training treatment. Physical mobilization was kept at the lowest possible level. Certainly the patients could not be prohibited from exceeding their prescribed extent of physical activity in their free time. The medication at the time of the first and second RNVA was also kept the same. In the control group, there is an improvement of the EF at rest. In the training group, no substantial change of the EF can be found at rest. The distinctly reduced heart rate at rest and after training can be discussed as a reason for this. A similar behaviour in trained sport students could be shown by Rerych et al. [24]. The dependence of the EF from the heart rate in healthy persons was described by Bauer et al. [3]. The lack of improvement of the EF at rest in the training group could be explained through the peripheral training effect with a reduction of the heart rate. Thus for the improvement of the ΔEF in the T-group due to the behaviour of the EF at rest a periphera mechanism of training has to be discussed. Changes of the left ventricular function over several months after a heart infarct are also described with other methods [4]. These facts must be kept in mind in the final evaluation of MI patients, and the use of RNVA in 8–9 weeks old MI should also be considered to control other treatment methods (such as the influence of medication, PTCA, coronary bypass surgery).

Behaviour of the ejection fraction during submaximal exercise

The EF during exercise clearly improves in the training group. This finding corresponds to the results of Jensen et al. [17]. In 19 patients, who had suffered a myocardial infarction more than 3 months earlier, they found an increase of the average ejection fraction during submaximal exercise after a 6 months training period. However, they did not examine a control group. It is recognizable in our control group, that the improvement of the EF during exercise is not a training effect alone. An equivalent result was found by Cobb et al. [13]. The difference between these reports and our series is, that the infarct age of our patients amounted to less than 3 months and we only carried out a 4 week training program. It also deals with different starting levels. It can be accepted that at this relatively early time period after a heart infarct, spontaneous changes in the left ventricular function could appear as a result of the adaptation mechanism of the remaining myocardium in the border district of the infarct region and in the infarct region itself. The behaviour of the EF in our C-group may show that the adjustment mechanism can last longer than 8 weeks after a myocardial infarction. Considerable deviations within a 4 week period were observed.

Through adequate physical exercise, also in patients with increased heart volumes, decreased ejection fractions at rest and in aneurysm patients, no recognizable damage is seen through the training treatment up to this time period [10]. This result corresponds to reports from Buchwalsky et al. [11]. They saw no damaging influence of the training in repeated floating catheter examinations on patients with increased heart volume after a heart infarct. This also holds true for the reports from Lee et al. [19], and Conn et al. [14].

The results observed indicate in contrast to the hypothesis above that through physical training in MI patients, not only the often described adaptation processes occur in the peripheral circulation, but also that cardiac mechanisms are probably directly affected. The hypothesis is being supported by the fact that the double product of systolic blood pressure and heart rate, at rest and during submaximal exercise (that is, during the measurement of the ejection fraction), were not statistically different between the T- and C-groups. However, the reaction of the ejection fraction changed from rest to exercise. Nevertheless, this observation is in contrast to other reports [13, 21, 23, 26].

Acknowledgement

We wish to thank the 'Verein zur Bekämpfung der Gefäßkrankheiten' e.V., Engelskirchen, for financial help and for help in preparation of this manuscript.

References

1. Bacharach SL, Green MV, Borer JS, Douglas MA, Ostrow HG, Johnston GS: Real time scintigraphic cineangiography, Computers in Cardiol. Proc IEEE Comp Soc St Louis 45–48, 1976.
2. Bachorach SL, Green MV, Borer JS, Douglas MA, Ostrow HG, Johnston GS: A real-time system for multi-image gated cardiac studies. J Nucl Med 18:79, 1977.
3. Bauer R, Sauer E, Truckenbrodt R, Langhammer H, Pabst HW, Sebening H, Wirtzfeld A, Blömer H: Die linksventrikuläre Herzfunktion in Ruhe und unter Ergometerbelastung. Herz 5, Nr 3, 156–157, 1980.
4. Blümchen G, Brandt D, Schlei W: Fülungsdruckmessungen (Einschwemmkatheterverfahren) bei Herzinfarktpatienten im chronischen Stadium unter Belastung. Herz/Kreislauf 10:479, 1981.
5. Bonanno JA, Lies E: Effects of physical training on coronary risk factors. Amer J Cardiol 33:760, 1974.
6. Borer JS, Bacharach SL, Green MV, Kent KM, Epstein SE, Johnston GS: Rapid evaluation of left ventricular function during exercise in patients with coronary artery disease. Circulation 54:suppl II, 1976.
7. Borer JS, Bacharach SL, Green MV, Kent KM, Epstein SE, Johnston GS: Realtime radionuclide cineangiography in the noninvasive evaluation of global and regional and regional left ventricular function at rest and during exercise in patients with coronary artery disease. New Engl J Med 296:839, 1977.
8. Borer JS, Kent KM, Bacharach SL, Green MV, Rosing DR, Seides SF, Epstein SE, Johnston GS: Sensitivity, specificity and predictive accuracy of radionuclide cineangiography during exercise in patients with coronary artery disease: comparison with exercise electrography. Circulation 60:572, 1979.
9. Borer JS, Rosing DR, Miller RH, Stark RM, Kent KM, Bacharach SL, Green MV, Lake CR, Cohen H, Holmes D, Donohue D, Baker W, Epstein SE: Natural history of left ventricular function during one year after acute myocardial infarction: Comparison with clinical, electrocardiographic, and biochemical determinations. Amer J Cardiol 46:1, 1980.
10. Grodzinski E, Kreutz F, Blümchen G, Borer JS: Über das Verhalten der Ruhe- und Belastungs-Auswurffraktion (EF) bei Herzinfarktpatienten vor und nach vierwöchigem Training. Vergleich zu einer Kontrollgruppe. Z Kardiol 72:105, 1983.
11. Buchwalsky R, Bahls J, Pinno D, Caliman J: Auswirkungen eines körperlichen Trainings auf die gestörte Hämodynamik nach Herzinfarkt. Verh Dtsch Ges inn Med 83:242, 1977.
12. Clausen JP, Trap-Jensen J: Heart rate and arterial blood pressure during exercise in patients with angina pectoris. Circulation 53:436, 1976.
13. Cobb FR, Sanders Williams R, McEwan P, Jones RH, Coleman RE, Wallace AG: Effects of exercise training on ventricular function in patients with recent myocardial infarction. Circulation Vol 66, No 1, 100–108, 1982.
14. Conn EH, Williams RS, Wallace AG: Exercise responses before and after physical conditioning in patients with severely depressed left ventricular function. Amer J Cardiol 49:296, 1982.

15. Ditchey RV, Watkins J, McKirnan MD, Froelicher V: Effects of exercise training on left ventricular mass in patients with ischemic heart disease. Amer Heart J 101:No 6, 1981.

16. Hung J, McKillop J, Goris M, De Busk R: The effects of exercise training on myocardial ischemia and left ventricular function soon after myocardial infarction: A randomized study. Circulation 64:Suppl IV, 748, 1981.

17. Jensen D, Atwood JE, Froelicher V, McKirnan MD, Battler A, Ashburn W, Ross J: Improvement in ventricular function during exercise studies with radionuclide ventriculography after cardiac rehabilitation. Amer J Cardiol Vol 46:770, 1980.

18. Lagerstrøm D, Rost R, Hollmann W: Ein neues Lauftraining für die Prävention und Rehabilitation. Sportarzt und Sportmed 26:169, 1975.

19. Lee AP, Ice R, Blessey R, Sanmarco ME: Long-term effects of physical training on coronary patients with impaired ventricular function. Circulation 60:No 7, 1979.

20. Leiß O, Bauer H, Murawski U, Egge H, Schumacher A, Blümchen: Effekt einer kombinierten Behandlung mit Diät und körperlichem Training auf die Lipoproteinlipide von Herzinfarktpatienten. Herz/Kreislauf 12:Nr 4, 174, 1980.

21. Letac B, Cribier A, Desplanches JF: A study of left ventricular function in coronary patients before and after physical training. Circulation 56:No 3, 375, 1977.

22. Marschall RC, Berger HJ, Reduto LA, Gottschalk A, Zaret BL: Variability in sequential measures of left ventricular performance assessed with radionuclide angiocardiography. Amer J Cardiol 41:531, 1978.

23. Nolewayka AJ, Kostuk WJ, Rechnitzer PA, Cunningham DA: Exercise and human collateralization: an angiographic and scintigraphic assessment. Circulation 60:114–121, 1979.

24. Rerych SK, Scholz PM, Sabiston DC, Jones RH: Effects of exercise training on left ventricular function in normal subjects: a longitudinal study by radionuclide angiography. Amer J Cardiol Vol 45, 1980.

25. Strauss HW, Zaret BL, Hurley PJ, Natarajan TK, Pitt B: A scintiphotography method for measuring left ventricular ejection fraction in man without cardiac catheterization. Amer J Cardiol 28:575–580, 1971.

26. Thompson PD, Cullinan E, Lazarus B, Carleton RA: Effect of exercise training on the untrained limb exercise performance of men with angina pectoris. Amer J Cardiol 48:844–850, 1981.

18. Adaptations to Prolonged Intense Exercise Training in Ischemic Heart Disease

A. A. EHSANI

Abstract

Endurance exercise training increases work capacity and the minimum work rate required to induce angina in patients with ischemic heart disease. To test the hypothesis that 12 months of high intensity exercise training can benefit the heart, 10 patients aged, 50 ± 9 (mean $\pm$ SD) with documented ischemic heart disease were studied. Exercise training consisted of endurance exercise at 50-70% of the measured maximal attainable O_2 uptake ($\dot{V}O_2$) 3 times per week for the first 3 months and at 70-85% of the maximal attainable $\dot{V}O_2$ 5 times per week. Heart rate (HR) at rest decreased from 60 ± 8 to 53 ± 6 beats/min. Maximal aerobic exercise capacity increased by 42% (24 ± 3 vs 34 ± 6 ml/kg/min; $p < 0.001$). Rate pressure product (RPP) at a constant absolute work rate was lower after training ($25.69 \times 10^3 \pm 5.9 \times 10^3$ vs $20.68 \times 10^3 \pm 3.46 \times 10^3$; $p < 0.001$) and was associated with (1) a lower plasma norepinephrine (1953 ± 606 vs 1142 ± 313 pg/ml; $p < 0.01$) and (2) lower ischemic ST segment depression (0.2 ± 0.1 vs 0.07 ± 0.08 mV; $p < 0.001$). At peak exercise, norepinephrine (2049 ± 654 vs 3408 ± 1454 pg/ml; $pp < 0.01$) and RPP ($25.34 \times 10^3 \pm 4.97 \times 10^3$ vs $27.64 \times 10^3 \pm 5.2 \times 10^3$, $p < 0.025$) were higher after training whereas ischemic ST segment depression did not change. Ejection fraction (EF), determined by equilibrium radionuclide ventriculography, at rest did not change after training (50 ± 11 vs 51 ± 12%). At peak cycle ergometer exercise EF remained unchanged (50 ± 11 at rest vs 50 ± 13% during exercise) before but increased from 51 ± 12 to 58 ± 12% ($p < 0.001$) after 12 months of training. At peak exercise, left ventricular end diastolic volume (LVEDV: 131 ± 28 vs 142 ± 27 ml; $p < 0.01$) and systolic blood pressure (175 ± 10 vs 200 ± 10 mm Hg; $p < 0.001$) were increased after training. Resting LVEDV also increased after training. However, endsystolic volume did not change. Thus, improvement in EF can not be attributed to changes in loading conditions. After low intensity exercise training, EF did not change even though rate pressure product at any given work rate was lower after training and maximal aerobic capacity increased. These data suggest that high intensity exercise training can induce intrinsic adaptations in the heart in patients with ischemic heart disease.

Introduction

Exercise training elicits a number of adaptations in patients with ischemic heart disease [1, 2]. These effects have been attributed to adaptations in skeletal muscles and autonomic nervous system and, until recently, the general consensus was that training does not appreciably affect the heart itself in patients with ischemic heart disease and that the improvement in symptoms and increased work capacity are due to lower myocardial O_2 requirements ($M\dot{V}O_2$) mediated through peripheral adaptations to training [2, 3].

Our hypothesis which was based on the data from the experimental animals, was that the failure to demonstrate direct cardiac effects by other investigators might have been due to inadequate training stimulus in terms of frequency, duration and intensity of the exercise. To test this hypothesis we conducted a number of studies using prolonged (12 months) exercise training with progressively increasing intensity in patients with documented ischemic heart disease [4–7]. The major and pertinent findings will be summarized below.

Methods

Exercise testing and measurement of maximal attainable O_2 uptake capacity

Each patient underwent the following exercise tests, 1 week apart, before and after 12 months of training: (1) A treadmill multistage exercise test

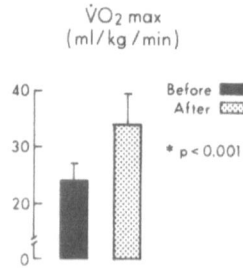

Figure 1. Effect of training in maximal attainable $\dot{v}O_2$ ($\dot{V}O_2$ max) before (solid bar) and after (stippled bar)

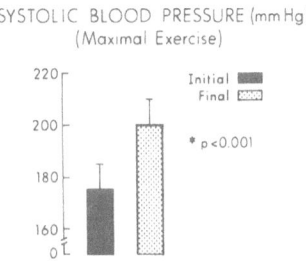

SYSTOLIC BLOOD PRESSURE (mmHg)
(Maximal Exercise)

Figure 2. Systolic blood pressure at maximal exercise was higher after (stippled bar) than before training (solid bar)

according to the Bruce protocol; (2) a maximal treadmill test for measurement of maximal oxygen uptake capacity using a modified Bruce protocol [4]. Patients who were not limited by angina attained their true maximal oxygen uptake capacity. In the patients with angina, symptom-limited maximal oxygen uptake was determined. The 'leveling off' criterion (that is, no further increase in oxygen uptake with increasing work rates) was used to define the true maximal aerobic power. For measurement of oxygen uptake, expired gas was collected in Douglas bags and analyzed for oxygen and carbon dioxide with a mass spectrometer (Perkin-Elmer MGA 1100). The volume of expired air was measured with a Tissot spirometer. The electrocardiogram was continuously monitored and blood pressure was measured with a mercury sphygmomanometer 30 seconds before the end of each stage of the exercise test.

Plasma lipid profiles

Plasma total triglyceride and cholesterol levels were measured directly, and very low density lipoproteins (VLDL) were separated from LDL and HDL at $d = 1.006$ by ultracentrifugation and measured as previously described [7]. Heparin manganese chloride was added to the infranatant to precipitate LDL, and HDL-C was measured directly.

Assessment of left ventricular function at rest and during exercise

Left ventricular performance was assessed using ECG-gated cardiac blood pool imaging with erythrocytes labeled *in vivo* by intravenous injection of 7.7 mg of stannous pyrophosphate followed in 20 minutes by 25 mCi of ^{99m}Tc given intravenously. The images were obtained with a standard field-of-view scintillation camera (Siemens LEM) equipped with a low-energy,

172

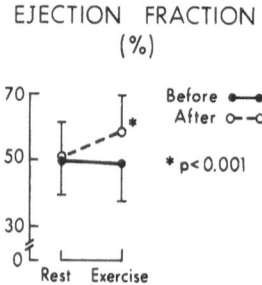

Figure 3. Resting ejection fraction did not change after training. Peak exercise ejection fraction, however, was higher after training.

medium-resolution, parallel-hole collimator. The patients were imaged supine with the scintillation camera positioned in the left anterior oblique projection (LAO) with 15° caudal angulation. A dedicated computer system (Technicare VIP 450) was interfaced to the scintillation camera. Data were collected in the frame mode (32 frames per R-R interval) in a 64×64 pixel matrix and were processed off line with a DEC PDP 11/34a minicomputer equipped with a Lexidata display unit. Ejection fraction (EF) was calculated as: $EF = (EDC - ESC \times 100)/EDC$ where EDC and ESC are background subtracted left ventricular end-diastolic and end-systolic counts respectively.

Following imaging at rest, each patient performed a graded supine bicycle exercise test with an electronically braked bicycle ergometer (Engineering Dynamics Corp.). The work rates were increased by 150 kpm/min every 3 minutes until severe fatigue or angina developed. In addition, M-mode echocardiogram was performed as previously described [5] on a selected number of patients to assess left ventricular size and characterize left ventricular hypertrophy in response to training.

Exercise training program

The duration of training was 12 months as described previously. Each exercise session consisted of 10 to 15 minutes of warm-up exercises followed by alternate walking and jogging, and continuous jogging on an indoor track or bicycle ergometer exercise, or both. Patients were expected to exercise 3 times a week during the first 3 months and 5 times a week thereafter. The duration of exercise was 30 minutes initially and was gradually increased until all patients were exercising continuously for 50 to 60 minutes (usually within 6 months). The intensity of exercise was adjusted to elicit 50 to 70 percent of the patient's maximal oxygen uptake capacity during the first 3 months. Subsequently it was progressively increased to 70 to 80 percent of

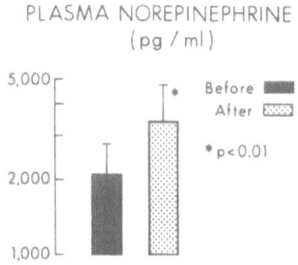

PLASMA NOREPINEPHRINE
(pg / ml)

Figure 4. Plasma norepinephrine concentration at maximal exercise was also higher after training.

maximal oxygen uptake capacity with two to three intervals of 2 to 5 minutes of training requiring 80 to 95 percent of maximal aerobic power interspersed throughout the training sessions. Each patient's clinical status was thoroughly evaluated at regular intervals before the intensity of training was increased. The heart rate was measured initially by radiotelemetry and subsequently by periodic electrocardiographic monitoring and palpation of the pulse. Measurements of maximal oxygen uptake capacity were repeated every 2 to 3 months in order to assess the patient's exercise tolerance and to adjust the training intensity to the desired percentage of maximal aerobic power.

Results

There was a marked improvement in exercise capacity and symptoms. Seven of the patients had effort angina. Of these 4 patients (57%) did not experience angina anylonger. Two patients raised their exercise threshold for angina and one patient continued to have effort angina after training with the same frequency as that before training. Most patients were able to run between 6.5 to 8 km per session averaging 25 to 32 km of running per week.

Maximal attainable O_2 uptake capacity (attainable $\dot{V}O_2$ max)

Attainable $\dot{V}O_2$max increased from 25 ± 3 (mean $\pm$ SD) to 37 ± 7 ml/kg/min ($p < 0.001$). There was an average of 3 kg weight loss after training ($p < 0.05$).

Adaptive responses to submaximal exercise

Heart rate at a given submaximal exercise intensity (absolute work rate) was significantly lower after training (108 ± 9 vs. 91 ± 10 beats/min; $p<0.01$). The product of systolic blood pressure and heart rate (RPP) decreased from $15.57\times10^3\pm3\times10^3$ to $11.23\times10^3\pm8\times10^3$ ($p<0.01$).

Adaptive responses to maximal exercise

In patients who were not limited by angina maximal heart rate during treadmill exercise did not change. However, in patients with effort angina, maximal heart increased after training. Systolic blood pressure at maximal exercise increased significantly (149 ± 25 to 169 ± 19 mm Hg; $p<0.001$). RPP increased from $22.97\times10^3\pm4\times10^3$ to $26.83\times10^3\pm4.3\times10^3$ ($p<0.02$). ST segment depression at maximal exercise, however, did not change after training.

Left ventricular contractile function

Ejection fraction (EF) at rest did not change (49 ± 14 vs. 51 ± 14) after training. At peak exercise (supine cycle ergometer exercise) EF increased from 49 ± 15 to 57.8 ± 15 ($p<0.01$). Left ventricular end-diastolic diameter determined echocardiographically increased from 47 ± 1 to 50 ± 1 mm ($p<0.01$). The posterior wall thickness at end diastole also increased from 8 ± 0.5 to 9 ± 0.5 mm ($p<0.01$). Therefore, the ratio of wall thickness to radius did not change (0.36 ± 0.02 vs. 0.37 ± 0.02).

Plasma lipid profiles

Plasma total cholesterol was 227 ± 36 before and 210 ± 31 mg/dl. The high density lipoprotein cholesterol (HDL-C) increased significantly from 37 ± 6 to 42 ± 9 mg/dl ($p<0.01$) The atherogenic index (total cholesterol/HDL-C) decreased from 6.3 ± 1.1 to 5.3 ± 1.6 ($p<0.01$) in response to training.

Comments

The results of these studies provide evidence that endurance exercise training may elicit adaptations in the heart itself in addition to the well known peripheral adaptations. It appears likely that if the training stimulus is sufficient it would be possible to detect favorable changes in the heart. These are characterized by (1) physiologic left ventricular hypertrophy, (2) improvement in left ventricular function as evidenced by an increase in ejection fraction at peak exercise, and (3) apparent improvement in myocardial ischemia as suggested by no significant change in the extent of ST segment depression at maximal exercise despite a large increase in rate pressure product. These data suggest that heart can raise its oxygen demand without any apparent deterioration in function or ischemia. Our data are compatible with the interpretation that low intensity exercise training elicits only peripheral adaptions causing improvement in symptoms and exercise capacity without any direct cardiac effect. On the other hand, high intensity training not only results in a larger improvement in exercise capacity and peripheral adaptations but also in cardiac adaptations. High intensity exercise training is only suitable for patients who are stable clinically and it should be used under medical supervision.

References

1. Mitchell JH: Exercise training in the treatment of coronary heart disease. Adv Intern Med 20:249, 1975.
2. Clausen JP: Circulatory adjustments to dynamic exercise and effect of physical training in normal subjects and patients with coronary artery disease. Prog Cardiovasc Dis 18:459, 1976.
3. Detry JM, Bruce RA: Effects of physical training on exertional ST segment depression in coronary heart disease. Circulation 44:390, 1971.
4. Ehsani AA, Heath GW, Hagberg JM, Sobel BE, Holloszy JO: Effects of 12 months of intense exercise training on ischemic ST segment depression in patients with coronary heart disease. Circulation 64:1116, 1981.
5. Ehsani AA, Martin WH III, Heath GW, et al.: Cardiac effects of prolonged and intense exercise training in patients with coronary artery disease. Am J Cardial 50:246, 1982.
6. Ehsani AA, Heath GW, Martin WH III, et al.: Effects of intense exercise training on plasma catecholamines in coronary patients. J Appl Physiol 57:154, 1984.
7. Heath GW, Ehsani AA, Hagberg J, et al.: Exercise training improves lipoprotein lipid profiles in patients with coronary artery disease. Am Heart J 105:889, 1983.

19. Physical Activity and Sudden Death

V. KALLIO

Abstract

Three important aspects of physical activity and sudden death are discussed in detail:
1. *Physical activity habits before the myocardial infarction and sudden death.* Data have been presented indicating improved survival in patients with myocardial infarction who have been physically active before the acute attack. Postulated mechanisms include reduction of cardiac adrenergic overactivity.
2. *Evidence of a protective effect of physical activity after myocardial infarction and the possible mechanisms involved.* Physical training has many positive effects on the heart and circulation and on the conventional risk factors. There is, however, no clear-cut scientific evidence on the protective effect on sudden death of physical activity programmes in myocardial infarction survivors. Some data of the results of a few controlled studies are presented.
3. *Physical activity after myocardial infarction and the risk of sudden death.* The incidence of sudden deaths connected with physical exercise training is rather low. It has been reported that the number of training hours per a case of sudden death is about 116,000 in survivors after myocardial infarction.

Sudden death is usually considered to be caused by ventricular arrhythmias leading to ventricular fibrillation. Ventricular arrhythmias are often precipitated by exertion and may be recorded in connection of exercise testing or continuous ECG-monitoring during physical activity. There is, however, no agreement on the prognostic significance of exercise-induced ventricular premature beats. Patients with exercise-induced 'Complex' ventricular arrhythmias should, nevertheless, be carefully monitored if included in physical training programmes.

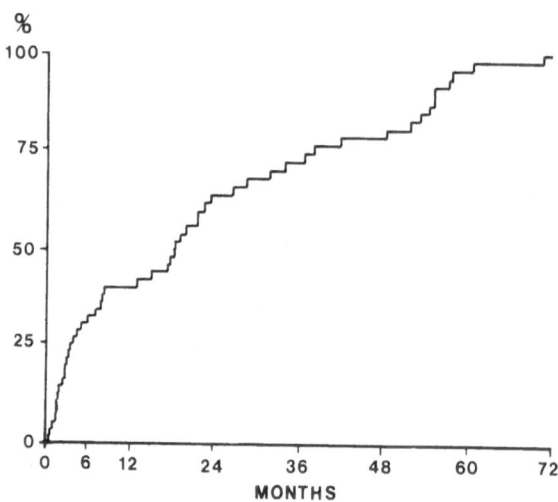

Figure 1. Sudden deaths expressed as percentage of their total number during 6 years' follow-up in patients after acute myocardial infarction. (Kallio et al., unpublished data).

Introduction

Sudden death accounts for some 30 to 50 per cent of all coronary deaths in acute myocardial infarction survivors. The most dangerous period for sudden death is during the first 6 months after discharge from hospital. According to the 6-year follow-up of our unselected material of 375 patients under 65 years with acute myocardial infarction 30% of the sudden deaths occurred during this period (Fig. 1). Sudden death is thus a major threat after myocardial infarction and at the same time a major challenge for preventive action to reduce the mortality in myocardial infarction survivors and individuals with ischemic heart disease.

It has been shown in the Framingham study that in individuals aged 45 to 74 years half of those with sudden death had a prior coronary heart disease (Kannel and Thomas, 1982). In patients with prior myocardial infarction nearly half of the deaths occurred outside the hospital and were predominantly sudden, often unwitnessed and without clear prodromal symptoms. It seems thus difficult to solve the problem by better organization of patient care. It has been pointed out that the risk of sudden death can be reduced only through primary and secondary prevention of coronary heart disease (Kannel and Thomas, 1982; Vuori et al., 1978).

According to a Finnish study (Vuori et al., 1978), on 2,606 autopsied cases of sudden deaths, 73% were caused by acute or chronic ischemic heart disease (Fig. 2). The authors showed that daily physical activity cannot be incriminated as an important contributory factor in sudden death from coronary heart disease in the general population. However, they found evi-

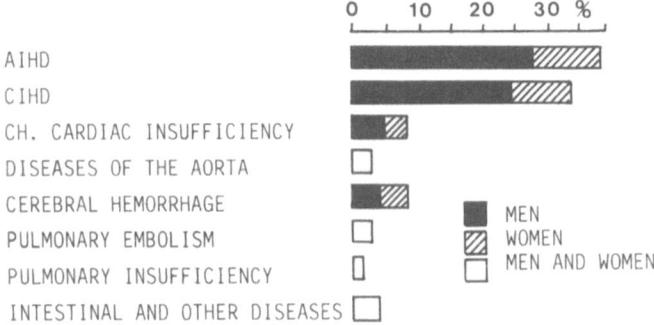

Figure 2. Causes of death in individuals who died suddenly (AIHD = Acute ischemic heart disease; CIHD = Chronic ischemic heart disease) (Vuori et al. 1978).

dence of a risk of sudden death in persons with manifest or latent coronary heart disease engaged in strenuous physical exertion. Identification of these persons before the attack seems difficult. The authors suggest, however, that the serious complications might be reduced through medical examination of persons engaged in strenuous physical activity and effective education of the public to avoid among all sudden bursts of activity without warming up, and competitive spirit leading to maximal effort.

Physical activity as a factor predisposing patients with ischemic heart disease to instantaneous death was studied in connection with the ischemic heart disease register in Helsinki (Kala et al., 1978). The survival of 1,056 subsequent men registered was studied with regard to their physical activity either at onset or immediately before the attack, within a day or within a week before the attack. It was found that the men with strenuous or unusual physical activity at the time of or immediately before the onset of the attack died instantaneously significantly more often than the rest of the group of all men with known activity (Fig. 3). The survival one month after the attack was, however, almost the same in both groups. The authors stress the

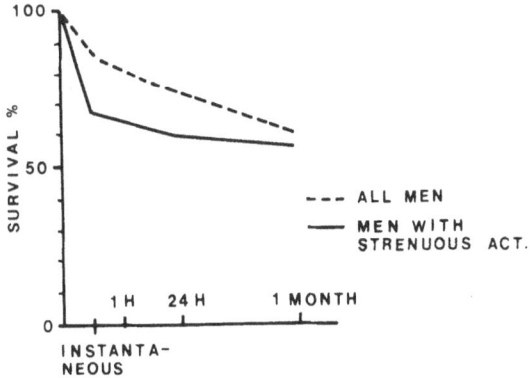

Figure 3. Strenuous physical activity related to instantaneous deaths (Kala et al., 1978).

importance of the readiness to resuscitate, especially among instructors supervising physical conditioning programmes for patients with ischemic heart disease.

Sudden Death and Exercise

The risk of sudden death related to vigorous exercise has been suggested to be associated with the level of habitual physical activity in the general population (Siscovick et al., 1984). It was estimated that the relative risk of sudden death during high-intensity physical activity among men engaged in low-level habitual activity was 56 (95% of confidence limits 23 to 131). In men with very high-intensity habitual activity the relative risk was clearly lower (5 with 95% of confidence limits, 2 to 14). The number of cases of primary cardiac arrest during exercise was, however, small. Thus the final conclusion of the authors was that even though intensive physical activity may be one of the factors that can precipitate primary cardiac arrest, habitual participation in such activity is in the general population associated with an overall reduction in the risk of primary cardiac arrest. The last part of this conclusion is consistent with a number of epidemiologic studies (Morris et al., 1)(%; Paffenbarger and Hale, 1975; Siscovick et al., 1982).

Sudden coronary death during supervised exercise training of patients participating in cardiac rehabilitation programmes has been reported to be relatively rare with one death occurring once in every 116,000 patient hours of training (Haskell, 1978) and more recently about once in every 250,000 patient hours of training (Haskell, 1980). According to Haskell (1982) the patients at greatest risk are often characterized by any one or more of the following: poor left ventricular function (ejection farction < 30%); exercise hypotension; multi-vessel disease (> 70% narrowing); very low exercise capacity; frequent complex PVCs; multiple myocardial infarctions and angina pectoris at rest or low level exercise. These patients should be identified and evaluated carefully with regard to proscription of vigorous exercise. Individuals with established risk factors of coronary heart disease should also be considered at increased risk of sudden coronary death. It was estimated that probably a third of the current events could be prevented in patients at high risk of sudden coronary death by more aggressive medical intervention and non-invasive evaluation of myocardial perfusion and ventricular function abnormalities during exercise.

Sudden death is in most cases due to malignant ventricular arrhythmias such as ventricular tachycardia leading to ventricular fibrillation (Schaefer and Cobb, 1975). Physical exercise has been shown to provoke complex ectopic beats and ventricular tachycardia in patients with coronary heart disease. The mechanism is likely to be a lowering of myocardial vulnerability threshold caused by local ischemia. On the other hand it has been shown by several authors that physical exercise causes a manifold increase in the circulating catecholamines which lower the threshold of myocardium to malignant arrhythmias and ventricular fibrillation (Dimsdale et al., 1984; Opie, 1975; Selvester et al., 1977).

The urinary excretion of catecholamines is similar in trained and untrained healthy individuals. Training may, however, reduce the sensitivity of the beta receptors and make the myocardium less vulnerable (Brundin and Cernigliaro, 1975). There is also some evidence to indicate that after a course of physical training the increase in the level of circulating catecholamines is less pronounced than before the training period (Cooksey et al., 1978; Winter et al., 1978). This could, at least theoretically, be an important aspect to advocate physical training in the prevention of sudden death in high risk individuals and in selected patients after myocardial infarction. In animals, physical training has been shown to reduce the susceptibility to sudden death (Billman et al., 1984).

Other theoretically interesting effects of physical training from the point of view of prevention of sudden death are abolition of angina pectoris in many patients and a greater submaximal workload at the onset of ischemic ST-segment depression and angina pectoris. Physical training also decreases heart rate and systolic blood pressure at a given work load. These effects are associated with considerable physiological and symptomatic improvement (DeBusk and Hung, 1982).

Evidence has been presented that the level of off-the-job physical activity prior to the acute myocardial infarction is related to survival during 3 years after the attack (Siltanen et al., 1982). It was demonstrated that the first-day survival figures in patients engaged in high-level leisure time physical activity was 88% contrasted to 75% in low activity patients (Fig. 4). The three-

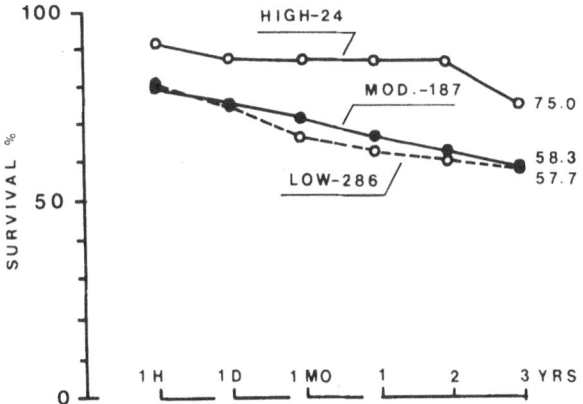

Figure 4. Survival after acute myocardial infarction related to habitual leisure time physical activity bevore the myocardial infarction (Siltanen et al., 1982).

182

year survival percentages were 75 and 58, respectively. The mortality figures include both sudden and non-sudden deaths. The authors suggest that the ability of physical activity and training to reduce cardiac adrenergic over-activity is the mechanism which mediates the beneficial effect of exercise on the fatality of an acute ischemic attack.

Several studies on myocardial infarction survivors indicate that improvements in physical condition through physical training even at maximal intensity can be brought about safely in carefully chosen subjects (Kallio, 1978; Saunamäki, 1978). These studies have, however, not been designed to answer the question whether physical exercise has a secondary preventive effect and, in particular, whether or not it reduces the occurrence of sudden death in myocardial infarction survivors.

Five controlled feasibility studies and clinical trials have been performed during the last 15 years on the effects of physical training in patients after myocardial infarction (Kentala, 1972; Palatsi, 1976; Shaw, 1981; Shephard, 1980; Wilhelmsen et al., 1975). These studies have included altogether 2,377 patients.

A trend towards better survival in the intervention group has been shown in all studies except the Canadian one, in which the high-intensity training group had a somewhat higher mortality compared with the low-intensity training group (Table 1). The mortality differences between the intervention and control group were, however, not significant in any of the studies. Neither was there a difference in the number of sudden deaths. Major problems connected with these studies were high drop-out rate, contamination of control group (drop-in), and relatively small number of cases in each study. The entry into the study was in some studies rather late. Physical activity was thus not shown to prevent sudden death in myocardial infarction survivors.

A Finnish study was performed in connection with the WHO-coordinated project aimed at studying the effects of a comprehensive intervention programme on mortality and morbidity in myocardial infarction survivors bel-

Table 1. Mortality figures in randomized clinical trials on survivors after acute myocardial infarction (I = Intervention group; C = Control group)

	Mortality per cent		
	I	C	p
Wilhelmsen et al. (1975)	17.7	22.3	0.38
Kentala (1972)	17.1	21.9	0.37
Palatsi (1976)	10.0	14.0	0.30
National Exercise and Heart Disease Project (Shaw 1981)	4.6	7.3	0.20
Southern Ontario Multicentre Exercise-Heart Trial (Shephard 1980)	9.5	7.3	0.36

ow the age of 65 randomized in an intervention (188 patients) and control group (187 patients) already in hospital (Kallio et al., 1979). Patients were well matched in the two groups. The intervention programme consisted of frequent contacts with an internist, optimal medical care, antismoking and dietary advice, advice on psychosocial problems and a physical exercise programme. 83% of all patients in the intervention group participated in the exercise programme tailored according to their physical capacity. The compliance in the intervention programme was good as judged from the clearly lower values in serum lipids, body weight and blood pressure determined at yearly check-ups. The patients of the control group were treated by physicians in the community and they did not participate in any organized rehabilitation programme.

The cumulative percentage of sudden deaths is shown in Figure 5. The number of sudden deaths in the intervention group was significantly smaller than in the control patients. This trend was still seen 6 years after the myocardial infarction.

The significant difference between the groups cannot be ascribed to a single component of the intervention programme. The study showed, however, that multifactorial intervention is feasible and safe and suggests that sudden death can be prevented in survivors of myocardial infarction participating in a comprehensive intervention programme including physical conditioning.

Another controlled study based on organized aftercare of myocardial infarction survivors has recently been performed in Helsinki. (Hakkila, personal communication). It has confirmed our findings in a material of some

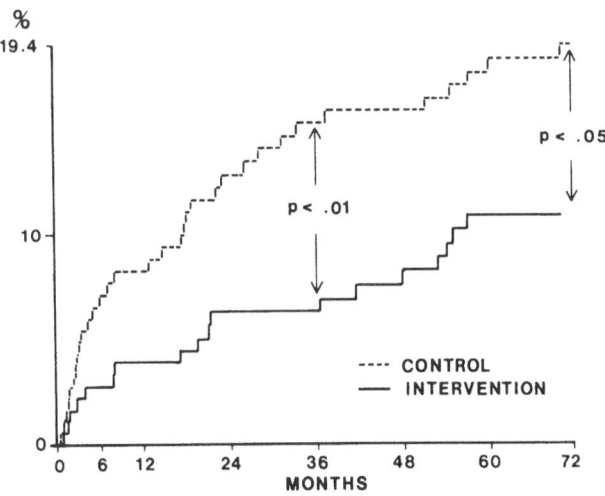

Figure 5. Cumulative percentages of sudden deaths during 6 Years' follow-up in patients with acute myocardial infarction participating in a controlled clinical study (Kallio et al., 1979).

800 patients and resulted in a significant reduction in the rate of sudden deaths and in total mortality.

Summary

1. 50 to 70% sudden deaths in the general population are caused by ischemic heart disease.

2. Strenuous or unusual physical exertion is associated with sudden, often instantaneous death in individuals with ischemic heart disease. Vigorous leisure-time habitual physical activity may, however, protect from death after the myocardial infarction.

3. Physical training of patients after myocardial infarction has many positive effects, which, theoretically, could diminish the risk of sudden death. It has, however, not been shown to reduce the number of sudden deaths, although a trend in this direction has been shown in controlled clinical trials.

4. Comprehensive multifactorial intervention including physical exercise programme and organized care after myocardial infarction have given promising results with regard to prevention of sudden deaths.

References

1. Billman GE, Schwartz PJ, Stone HL: The effects of daily exercise on susceptibility to sudden cardiac death. Circulation 69(6):1182–1189, 1984.
2. Brundin T, Cernigliaro C: The effect of physical training on the sympathoadrenal response to exercise. Scand J Clin Lab Invest 35:525, 1975.
3. Cooksey JD, Reilly P, Brown S, Bomze H, Cryer PE: Exercise training and plasma catecholamines in patients with ischemic heart disease. Am J Cardiol 42:372–376, 1978.
4. DeBusk RF, Hung J: Exercise conditioning soon after myocardial infarction: Effects on myocardial perfusion and ventricular function. In: Greenberg HM, Dwyer EM (eds) Sudden coronary death. Ann NY Acad Sci 382:343–354, 1982.
5. Dimsdale JE, Hartley LH, Guiney T, Ruskin JN, Greenblatt D: Postexercise peril. Plasma catecholamines and exercise. JAMA 251:630–632, 1984.
6. Haskell WL: Cardiovascular complications during exercise training of cardiac patients. Circulation 57:920, 1978.
7. Haskell W: Cardiovascular complications during medically supervised exercise training. In: physical conditioning and cardiac rehabilitation. John Wiley and Sons, New York, p 159–168, 1980.
8. Haskell WL: Sudden cardiac death during vigorous exercise. Int J Sports Med 3:45–48, 1982.
9. Kala R, Romo M, Siltanen P, Halonen PI: Physical activity and sudden cardiac death. In: Manninen V, Halonen PI (ed) Sudden coronary death. Adv Cardiol 25:27–34, Karger, Basel, 1978.
10. Kallio V: Results of rehabilitation in coronary patients. Adv Cardiol 24:153–163, 1978.

11. Kallio V, Hämäläinen H, Hakkila J, Luurila OJ: Reduction in sudden deaths by a multi-factorial intervention programme after acute myocardial infarction. Lancet 2:1091–1094, 1979.

12. Kannel WB, Thomas HE: Sudden coronary death: The Fragmingham study. In: Greenberg HM, Dwyer EM (eds) Sudden coronary death. Ann NY Acad Sci 382:3–21, 1982.

13. Kentala E: Physical fitness and feasibility of physical rehabilitation after myocardial infarction in men of working age. Ann Clin Res 4(Suppl 9):1–84, 1972.

14. Morris JN, Everitt MG, Pollard R, Chave SPW: Vigorous exercise in leisure-time: protection against coronary heart disease. Lancet 2:1207–1210, 1980.

15. Opie LH: Long-distance running and sudden death. New Engl J Med 293:941, 1975.

16. Paffenbarger RS Jr, Hale WE: Work activity and coronary heart mortality. N Engl J Med 292:545–550, 1975.

17. Palatsi I: Feasibility of physical training after myocardial infarction and its effect on return to work, morbidity and mortality. Kaleva. Oulu, 1976.

18. Saunamäki KI: Feasibility and effect of physical training with maximum intensity in men after acute myocardial infarction. Scand j Rehab med 10:155–162, 1978.

19. Schaefer WA, Cobb LA: Recurrent ventricular fibrillation and modes of death in survivors of out-of-hospital ventricular fibrillation. N Engl J Med 293:259–262, 1975.

20. Selvester R, Camp J, Sanmarco M: Effects of exercise training on progression of documented coronary arteriosclerosis in men. In: Milvy P (ed) The marathon: physiological, medical, epidemiological, and psychological studies. Ann NY Acad Sci 301:495–508, 1977.

21. Shaw LW: Effects of a prescribed supervised exercise program on mortality and cardiovascular morbidity in patients after a myocardial infarction. The National Exercise and Heart Disease Project. Am J Cardiol 48:39–46, 1981.

22. Shephard RJ: Recurrence of myocardial infarction. Observations on patients participating in the Ontario Multicentre Exercise-Heart Trial. Eur J Cardiol 11:147–157, 1980.

23. Siltanen P, Tomo M, Haapakoski J: The influence of previous physical activity on survival and reinfarction after first myocardial infarction. Acta Med Scand (Suppl) 668:34–48, 1982.

24. Siscovick DS, Weiss NS, Fletcher RH, Lasky T: The incidence of primary Cerdiac Arrest during vigorous exercise. N Engl J Med 311:874–877, 1984.

25. Siscovick DS, Weiss NS, Hallstrom AP, Inui TS, Peterson DR: Physical activity and primary cardiac arrest. JAMA 248:3111–3227, 1982.

26. Wilhelmsen L, Sanne H, Elmfeldt d, Grimby G, Tibblin G, Wedek H: A controlled trial of physical training after myocardial infarction, effects on risk factors, nonfatal reinfarction and death. Prev Med 4:491–508, 1975.

27. Winder WW, Hagberg JM, Hickson RC, Ehsani AA, McLane JA: Time course of sympathoadrenal adaptation to endurance exercise training in man. J Appl Physiol 45:370–374, 1978.

28. Vuori I, Mäkäräinen M, Jääskeläinen A: Sudden death and physical activity. Cardiology 63:287–304, 1978.

20. Physical Exercise and Sympathetic Drive

M. LEHMANN and J. KEUL

Abstract

Endurance training influences 3 main systems of the human organism:
1. Vegetative tonus, sympathoadrenergic response and hormonal regulation.
2. Hemodynamics of the heart.
3. Metabolism and energy turnover especially of the muscle.
In well-trained persons the catecholamine level in blood is reduced in rest and during exercise. According to the reduction of the catecholamine level and the increase in performance and oxygen uptake a decrease of heart rate, blood pressure, myocardial contractility, lactate production and acidosis is observed. There is a significant correlation between the decrease of the catecholamine level and the increase of adrenoreceptors and the change in heart volume ($P < 0.005$), oxygen uptake, physical performance ($P < 0.001$) and metabolic values.

In patients with myocardial or coronary insufficiency an increase in catecholamine level and a decrease in adrenoreceptors are found depending of the stage of heart disease and the reduction in hemodynamic parameters. In post-infarct-patients after physical therapy a decrease in sympathetic drive and an increase in adrenoreceptors corresponding with an increase in physical performance are observed. Furthermore the metabolic and hormonal regulation are improved. After static training these adaptations and advantages are not observed.

Introduction

The negative correlation between pumping capacity of the heart and sympathetic activity at rest and at identical work loads [1, 11, 22–24, 9, 31] is of increasing interest for diagnostic and prognostic reasons in cardiac patients [6, 11, 22–24, 29]. Determinations of free plasma catecholamines as biochemical indicators of the overall sympathetic drive enable an estimation of the symathetic activity [17, 42]. Subject of this paper is the influence of age, training and heart failure on sympathetic activity.

Methods

Free plasma and urinary catecholamines were determined radioenzymatically [7]. The influence of age was investigated in 126 healthy men, based on urinary catecholamine excretion, and in 9 old (66 ± 6 years) and 11 young subjects (26 ± 3 years) during incremental ergometric exercise, based on plasma catecholamine responses. Oxygen uptake (open system), heart rate responses (ECG) and blood lactate levels [13] were additionally determined. The influence of training was investigated in 8–10 weight lifters (static training), 11 cyclists (dynamic training) and 10 healthy control subjects, and additionally in 20 CHD-patients (postinfarct patients). The influence of heart failure on haemodynamic data and sympathetic activity was studied in 106 men. 47 of them were healthy control subjects, 59 CHD-patients (post-infarction patients). Haemodynamic data were determined by Swan-Ganz-catheter at rest and during graded exercise in supine body position. Cardiac output was measured by thermodilution technique [10]. Statistical methods used were analysis of variance and Scheffé's test, t-test for paired and unpaired data. Correlations were calculated by least squares analysis. Level of significance was set at $p < 0.05$.

Results and discussion

It is not at all possible to consider all points of view in this short summary. We therefore refer to the extensive literature on this field. Free urinary noradrenaline ($r = 0.37$, $p < 0.001$) (Fig. 1), correlates positively with age, according to basal and exercise-induced plasma noradrenaline, in contrast to adrenaline and dopamine [18, 19, 25]. Circulating or excreted free noradrenaline therefore increases related to age and adrenaline or dopamine. The age-dependent influence is mainly recognizable during physical exercise [19, 25, 38]. Thus noradrenaline responses are up to 700 % higher in older subjects than in younger individuals at identical work loads, adrenaline responses however approximately 300 % (Fig. 2), indicating an age-related change of the adrenaline-noradrenaline ratio [19]. Both negative age-correlation of physical fitness and aging of structures such as adrenoreceptors may contribute to a disproportionate increase of sympathoneuronal

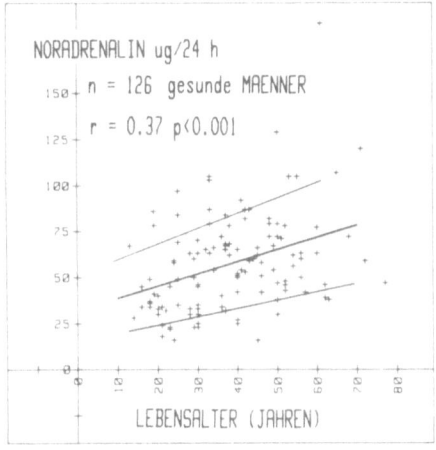

NORADRENALIN ug/24 h

n = 126 gesunde MAENNER

r = 0.37 p<0.001

LEBENSALTER (JAHREN)

Figure 1. 24-h-urinary excretion of free noradrenaline correlates positively with Age (Lebensalter, x-axis) in contrast to adrenaline and dopamine

activity. An age-associated reduction of sensitivity to catecholamines consequently is observed, as indicated by a decreased sensitivity to isoproterenol [16, 36, 40] and a reduced density of beta-adrenoreceptors [37, 40]. Sensitivity of human arteries and veins to noradrenaline, however, seems to be unchanged [39]. Age-related change of adreno-receptor density and sensitivity of the organism to catecholamines can be one cause of altered sympathetic activity, but can also be caused by higher sympathetic drive in old subjects. This question is open at present. Despite this problem, we suppose, that the described age-associated change of sympathetic activity participates in the age-dependent alterations of haemodynamics [8, 14, 15, 32, 36].

Both dynamic and static training results in a control of sympathetic activity at identical work loads (Fig. 3) [12, 20, 24, 26, 34, 41]. This control is seen to depend on the training state of the sceletal muscles [35]. That means, that both an increased aerobic capacity and changed muscle fiber composition (dynamically trained subjects) and an increased muscle mass and strength (statistically trained subjects) are responsible for this control. Despite low sympathetic drive, strength trained subjects, however, show tachycardia during exercise as compared with untrained and endurance trained subjects (Fig. 3), thus pointing to a reduced vagal influence on cardiac sinus rate. Therefore, we can assume, that only dynamic endurance sports cause an increase of aerobic capacity and vagal tone, combined with a control of sympathetic drive. Effects, which are also of high interest for physical therapy in cardiac patients. Beside, the training-dependent change of sympathetic activity, endurance trained subjects show higher density of beta-receptors on intact blood cells [2, 26] – results, however, are contradictory [5] – and a controlled alpha-receptor density [28], which on the other

190

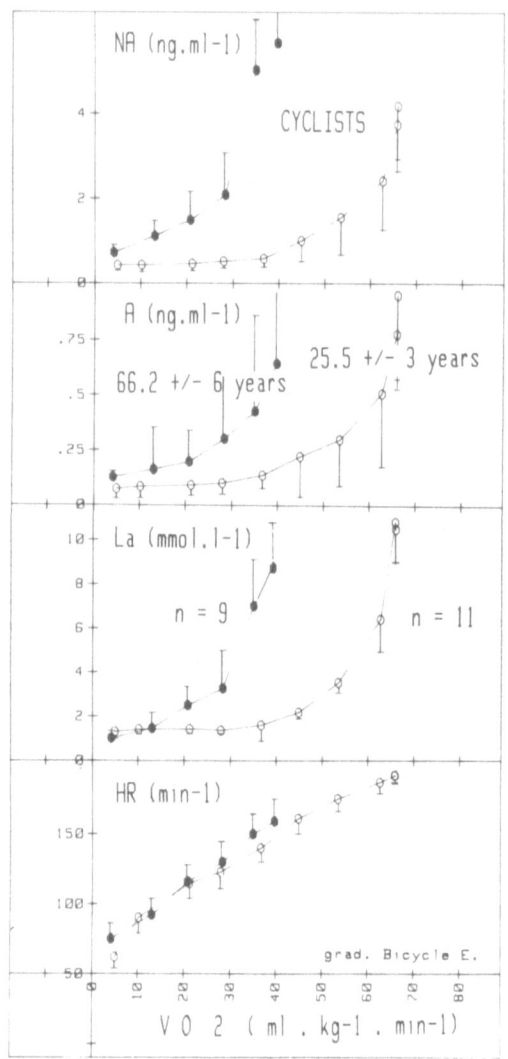

Figure 2. Exercise-induced noradrenaline, adrenaline and lactate responses in the blood are higher in old cyclists as compared with young cyclists at identical work loads

hand seems to be higher in statically trained subjects [27, 28]. It is open at present, if they are transferable from blood cells to other sympathetic target organs. What however can be proven is a possible control of the overproportional sympathetic drive in postinfarction patients, dependent on physical therapy (Fig. 4) [30].

Free plasma [9, 11, 22] and urinary noradrenaline – less adrenaline and dopamine [22, 29] – are negatively correlated with cardiac pumping capacity, performance ability [11, 22–24, 29] and the prognosis of high risk cardiac

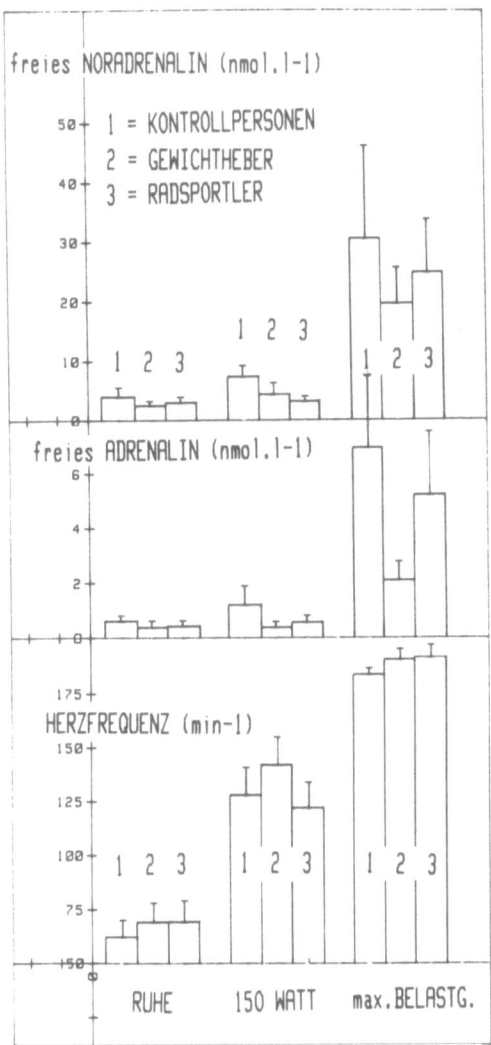

Figure 3. Strength trained subjects (Weight lifters, Gewichtheber, index 2) and endurance trained individuals (Cyclists, Radsportler, index 3) show a control of plasma adrenaline and noradrenaline responses at identical work load (150 Watt) as compared with untrained control subjects (Kontrollpersonen, Index 1). At rest (Ruhe) and at exhaustion (max. Belastg.) only slight differences exist between the three groups, except for the lower adrenaline responses of weight lifters at exhaustion and a higher heart rate of strength trained subjects at submaximal work loads (150 Watt)

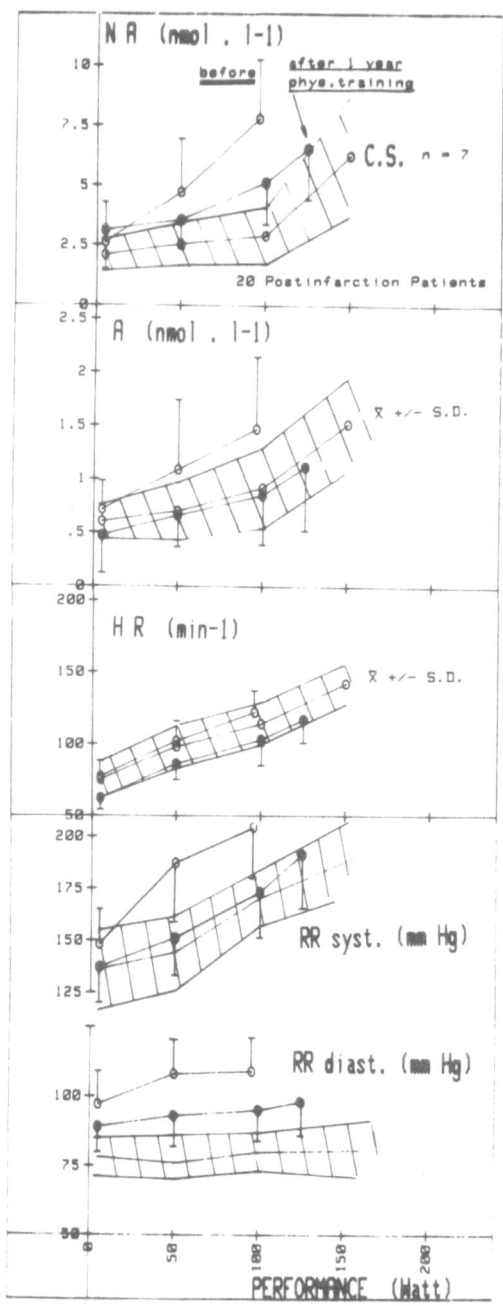

Figure 4. Noradrenaline, adrenaline, heart rate, and blood pressure responses of 20 postinfarction patients were lower after 1 year of physical therapy, performance ability was higher

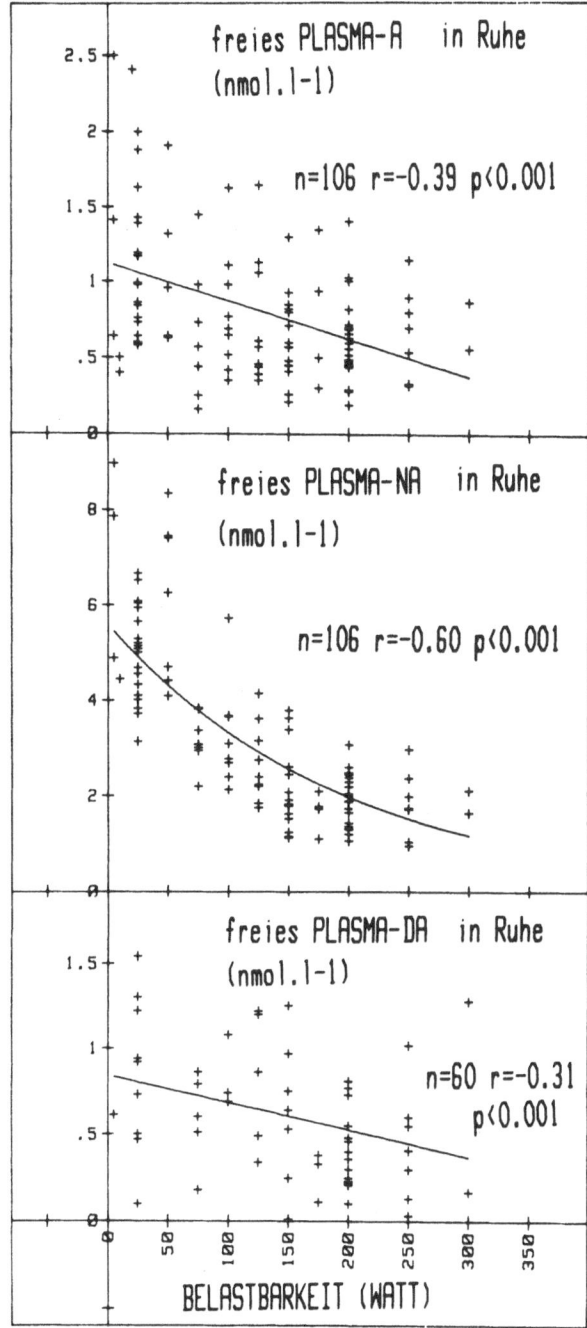

Figure 5. Free plasma catecholamines Adrenaline (A), Noradrenaline (NA) and Dopamine (DA), (basal concentrations), correlate negatively with the performance ability of 106 men, (47 healthy individuals and 59 CHD-patients, grade I-IV according to NYHA classification)

patients [6]. The higher the performance ability and left ventricular functional capacity, the lower are the basal free plasma catecholamines (Fig. 5), according to earlier results [22–24] and other research groups [11]. The prognostic quality of the basal noradrenaline levels ($r = -0.60$, $n = 106$) shows no decisive disadvantages as compared with the prognostic validity of relevant haemodynamic parameters, such as stroke volume index ($r = 0.71$, $n = 106$). Negative relationships between sympathetic drive, sensitivity of the organism to catecholamines and the cardiac functional state have to be taken into account, which can influence the cardiac function in a negative manner and amplify heart failure in cardiac patients, exceeding the primarily morphologically conditioned state [1, 3, 4, 23, 27, 29].

Summary

We evaluated the influence of age, training and heart failure on free noradrenaline and adrenaline. 24-h-urinary noradrenaline ($r = 0.37$, $n = 126$) basal plasma noradrenaline ($r = 0.54$, $n = 11$) and exercise-induced noradrenaline responses (at identical work loads), ($r = 0.69$, $n = 20$) are positively age-correlated in contrast to 24-h-urinary and basal plasma adrenaline. Exercise-induced maximal adrenaline-responses are approximately 50% lower in old subjects than in young individuals, in contrast to similar noradrenaline responses, indicating a age-associated change of adrenaline-noradrenaline-ratio. Negative age-correlation of both physical fitness as well as sensitivity to catecholamines (beta-adrenergic agonists) are seen as main factors of the age-dependent change in sympathetic activity. Endurance and strength training result in a control of noradrenaline and adrenaline responses at identical work loads. Increased vagal tone and aerobic capacity, however, coincide only with dynamic endurance training. Negative training-correlation of noradrenaline occurs also in healthy old subjects ($r = -0.72$, $n = 11$) and in cardiac patients (postinfarction patients) after one year of physical therapy. There is a negative correlation between left ventricular function as indicated by stroke volume index, and basal free plasma noradrenaline ($r = -0.67$) in 47 healthy subjects and 59 CHD-patients, grade I-IV according to NYHA classification. The prognostic validity of basal free noradrenaline ($r = -0.66$, $n = 59$ CHD patients) and stroke volume index ($r = 0.62$, $n = 59$) is similar with regard to the performance ability and the left ventricular capacity.

References

1. Baumann G, Rieß G: Verhalten kardialer ß-Rezeptoren bei akutem Myokardinfarkt und chronischem Herzversagen. Mögliche Rolle von H_2-Rezeptor-Agonisten im katecholamin-refraktärem Myokard. Herz Kreisl 14:169–178, 1982.
2. Bieger W, Zittel R: Effect of physical activity on beta-receptor activity. In: Knuttgen HG, Vogel JA, Poortmans J (eds) Biochemistry of exercise. Human Kinetics Publishers Champain Ill:715–722, 1982.
3. Braunwald E: The control of ventricular function in man. Br Heart J:27–1, 1965.
4. Bristow MR, Ginsburg R, Minobe W et al.: Decreased catecholamine sensitivity and β-adrenergic receptor density in failung human hearts. N Engl J Med 307:205–211, 1982.
5. Butler J, O'Brien M, O'Malley K et al.: Relationship of β-adrenoceptor density to fitness in athetes. Nature 298:60–61, 1982.
6. Cohn JN, Levine TB, Olivari MT et al.: Plasma norepinephrine as a guide to prognosis in patients with chronic congestive heart failure. N Engl J Med 311:819–823, 1989.
7. DaPrada M, Zürcher G: Simultaneous radioenzymatic determination of plasma and tissue adrenaline, noradrenaline and dopamine within the fentomole range. Life Sci 19:1161–1174, 1976.
8. Ekelund LG, Holmgren A: Central hemodynamics during exercise. Circ Res 20/21 (Suppl):33–43, 1967.
9. Fischer-Hansen J, Christensen NJ, Hesse B: Determination of coronary sinus noradrenaline in patients with ischarmic heart disease: Coronary sinus catecholamine concentration in relation to arterial catecholamine concentration, Pulmonary artery ocygen saturation and left ventricular end-diastolic pressure. Cardiovas Res 12:415–421, 1978.
10. Forrester JS, Ganz W, Diamond G et al.: Thermodilution, cardiac output determination with a single flow directed catheter. Am Heart J 33:306–311, 1972.
11. Francis GS, Goldsmith SR, Cohn JN: Relationship of exercise capacity to resting left ventricular performance and basal plasma norepinephrine levels in patients with congestive heart failure. Am Heart J 104:725–731, 1982.
12. Hartley LH, Mason JW, Hogan RP et al: Multiple hormonal responses to graded exercise in relation to physical training. J Appl Physiol 33:602–606, 1972.
13. Hohorst HJ: L-(+)-Laktat. Bestimmung mit Laktatdehydrogenase und DPN. In: Bermeyer HU (ed) methoden der enzymatischen Analyse. Verlag Chemie Weinheim:266–277, 1962.
14. Hollmann W, Barg W, Weyer G et al.: Der Alterseinfluß auf spiroergometrische Meßgrößen im submaximalen Arbeitsbereich. Med Welt 21:1280–1288, 1970.
15. Hollmann W, Liesen H: Der Trainingseinfluß auf die Leistungsfähigkeit vonHerz, Kreislauf und Stoffwechsel im Alter. MMW 114:1336–1342, 1972.
16. Lakatta EG, Gerstenblith G, Angell CS et al.: Diminished inotropic response of aged myocardium to catecholamines. Circ Res 36:262–268, 1975.
17. Lake CR, Ziegler MG, Kopin IJ: Use of plasma norepinephrine for evaluation of sympathetic neuronal function in man. Life Sci 18:1315–1326, 1978.
18. Lake CR, Ziegler MG, Coleman D et al.: Age-Adjusted plasma norepinephrine levels are similar in normotensive and hypertensive subjects. N Engl J Med 4:208–209, 1977.
19. Lehmann M, Keul J, Huber G et al.: Alters- und belastungsbedingtes Verhalten der Plasmakatecholamine. Klin Wochenschr 59:19–25, 1980.
20. Lehmann M, Keul J, Huber G et al.: Plasma catecholamines in trained and untrained volunteers during graded exercise. Int J Sports Med 2:143–147, 1981.
21. Lehmann M, Eschenbruch E, Tollenaere P et al.: Simultane Mehrfachbestimmung von Dopamin, Noradrenalin und Adrenalin im koronarvenösen und aortalen Blut sowie im rechtsatrialen Gewebe des suffizienten Herzens während Bypass- Chirurgie. Herz 8:47–54, 1981.

22. Lehmann M, Keul J: Die Beziehung der Plasmakatecholamine zur Herzgröße, Förderleistung und zum Füllungsdruck des insuffizienten Herzens. Herz Kreisl 14:142–148, 1982.
23. Lehmann M, Rühle K, Schmid P et al.: Hämodynamik, Plasmakatecholaminverhalten und β-Adrenozeptorendichte bei Trainierten, Untrainierten und Herzinsuffizienten. Z Kardiol 72:529–536, 1983.
24. Lehmann M, Dickhuth HH, Huber G et al: Simultane Bestimmung von zentraler Hämodynamik und Plasmakatecholaminen bei Trainierten, Untrainierten und Kontraktionsstörung des Herzens in Ruhe und während Körperarbeit. Z Kardiol 72:561–568, 1983.
25. Lehmann M, Spöri U, Keul J: Ausscheidung an freiem Dopamin, Noradrenaline und Adrenalin bei 190 Männern in Beziehung zum Alter und Blutdruck. Klin Wochenschr: In Druck, 1985.
26. Lehmann M, Dickhuth HH, Schmid P et al.: Plasma catecholamines, β-adrenergic receptors, and isoproterenol sensitivity in endurance trained and non-endurance trained volunteers. Eur J Appl Physiol 52:362–369, 1984.
27. Lehmann M, Schmid P, Bergdolt E et al.: Ist die Alpha-Adrenorezeptorendichte an intakten Thrombozyten bei statisch trainierten Athleten erhöht? Klin Wochenschr 62:992–995, 1984.
28. Lehmann M, Bergdoldt E, Keul J: Verhalten von Alpha- und Beta-Adrenorezeptoren an intakten Blutzellen bei statisch und dynamisch trainierten Personen. Klin Wochenschr: In Druck, 1985.
29. Lehmann M, Keul J: Güte hämodynamischer Größen und basaler freier und konjugierter Plasmakatecholamine für die Prognose der Belastbarkeit von 106 gesunden und herzkranken Männern. Z Kardiol: In Druck, 1985.
30. Lehmann M, Berg A, Keul J: Änderung der sympathischen Aktivität bei 18 Postinfarktpatienten nach 1 Jahr Bewegungstherapie. Z Kardiol: In Druck, 1985.
31. Mäurer W, Yoshida Y, Kübler W: Die Urinausscheidung der Katecholamine Adrenalin, Noradrenalin und Dopamin sowie der Abbauprodukte Metanephrin und Normetanephrin bei Herzkranken. Z Kardiol 65:1124–1138, 1976.
32. Palmer CJ, Ziegler MG, Lake CR: Response of norepinephrine and blood pressure to stress increases with age. J Gerontol 33:482–487, 1978.
33. Péronnet F, Cléroux J, Perrault H et al.: Plasma norepinephrine response to exercise before and after training in humans. J Appl Physiol 51:812–815, 1981.
34. Roskamm H, Samek L: Kardiozirkulatorische Anpassung an körperliche Belastung. In: Kindermann W, Hort W (eds) Sportmedizin für Breiten- und Leistungssport. Demeter Gräfelfing:169–178, 1980.
35. Roth GS: Changes in hormone action during aging: Glucocorticoid regulation of adipocyte glucose metabolism and catecholamine regulation of myocardial contractility. Proc Soc Ex Biol Med 165:188–192, 1980.
36. Schocken DD, Roth GS: Reduced β-adrenergic receptor concentratton in aging man. Nature 267:856–858, 1977.
37. Sowers JR: Plasma norepinephrine responses to posture and isometric exercise increase with age. J Gerontol 38:315–317, 1983.
38. Stevens MJ, Lipe S, Moulds RF: The effect of age on the responses of human isolated arteries and veins on noradrenaline. Br J Clin Pharmacol 14:750–752, 1982.
39. Vestal RE, Wood AFF, Shand DG: Reduced β-adrenoceptor sensitivity in the elderly. Clin Res 26:488A, 1978.
40. Winder WW, Hickson RC, Hagberg JM et al.: Training-induced changes in hormonal and metabolic responses to submaximal exercise. J Appl Physiol 56:766–771, 1979.
41. Yamaguchi N, deChamplain J, Nadeau R: Correlation between the respooses of the heart to sympathetic stimulation and the release of endogenous catecholamines into the coronary sinus of the dog. Circ Res 36:662–667, 1975.

21. Physical Exercise in Comprehensive Care

J. J. KELLERMANN

Abstract

The discussion of the subject of physical exercise as a secondary preventive measure may make the impression of being superfluous because such discussions have been held many times before with rather disappointing results. Nonetheless, newer studies have again renewed the interest and deepened the challenge in dealing with this subject. The implementation of Comprehensive Coronary Care (CCC) including multiple measures involving physical, psychological and pharmacological procedures together with a new concept of pharmacological and surgical re-vascularization have caused a remarkable improvement in the management of coronary heart disease.

When discussing the role of physical training per sé as one measure of CCC one must observe the fact that a single factor cannot be expected to influence a multi-factorial disease. In my opinion the irrefutable evidence that shows that physical training has an effect on the longevity is lacking and will not be available for many years to come, if at all. On the other hand a number of important physiological and psychological benefits have been found to be accompanying prolonged physical training programme in a selected patient population suffering from coronary heart disease. The effect of training are an improvement of cardio-circulartory performance for given work tasks. This includes a decrease of heart rate, systolic blood pressure, the double product, an increase of stroke volume, overall physical work performance, oxygen pulse and in some instances the rise of the angina pectoris threshold heart rate and threshold rate-pressure product in patients with angina pectoris.

Of late there is additional evidence, mostly in the experimental animal, which show that daily exercise effect beneficially the susceptibility of sudden cardiac death and increases the threshold for ventricular fibrillation. Moreover, nuclear studies have shown that at least, in selected patients physical training may improve the left ventricular systolic performance and increase left ventricular ejection fraction. However, in summarizing the results of a large number of studies concerning the left ventricular performance and myocardial perfusion it must be concluded that the outcome is equivocal.

Recent analysis of prospective randomized trials concerning physical exercise training as a secondary measure have shown that from 6 studies 5 indicated that there may be a benefit from physical training for post-myocardial infarction patients. Unfortunately all these trials were too short and the sample size too small. This fact together with a number of difficulties concerning drop-out and drop-in rates make it impossible to reach a clear scientific verdict.

In my opinion important data is accumulating, especially in the field which was rarely discussed in the past namely, 'The Importance of Exercise Performance in Patients with Left Ventricular Dysfunction' and cardiac failure. This information, when available, may add substantially to a more profound knowledge of the benefits and the long term effects of a single procedure in the management of chronic multi-factorial disease.

Introduction

A discussion on the subject of Physical Exercise as a Secondary Preventive Measure may seen superfluous because many such discussions have been held in the past and a large number of scientific papers on the subject have been published in the last 2 decades. Unfortunately ill-defined hypothesis, and unachievable goals, have not only complicated research in this field in the past, but sometimes it was felt that the authors were fighting Don-Quixote wars in order to find scientific proof that exercise therapy indeed can be considered as a measure of secondary prevention. Before going into a more detailed analysis of what has been established and what remains scientifically unproven one should stress immediately that the possibility that a single therapeutic measure can directly influence the prognosis of a multi-factorial disease seems almost to be a 'mission impossible'. Nonetheless, a great number of expensive randomized trials have so far failed to produce meaningful results concerning the effect of physical training on longevity. The reason for reaching any conclusive outcome were the number of unavoidable biases involved in long term randomized prospective studies including high drop-out and drop-in rates, patients compliance and contaminations [1]. On the other hand a great number of non-randomized controlled studies with a follow-up of 15 years and longer have repeatedly shown lower mortality rates in the intervention group but because of the lack of randomization they are being considered an 'anecdotal experience' [2].

Hemodynamic response to physical training

In the late nineteen sixties, Frick and Katila [3] found that in a trained group of patients there was a trend to larger stroke volumes and better left ventricular functions when compared to controls. They found smaller A-V oxygen differences during exercise which, they presumed, reflects enhanced forward flow due to a better L.V. function. It was that the mechanism evoking larger stroke volumes and improved L.V. functions is myocardial hypertrophy and/or more synchronous contractile pattern. Hagberg et al. [4] found in a recently published study an increase in left ventricular stroke volume and storke work in patients with CHD. At the same time, percentage of VO_2 maximal and mean B.P. was the same before and after training, while left ventricular stroke work increased by 18 %. The authors concluded that in patients with CAD, prolonged intensive exercise causes an increase in stroke volume and this as a result of cardiac rather than of peripherial adaptations.

Varnauskas [5] examined the coronary circulation during heavy exercise in controls and coronary patients. He found that the coronary flow response to *moderate exercise* was identical in patients and controls. It was found, that during heavy exercise the increase of coronary flow was lower in relation to $HR \times SBP$ product in the patients group when compared to the control subjects. Also vascular resistance did not decrease to the same levels as in the controls. Others have found that patients with CAD can exhibit signs of left ventricular failure during exercise including a decrease in stroke volume at higher work loads, reduce myocardial contractility and increase LVEDP. There is little doubt that peripheral circulation plays a decisive role in the effectiveness of physiologic training effect. The reduction in cardiac output/oxygen consumption relation, observed especially under submaximal conditions in coronary patients, may be considered as a peripherial training effect. It has been shown that exercise therapy can result in a precipitation of cardiac failure. Scheuer [6] has indicated that there is unequivocal evidence that in experimental animals chronic physical exercise resulted in an increased capillary growth in the myocardium which in turn caused an enlargement of the extramural vessels. He further states that the evidence that physical training enhances collateral vessel formation in humans with Cardiac Heart Disease is at best equivocal.

It is believed that physical training is a stimulus for a coronary collateral development and that exercise may induce or accelerate coronary collateral circulation [6]. It is questionable, however, whether collateral circulation can be stimulated by severity of hypoxia or by physical training per se. Needless to underline that *there certainly may be a causal influence of both stimuli.* In animals physical training was shown to increase coronary collateral growth. However, such influences has never been clearly demonstrated in men. Noakes and co-workers [7] found an increase, as a consequence of training, in the ventricular fibrillation threshold of isolated rat hearts. Authors stated, however, that the findings that exercise training increased myocardial resistance to ventricular fibrillation occurs spontaneously and has no response to exogenous electrical stimulus. Another study which should be mentioned is that of Billman and co-workers [8] who found that exercise altered the autonomic control of the heart possibly decreasing sympathetic or increased para-sympathetic tone. They came to the conclusion that daily exercise can prevent sudden cardiac death in a sub-population of animals previously identified to be particularly vulnerable to ventricular fibrillation.

Physiological benefits of a physical training programme

It is generally accepted that physical training improves circulatory conditions and diminishes cardiac work [9]. As a response to effective physical training heart rate and rate-pressure product for given work levels decrease. The proper training effect includes: (a) decrease of H.R., Systolic blood pressure, muscular blood flow, lactic acid concentration and myocardial oxygen demands (for given tasks). (b) increases in the arteriovenous oxygen difference at maximal work levels, stroke volume, maximal oxygen uptake, maximal work performance and the concentration of oxydative enzyms. (c) improvement in the maximal oxygen potential, indicated by a larger mitochondrial mass. In healthy individuals vigorous training may increase maximal oxygen uptake by 15% or more. *The implementation* of physical training in patients with coronary heart disease must be based on clinical and conceptual considerations. Contra-indications should be strictly observed and an effective follow-up should always be available. The aim of physical training in the coronary patient is the improvement of work performance and the achievement of a training effect. It has been found that training effect is not limited to the central circulation only, but that there are also peripheral circulatory alternations as a result of training. Furthermore, it should be mentioned that there is accumulating evidence that physical training does not change left ventricular end-diastolic pressure, end-diastolic volume or ejection fraction. Segmental contractility was found uneffected. No deterioration after training has been observed in patients with end-diastolic pressures above 20 mm Hg and ejection fraction below 45%. These latter observations have been made after short term training. Interestingly, it was found that the coronary patient has a much better tolerance for physical exertion than believed. Certainly, in assessing the physiological response of training one must differentiate between the various types of training. The effect of physical training is dependent on sufficient intensity, duration and frequency, in order to produce measurable effects and enhanced overall performance. We have found that the cardiocirculatory response in arm training is especially beneficial in patients with angina pectoris. In our experience physical training in coronary patients should be supervised and implemented only according to possible benefits.

Exercise therapy in impaired ventricular function

Data available to-date point to wide range of conclusions concerning the effect of physical training in patients with impaired ventricular function. While some authors speculate that ventricular function is being improved after training, others found unchanged left ventricular dimensions and concluded that training has no direct influence on the myocardium, either beneficial or detrimental [10]. It seems that a controlled well dosed physical training applied in coronary patients with mild to moderate impaired ventricular function has no deteriorating effect on the myocardium. While there is doubt as to whether exercise has a beneficial influence on myocardial perfusion, i.e. increase of coronary blood flow, one can, in our experience, safely recommend an individually adapted supervised exercise training in selected patients with coronary artery disease. Most authors found unchanged E.F. left ventricular end-diastolic pressure and volume after train-

Table 1. Review of literature

Author	N	Duration of training	Training effect	Initial E.F. percentage
Denniss et al. (18)	32	short term	Positive	18 (mean)
Lee et al. (19)	18	12–42 (months)	Positive	40 or less unchanged also other dim.
Jensen et al. (20)	16	6 (months)	Positive	Unchanged 6 pts. incr.
Verani et al. (21)	16	12 (weeks)	15 out of 16 positive	.52.4 (mean) increase $p < 0.02$
Letac et al. (22)	15	2 (months)	Positive	Unchanged
Conn et al. (23)	10	4–37 (months)	Positive	Less than 27
Williams et al. (17, 24)	53	6–12 (months)	Positive	50 (mean) increase ($p < .002$)
Sklar et al. (25)	21	12 (weeks)	Positive	MBFD + E.F. Unchanged

ing. It must be emphasized that methods to measure distinctive changes in left ventricular dimensions and especially of regional function still remain somewhat unsatisfactory.

Upon reviewing the literature (see Table 1), we have quoted eight studies in which physical training was used in small groups of patients with C.A.D. in whom the ejection fractions were low. The aim of all these studies was to examine the effect of physical training on left ventricular performance. In all of the eight studies there was a positive training effect to physical training with duration from 2 months to 42 months and this was also the case in patients with quite severely impaired left ventricular function. The recently published article by Carrol and co-workers [11] on Systolic Function During Exercise in Patients with CHD seems to be of special interest. The authors found that systolic function in coronary artery disease is determined by acute and chronic alterations in regional function. During exercise, there is an interplay between regional dysfunction from ischemia or infarction and regional hyperfunction of nonischemic myocardium which determines global performance.

The concept of comprehensive coronary care

As has been pointed out earlier scientific evidence is missing which would prove that exercise therapy has an effect on secondary prevention [12]. Randomized trials have failed to produce meaningful results while non-randomized controlled trials have shown a lower mortality in the intervention group. In our experience rehabilitation programmes should be considered an integral part of CCC. The early initiation of such comprehensive interventions in the acute convalescent and maintenance phase, after cardiac infarction, may well have contributed to the decline in death rates in some countries. It should not be forgotten, however, that exercise training is only one component and this must be repeatedly underlined in order to avoid any misconceptions about the possible role of exercise therapy in the general concept of coronary care [13].

It is possible to prescribe a special physical training programme on an individual basis and to achieve a maximal effect on functional capacity and work performance in accordance with the patients functional capacity and reserves. We have used a number of different training activities in the past two decades and of late we have introduced an additional intensive arm training in patients with angina pectoris. In our experience such a training, lasting for at least 16 weeks, will have a striking effect on the subjective feeling of patients with angina, e.g. in one of our studies involving 19 patients 18 did not have complaints during arm egometry or any further anginal pain. Interestingly, out of the 19 patients who had angina during leg egometry as well, only 5 complained of angina during leg egometry after the 16 week period in which they actually underwent arm training. It should be noted that the medication was not changed prior to or during the training period [14].

Psychological benefits of physical training

Evidence was given that physical training improves the emotional stability of an individual. It has been found that there is no correlation between training intensity, i.e. physiological improvement and the psychological effect. In coronary patients fear, anxiety and frustration decreases as a consequence of training. Furthermore, it enhances the return to work of the patient, his self-esteem and his general motivation to life also improves [15]. It is our experience that in patients undergoing prolonged physical training programmes there is a significant drop in absence at work and they are also less dependent on drugs. Psychological stresses experienced during normal daily life activities may result in a sudden increase in heart rate which has been shown to be associated with a large increase in circulating catecholamines. It is quite difficult to measure emotional stress in laboratory conditions and in a continuous 24 hour ECG monitoring one can make only indirect assessments when sudden appearance of tachycardia and/or arrhythmia concur with a patients protocol indicating stressful situation. In most of our patients these comparisons suggest that the appearance of tachycardia was often accompanied by ventricular ectopic activity only. In a very few patients the recorded ectopy showed R on T, premature contractions and couples and short runs. We agree with others that the neural and psychological inputs, as well as different environmental factors, may trigger the development of dangerous arrhythmias and these mechanisms are unpredictable and uncontrolable [16].

In our experience beta blocking compounds proved to have a beneficial effect in patients suffering from high frequency induced ventricular ectopy and tachycardia. One of the most interesting findings we had was the point that the ventricular premature contractions were more common in a variety of daily life activities or situations during continuous monitoring as compared to the ECG recording during exercise stress testing. This latter observation may justify special attention in order to differentiate between a direct sympathetic action of exercise performance and the possible vagal withdrawal which may be predominant in sudden environmental and emotional stresses. An effective beta blockade may reduce the danger of sudden increase in heart frequency and the possible ectopy accompanied by it. The possible use of beta blockade in Type A personalities seems also quite promising.

In our experience compulsory coronary care has a beneficial effect on behavioural patterns. At our Institute the patient population does not consist mainly of the so-called 'A' Type Personality and therefore we have no personal experience of the effect of beta-blockade in this group of coronary patients. Nonetheless, there is no doubt that psychosocial stresses and especially uncontrolled emotional events may be responsible for deterioration of the disease.

Summary

Exercise therapy is only one component of comprehensive coronary care. It should be part of a general therapeutic concept which must be based on a proper balance and timely initiation of drug therapy and/or coronary surgery, if indicated. Risk factor modifications, prevention of arrhythmias together with a possible change in life style and behaviour patterns, is to our knowledge, the best available synthesis in the management of coronary heart disease and may have a direct effect on the quality of survival in coronary patients.

References

1. Kellermann JJ: Cardiac Rehabilitation as a secondary preventive measure – endpoints. The logic of desirability and availability. In: Kellermann JJ (ed). Comprehensive Cardiac Rehabilitation. Advances in Cardiology, Vol 31. S. Karger, Basel, London, New York, 134–137, 1982.
2. Spodick DH: The randomized controlled clinical trials. American Journal of Medicine, 73:420–425, 1982.
3. Frick M, Katila M, Sjogren A: Cardiac function and physical training after myocardial infarction. In: Larsen OA, Malmborg RO (eds): Patients in CHD and Physical Fittness. Copenhagen, Munksgaard, 43–47, 1971.
4. Hagberg JM, Ehsani A, Holloszy JO: Effect of 12 months of intense exercise training on stroke volume in patients with coronary artery disease. Circulation 67:No 6:1194–1199, 1983.
5. Varnauskas E, Bergman H, Houk P et al.: Hemodynamic effects of physical training in coronary patients. Lancet Vol 2:8, 1966.
6. Scheuer J: Effects of physical training on myocardial vascularity and perfusion. Circulation 66 No 3:491–495, 1982.
7. Noakes TD, Higginson L, Opie LH: Physical training increases ventricular fibrillation threshold of isolated rat hearts during normoxia, Hypoxia and regional ischemia. Circulation 67, No 1:24–30, 1983.
8. Billman GE, Schwartz PJ, Stone HL: The effects of daily ecercise on susceptibility to sudden cardiac death. Circulation 69, No 6:1182–1189, 1984.
9. Kellermann JJ: Rehabilitation of patients with coronary heart disease. Progress in Cardiovascular Disease, Vol XVII, 4:303–328, 1975.

10. Kellermann JJ: Exercise in impaired ventricular function in Kellermann, Raineri, Litchman (eds). In Assessment of Ventricular Function. Plenum Press, London – New York (to be published), 1985.

11. Caroll JD, Hess OM, Studer NP et al.: Systolic function during exercise in patients with coronary artery disease. Journal of the American College of Cardiology, Vol 2, 2:206–216, 1983.

12. Kellermann JJ: The secondary preventive effect of comprehensive coronary care (CC). In: Raineri A, Kellermann JJ (eds).Selected Topics in Preventive Carciology. Ettore Majorana International Science Series, Plenum Press, New York & London: 165–172, 1983.

13. Kellermann JJ, Denolin H (eds): Critical Evaluation of Cardiac Rehabilitation. Bibliotheca Cardiologica No.26. S. Karger, Basel – london – new York, 1977.

14. Ben-Ari E, Kellermann JJ: Comparison of Cardiocirculatory responses to intensive arm and leg training in patients with angina pectoris. Heart and Lung, Vol 12, No. 1:337–341, 1983.

15. Wintner I, Kellermann JJ: Psychological factors involved in cardiac rehabilitation. In: Stocksmeier U (Editor): Psychological Approach to the Rehabilitation of Coronary Patients. Berlin, Heidelberg, New York, Springer Varlag. 156–172, 1976.

16. Kellermann JJ: Modulation sympathetic stimulation as a desirable feature within the framework of comprehensive rehabilitation in patients with coronary heart disease. In: Gross F (ed). Modulation of Sympathetic Tone in the Treatment of Cardiovascular Disease, Hubert, Basel:292–299, 1979.

17. Williams RS, Mckinnis RA, Cobb FR, Higginbotham MB, Wallace AG, Coleman RE, Califf RM: Effects of physical conditioning on left ventricular ejection fraction in patients with coronary artery disease. Circulation 70, .no. 1:69–75, 1984.

18. Denniss AR, Ross DA, Russell PA, et al.: Early exercise testing physical training and mortality inpatients with severe left ventricular dysfunction. Journal of the American College of Cardiology, Supp 1, 717, 1983.

19. Lee AP, Ice R, Blessey R, Sanmarco ME: Long term effects of physical training on coronary patients with impaired ventricular function. Circulation 60, No. 7:1519–1526, 1979.

20. Jensen D, Atwood JE, Froelicher V et al.: Improved in ventricular function during exercise studies with radionuclide ventriculography after cardiac rehabilitation. The Am J Cardiol Vol 46:770–777, 1980.

21. Verani MS, Hartung GH et al.: Effects of exercise training on left ventricular performance and myocardial perfusion in patients with coronary artery disease. The Am J of Cardiol Vol 47:797–803, 1981.

22. Letac B, Cribier A, Desplanches JF: A study of left ventricular function in coronary patients before and after physical training. Circulation, vol 56:375–378, 1977.

23. Conn EH, Williams RS, Wallace AG: Exercise responses before and after physical conditioning in patients with severely depressed left ventricular function. The Am J of Cardiol Vol 49:298–300, 1982.

24. Williams Rs, Conn EHK, Wallace AG: Enhanced exercise performance following physical training in coronary patients stratified by left ventricular ejection fraction. Circulation, Supp IV. 186, 1983.

25. Sklar J, Niccoli A, Leithner M, Groves B, Brammell H: Changes in ventricular function after cardiac rehabilitation are not related to changes in myocardial perfusion. Circulation. Abstracts, Vol. 66, 4:II-187, 1982.

22. Exercise Capacity and Regional Myocardial Perfusion Distribution in Ischemic Heart Disease With and Without Collaterals

R. WOLF, P. PRETSCHNER, H. HUNDESHAGEN and P. R. LICHTLEN

Abstract

The functional role of collaterals (COLL) remain a subject of debate, thus, out of 43 PTS with angina pectoris and ischemic ST depressions 2 groups were identified by angiographic criteria: GR, A, proximal occlusion of one major coronary artery (7 LAD, 8 LCX, 3 RCA) and complete filling by non compromised COLL; GR, B, subtotal proximal stenosis (> 75%) of one major branch (14 LAD, 2 LCX, 9 RCA) without COLL, contralateral vessels were free of significant lesions, poststenotic LV wall motion was normal. After an initial (INIT) symptom-limiting bicycle ergometry both groups were reexamined after a systematic 6 week exercise (EX) program. Using the 201-TL stress scintigraphy, regional myocardial perfusion was analyzed in 12 PTS with 54 poststenotic areas (PA) perfused entirely by COLL and 30 PA supplied by > 75% stenosed coronary arteries without COLL. Quantitative regional tracer uptake in PA and corresponding normal areas (NA) was evaluated by a computer program. Results:

Table 0.

		Ergometry					Counts
		Max HR	DUR (min)	CAP (W)	SPRP	EF	PA/NA
A	Init	123	5,8	100	211	63%	8,1/11,3+
	Ex	134	7,4+	136+	226	–	– –
B	Init	137	5,9	116	235	64%	8,9/12,4
	Ex	139	7,5+	134	240	–	– –

+ $p < 0,02$; HR: heart rate; DUR: Duration; CAP: Exercise capacity.

The relative size of perfusion defects was comparable in PTS with and without COLL (LAD 27.1 vs 24.7%, LCX and RCA 13.6 vs 15.7%). Comment: in this specific anatomic situation COLL show a significant but clearly limited protective effect during stress even after a short time exercise program, regional 201-TL uptake indicates a comparable reduction of blood flow in poststenotic areas supplied by coll or > 75% stenosed coronary arteries.

Introduction

The functional role and clinical relevance of coronary collaterals in ischemic heart disease remain controversial [17, 39]. From experimental and clinical studies it is generally accepted, that myocardial blood flow through angiographically well developed collateral channels may be sufficient to maintain a normal oxygen supply and regional left ventricular wallfunction at rest [5–7, 23, 27, 29, 37, 38]. This, however is not representative for ischemic conditions with increased oxygen demand. Additionally, it was assumed, yet not proven, that physical training may stimulate the development of coronary collateral vessels [19, 22, 29, 35, 39]. Conflicting results are primarily due to the fact, that the quantification of collateral blood flow in humans is limited by methodological reasons, usually requiring intracoronary application of radioisotopes [15, 16]. Previous investigations have indicated, that 201-Thallium imaging is a reliable noninvasive method for analyzing myocardial perfusion distribution and detecting areas of transient relative hypoperfusion during exercise compared to resting conditions [3, 14, 20, 21, 31]. However, most clinical, scintigraphic, and angiographic studies have analyzed collateral circulation in vessels that are not completely occluded. Thus, the contributions of the antegrade and collateral flow cannot be separated. The human analog to experimental studies is a completely obstructed coronary vessel without infarction, which permits the investigation of isolated collateral supply at rest and during stress.

Hence, this investigation tries to answer the following question:

Can an exclusive collateral perfusion of obstructed coronary branches prevent stressinduced ischemia or is this comparable to subtotally stenosed coronaries without collateral supply?

This was tested in two ways:

1. Comparison of collateral myocardial perfusion with antegrade flow through subtotally stenosed vessels, quantitatively analyzed by regional 201-Thallium uptake of poststenotic areas and qualitatively investigated by the number of ischemic perfusion defects.

2. Comparison of exercise capacity and ischemic threshold in coronary patients with and without collateral vessels, estimated by clinical and electrocardiographic parameters.

Methods

1. 201-Thallium (Tl) perfusion scintigraphy

Regional myocardial perfusion studies were performed in 14 patients with angiographically proven coronary artery disease. In 8 patients 8 poststenotic areas were identified, supplied by subtotally stenosed coronary vessels (4 LAD, 4 RCA; > 75–90 % obstruction of the luminal diameter) without collateral filling of the poststenotic vessel segment. In 6 patients a proximally occluded LAD could be demonstrated, perfused entirely by large collaterals from nonobstructed coronary branches. In both groups the remaining coronary vessels were free of stenotic lesions. Poststenotic regional wall motion, assessed by biplane left ventricular angiography, was normal or slightly reduced in all cases.

201-Thallium imaging was performed after bicycle ergometry with increasing work-loads. When ischemic symptoms appeared or the age-predicted maximal heart rate was attained, 2 mCi 201-Tl were injected intravenously and exercise was continued for 2 min. Immediately after stress testing, 201-Tl scintigraphy was initiated. A redistribution study at rest was performed after 4 h.

Scintigraphy was performed with a PICKER DYNA CAMERA 4/15 (low-energy general purpose collimator, 20 % energy window) and a DEC pdp 11/34 computer in 4 projections (anterior, LAO 30°, 60°, left lateral). Analog and digital displays of 201-Tl distribution (64×64 matrix, 30 % background subtraction with contrast enhancement, 16 shades of gray) were judged by three independent observers. A significant ischemic perfusion defect was defined as a reduction of activity > 25 % by visual inspection and positive redistribution at rest. Because 6 anatomically defined left ventricular regions (anterior, apical, inferior, septal, lateral, posterior) can be identified in 4 scintigraphic projections, a poststenotic ischemic clearly can be related to the corresponding stenosed artery.

A quantitative evaluation of regional 201-Tl uptake was performed by a computer program. After visual identification, each myocardial area was divided automatically into 8 segments. Mean 201-Tl activity of each segment, localized in a normally perfused or poststenotic region, was calculated and expressed as counts/minute/matrix point.

2. Exercise studies and estimation of the ischemic threshold before and after training

Clinical exercise studies were performed in two patient groups, characterized by one of the following angiographic criteria:

1. Proximal occlusion of one major coronary artery and complete perfusion by non compromised large collaterals.

2. High-grade (> 75–90%) obstruction of the luminal diameter in one coronary vessel without collateral filling.

The remaining contralateral branches were without significant lesions; the poststenotic LV wall motion was normal or minimally reduced.

Both patient groups underwent upright bicycle ergometry with increasing workloads on an electrically braked ergometer. Workload increments of 25 watt were added every 2 minutes until the appearance of limiting chest pain, dyspnoe, fatigue, ischemic ST segment depressions or the age-predicted maximal heart rate was achieved. Heart rate, systolic blood pressure, and the electrocardiogram were recorded at the end of each minute of exercise and at the onset of ischemia. The onset of an ischemic reaction was defined as the moment a subject developed significant ST segment depressions > 0.1 mV in at least 2 leads independent from the occurrence of angina pectoris. Maximally reached workload, exercise duration, heart rate, and systolic pressure rate product were documented.

Subsequently, both patient groups were referred to a 6 weeks exercise training program. Subjects trained for 40 minutes twice a day, 5 times/week. Each training session consisted of a warm-up and cool-down period, jogging or ergometer cycling. Patients exercised at or near the maximal achieved heart rate before the onset of ischemic ST depressions. During the training period each patient received nitrates and, if necessary calcium antagonists in an individual dosage to permit exercise without anginal pain. No patient required additional treatment with beta blockers. At the end of the exercise training period each patient underwent a second symptomlimited bicycle stress test, using the initial exercise protocol. All antianginal drugs except nitrogyclerin were withheld for 48 hours prior to the first and second exercise test.

Results

1. 201-Thallium perfusion studies

Proximal coronary occlusions and complete filling by large collaterals were present in the left anterior descending artery (LAD) in 6 cases (Fig. 1).

The total number of myocardial segments in the distribution area of each coronary artery and clinical and angiographic data in the scintigraphically studied patients are summarized in Table 1 and 2.

There was no significant difference in the incidence of ischemic and normal myocardial segments in coronary patients with and without collaterals (Table 3). Regional 201-Thallium uptake is indicated in Fig. 2. During exer-

THALLIUM-201 SCINTIGRAPHY LAD-OCCLUSION WITH RETROGRADE COLLATERAL FILLING

(R.W., m, 43 yrs.)

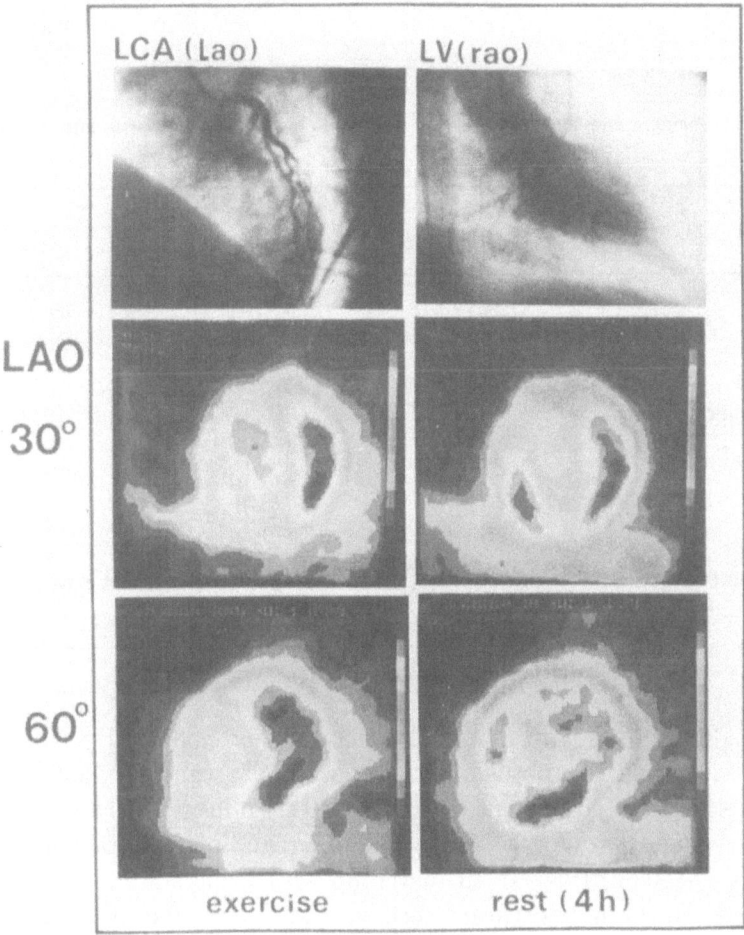

Figure 1. 201-Tl scintigraphy in a patient with proximal occlusion of the LAD and complete filling by the RCA. Top, left side: left coronary angiogram with proximal LAD occlusion. Right side: left ventricular endsystolic angiogram, revealing a hypokinetic anterior wall motion. In the mid and bottom, left side: 201-Tl scintigraphy in LAO 30° and 60° projections, respectively, indicating a transient perfusion defect of the septal, anterior and apical region with positive redistribution at rest (right side)

Table 1. Number of myocardial segments (201-thallium scintigraphy) in the distribution areas of the left and right coronary artery

Projection	LAD	LCX	RCA	
Anterior	4 anterior	–	3 inferior	Segments
LAO 30°	3 septal	3 posterolateral	2 inferior	Segments
LAO 60°	4 anterior	2 anterolateral	3 inferior-posterior	Segments
Total	11	5	8	Segments

Table 2. Clinical, angiographic, and scintigraphic results in coronary patients with and without collateral vessels

	Collaterals (n = 6)	No collaterals (n = 8)	
Age (yrs)	45,7±4,0	51,5±10,8	2 P = ns
Men	6	8	
Diseased vessel (no of poststenotic segments)			
LAD	6 (66)	4 (44)	
LCX	– –	– –	
RCA	– –	4 (26 [a])	
Total	6 (66)	8 (70)	
Ejection fraction (%)	62,3±8,6	64,8±5,7	2 P = ns
Grade of obstruction (%)	100	90,0±9,8	

[a] In 2 patients with RCA-obstructions no anterior projections were available.

cise in the patient group with proximal occlusions and collateral perfusion 201-Tl activity in 10 poststenotic myocardial segments achieved 8.00 ± 1.73 cts/min/mp compared to 11.31 ± 2.19 cts/min/mp in 16 normally perfused segments, resulting in a mean difference of 29% of regional tracer uptake ($p < 0.02$) (Fig. 3). In the group with highgrade obstructions 201-Tl activity in 14 hypoperfused segments was 8.96 ± 0.46 cts/min/mp during stress compared to 13.05 ± 1.25 cts/min/mp in 16 normal segments (31% difference; $p < 0.001$). Both segments were significantly different, whereas no significant differences of activity in both normal and poststenotic segment between the two groups could be demonstrated.

2. Exercise studies before and after physical training

Clinical and angiographic data of the two patient groups with and without collaterals are summarized in Table 4. There were no significant differences

REGIONAL 201 TI UPTAKE OF NORMAL AND
POSTSTENOTIC LV SEGMENTS DURING STRESS

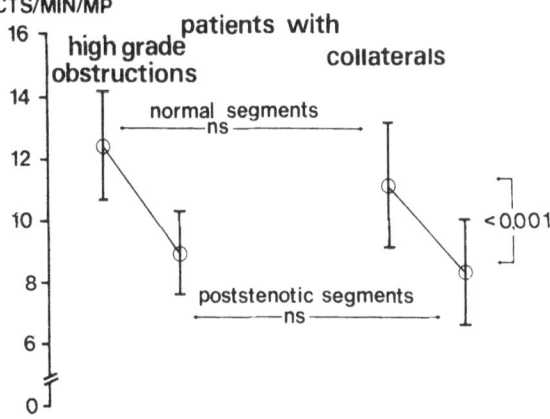

Figure 2. Regional 201-Tl uptake (Counts/minute/matrix point) of normal and poststenotic myocardial segments in patients with high grade obstructions without collaterals and occlusions with complete collateral filling

Table 3. Number of ischemic and normally perfused myocardial segments in 201-thallium scintigraphy in coronary patients with and without collaterals

	Ischemic	Normally perfused
Collaterals	10	56
No collaterals	14	56

$x^2 = 0,55$ 2 P = ns

Table 4. Clinical and angiographic results in coronary patients with and without collateral vessels

	Collaterals (n = 26)	No collaterals (n = 21)	
Age (years)	52,5±7,4	53,2±6,3	2 p = ns
Men	22	21	
Diseased vessel			
LAD	15	9	$x^2 = 1,02$
LCX/RCA	11	12	2 P = ns
Grade of obstruction (%)	100	88,3±8,6	
Ejection fraction (%)	63,7±8,1	64,0±9,7	2 P = ns

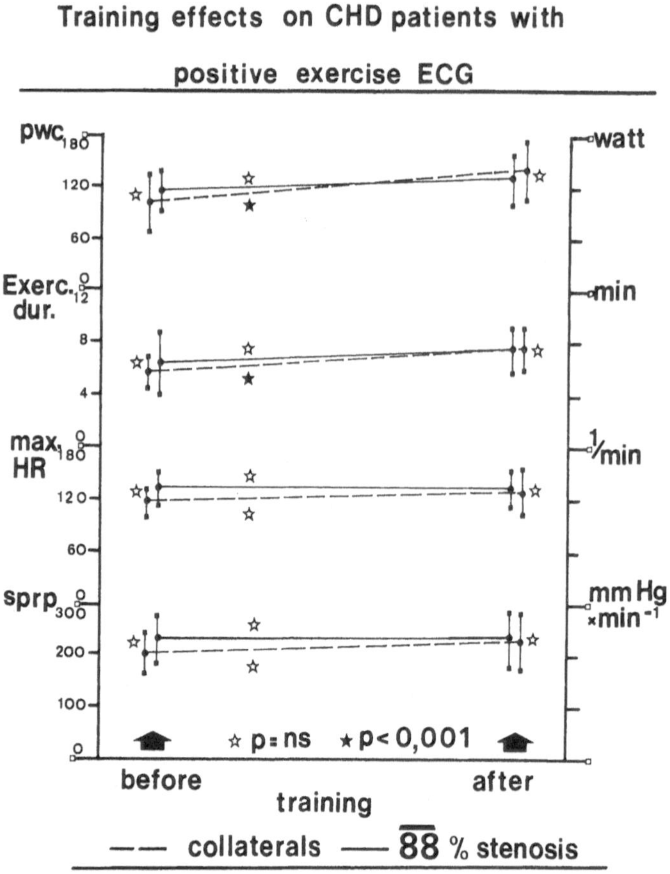

214

Figure 3. Effect of 6 week exercise training on patients with high grade obstructions without collaterals and occlusions will complete collateral filling (pwc = physical working capacity; exerc. dur. = symptom-free exercise duration; max. HR and sprp = maximal achieved heart rate and systolic pressure rate product, respectively, ad the onset of ischemia)

in age, sex distribution, distribution of diseased vessels and left ventricular ejection fraction. The grade of obstruction in the collateral group was 100% according to the definition of an entire collateral perfusion of the poststenotic area. The angiographically estimated grade of obstruction in the group without collaterals achieved 88.3±8.6% of the luminal diameter.

Predicted physical working capacity (PWC) observed PWC and maximal exercise duration both before and after training are summarized in Table 5. After a 6 week training period a significant increase of exercise tolerance and duration could be observed. The incidence of positive (ST segment depression > 0.1 mV), negative or questionable results of exercise ECG in patients with and without collaterals is indicated in Table 6. Both before and after training there was no significant difference between the 2 groups or a shift from a positive to a negative result or viceversa. The results of bicy-

Table 5. Results of bicycle ergometry in coronary patients with and without collateral vessels before and after physical training

	Collaterals (n = 26)	No collaterals (n = 21)	
Predicted PWC	147,12±24,87	150,95±13,75	2 P = ns'
Observed PWC before training	98,24±32,70	117,14±21,88	2 P<0,05
	2 P<0,001	2 P<0,05	
Observed PWC after training	135,81±34,75	130,0±24,95	2 P = ns
Exercise duration before training (min)	5,76±1,33	6,29±1,95	2 P = ns
	2 P<0,001	2 P<0,025	
Exercise duration after training (min)	7,46±1,63	7,38±1,69	2 P = ns

PWC = Physical working Capacity (WATT).

Table 6. Results of exercise ECG (bicycle ergometry) in coronary patients with and without collateral vessels

	Collaterals	No collaterals
Positive	14	12
Negative	7	5
Questionable	5	4

$x^2_{2DF} = 0,07$ 2 p = ns

cle ergometry in the subgroups with and without collaterals and positive exercise ECG both before and after physical training are summarized in Fig. 3. Physical working capacity and exercise duration increased in both groups, however this increase was not significant in the patient group without collateral vessels. Maximal heart rate and systolic pressure rate product at the onset of ischemic ST depressions were not significantly changed after training in both groups. No significant differences of these parameters both before and after physical training could be demonstrated between the two groups.

Discussion

Several investigations have dealt with the protective effect of coronary collaterals in chronic ischemic heart disease [39]. In most studies left ventricular global or regional poststenotic wall motion was correlated with the presence or absence of angiographically well developed collateral vessels [12a, 13, 17, 22, 38]. However, a normal resting function of a poststenotic wall segment, supplied entirely by non-compromised collaterals, does not exclude a limited increase of blood flow and metabolic imbalance during stress [26]. Recent experimental, clinical, and intraoperative data during coronary bypass surgery have suggested, that the conductivity of collaterals during maximal pharmacologic or hyperemic vasodilatation correspond to one third of the normal coronary conductivity and equals a high grade stenosis [2, 5, 6, 12, 15, 16, 23, 28, 33, 37–39]. In contrast, myocardial perfusion studies with 201-Thallium during exercise have led to conflicting results. However, this is primarily due to different patients selection, experimental study design, and methodologic limitations [2, 5, 12, 23, 33, 37, 40].

One relevant/limitation of 201-Thallium myocardial imaging is, that perfusion scintigrams display relative distributions rather than absolute values for myocardial blood flow [3, 14, 20, 21, 24, 31]. Thus, in multivessel disease 201-Thallium scintigraphy reveal only the most severe ischemic area despite a significant reduction of the absolute flow in different poststenotic areas [24]. To eliminate this disadvantage, we have preferred a quantitative approach of segmental analysis of exercise 201-Thallium scintigraphy in the anatomically well defined situation of exclusively antegrade or collateral blood supply of an isolated poststenotic region.

Moreover, the scintigraphic identification of ischemic perfusion defects is related to the muscle mass at risk [18]. Thus, non-occurrence of a perfusion defect is determined by the mass of hypoperfused myocardium and does not exclude a significant reduction of the conductance properties of collateral channels. Our results are not at variance with data from Rigo et al. [23], who demonstrated an at least relative protection of collaterals from exercise-induced ischemic perfusion defects. A collateral supply of areas at risk may significantly improve myocardial preservation in contrast to a high grade stenosed or occluded vessel without collaterals. However, this concept permits no quantification of the limited flow reserve of collateral vessels. Recent data from Tubau et al. [33] have shown, that large intercoronary collaterals significantly reduce the frequency of exercise-induced perfusion defects compared to subtotally stenosed arteries without collateral supply. However, the presence of ischemic ST depressions, maximal exercise time, and maximal pressure-rate-product did not significantly differ in both groups. The functional similarity of subtotally stenosed coronary arteries and collateral vessels, as indicated by 201-Thallium perfusion studies, brought up the question of its clinical relevance. In both exercise groups with either one isolated high grade coronary obstruction or complete occlusion and exclusive collateral poststenotic perfusion, resting ventricular function, hemodynamics, and stress tolerance up to an ischemic reaction were comparable. A six week exercise training program revealed no significant effects on the maximally achieved heart rate and double product at the onset of ischemic symptoms, indicating no increase of poststenotic oxygen supply by new developed or functionally improved collaterals [1, 9, 25, 30].

Improved exercise capacity and duration have to be attributed to adaptation in training skeletal muscles because the onset of ischemia in response to a given work load is delayed but not associated with a significant increase in the ischemic threshold [4, 8, 11, 19, 22, 32, 34, 35]. This is in agreement with previous results from Schaper [29], indicating no effect of physical training on collateral resistance in chronic coronary artery occlusion in the dog. In our study patients with well developed collaterals were untrained before angiography. Thus, the absence or presence of collaterals is primarily determined by the progression and severity of the underlying coronary obstructive disease. From our study the following conclusions may be stated:

1. Large collaterals show a significant but clearly limited protective effect during stress.
2. Regional 201-Thallium uptake and the clinically estimated ischemic threshold indicate a comparable reduction of flow in poststenotic areas perfused by collaterals or subtotally stenosed coronary arteries.
3. A short time exercise program did not improve ischemic threshold in patients with performed collaterals, but increased exercise capacity by peripheral circulatory effects.

References

1. Amsterdam EA, Hughes EA, DeMaria AN, Zelis R, Mason DT: Indirect Assessment of Myocardial Oxygen Consumption in the Evaluation of Mechanisms and Therapy of Angina Pectoris. Amer J Cardiol 33:737, 1974.
1a. Amende I, Simon R, Lichtlen P: Die Wirkung von Röntgenkontrastmittel auf die linksventrikuläre Dynamik. In: P.R. Lichtlen: Koronarangiographie (Perimed), 291, 1979.
2. Banka VS, Bodenheimer MM, Fouche CM, Agarwal JB, Helfant RH: Relationsship between coronary collaterals and zonal ischemia in an. Circulation 59 and 60 (Suppl II):II–134, 1979.
3. Blood DK, McCarthy DM, Sciacca RR, Cannon PJ: Comparison of Single-Dose and Double-Dose Thallium-201 Myocardial Perfusion Scintigraphy for the Detection of Coronary Artery Disease and Prior Myocardial Infarction. Circulation 58:777, 1978.
4. Ehsani AA, Heath GW, Hagberg JM, Holloszy JL: Influence of exercise training on ischemic ST segment response in patients with coronary artery disease. Circulation 59 and 60 (Suppl II):II–245, 1979.
5. Eng C, Patterson R, Halgash D, Horowitz S, Gorlin R, Herman M: The regional nature of collateral protection in exercise. Circulation 59 and 60 (Suppl II):II–245, 1979.
6. Flameng W, Schwarz F, Hehrlein F, Boel A: Functional significance of coronary collaterals in man. Basic Res Cardiol 73:188, 1978.

218

7. Frick MH, Valle M, Korhola O, Riihimäki E, Wiljasalo M: Analysis of coronary collateral in ischemic heart disease by angiography during pacing induced ischemia. Brit Heart J 38:186, 1976.

8. Ferguson RJ, Charlebois J, Taylor AW, Coté P, Péronnet F, Champlain J, Bourassa MG: Peripheral adaptations with training in patients with angina pectoris. Circulation 59 and 60(Suppl II):II-235, 1979.

9. Hoffmann JI, Buckberg GD: The Myocardial Supply: Demand Ratio – A Critical Review. Amer J Cardiol 41:327, 1978.

10. Holmberg S, Serzysko W, Varnauskas E: Coronary circulation during heavy exercise in control subjects and patients with coronary heart disease. Acta med scand 190:465, 1971.

11. Hung J, McKillop J, Goris M DeBusk R: The effects of exercise training on myocardial ischemia and left ventricular function soon after myocardial infarction: a randomized study. Circulation 64(Suppl II):II-198, 1981.

12. Haaz W, Iskandrian S, Segal BL: Effects of the degree of coronary narrowing, collarerals and ventricular function on myocardial perfusion. Circulation 59 and 60:II-62, 1979.

12a. Kober G, Kuck H, Großmann R, Kaltenbach M: Bedeutung von Kollateralen für die Protektion des Myokards bei der koronaren Herzerkrankung. Z Kardiol 70:81, 1981.

13. Langou RA, Peilen KC, Goodyer AVN: Effect of Coronary collateral vessels on ventricular wall motion in single vessel Coronary artery diesease. Circulation 59 and 60:II-89, 1979.

14. L'Abbate A, Biagini A, Michelassi C, Maseri A: Myocardial Kinetics of Thallium and Potassium in Man. Circulation 60:776, 1979.

15. Lichtlen PR, Wolf R, Engel HJ, Hundeshagen H: Coronary dilatarory reserve of severly obstructed coronary arteries and collaterals. Circulation 58(Suppl II):II-750, 1978.

16. Lichtlen PR, Engel JH: Assessment of Regnional Myocardial Blood Flow Using the Inert Gas Washout Technique. Cardiovasc Radiol 2:203, 1979.

17. McGregor M: The Coronary Collateral Circulation. Circulation 52:529, 1975.

18. Mueller TM, Marcus ML, Ehrhardt JC, Chaudhuri T, Abboud FM: Limitations of Thallium-201 Myocardial Perfusion Scintigrams. Circulation 54:640, 1976.

19. Neill WA, Oxendine JM: Exercise Can Promoto Coronary Collateral Development Withaut Improving Perfusion of Ischemic Myocardium. Circulation 60:1513, 1979.

20. Nichols AB, Blood DK, Weiss MB, Chen PH, Cannon PJ: Relationshup of Thallium-201 perfusion images to regional myocardial blood flow in man. (abstr) Amer J Cardiol 47:484, 1981.

21. Nielsen A, Morris KG, Murdock RH, Bruno FP, Cobb FR: Linear relationsship between districution of Thallium-201 and blood flow in ischemic and non-ischemic myocardium durin exercise. Circulation 59 and 60 (suppl II):II-148, 1979.

22. Nolewajka AJ, Kostuk WJ, Rechnitzer PA, Cunningham DA: Exercise and Human Collateralization: An Angiographic and Scintigraphic Assessment. Circulation 60:114, 1979.

23. Rigo P, Becker LC, Griffith LSC, Alderson PO, Bailey IK, Pitt B, Burow RD, Wagner HN: Influence of Coronary Collateral Vessels on the Results of Thallium-201 Myocardial Stress Imaging. Amer J Cardiol 44:482, 1979.

24. Rigo P, Bailey IK, Griffith LSC, Pitt B, Burow RD, Wagner HN, Becker LC: Value and Limitations of Segmental Analysis of stress Thallium Myocardial imaging for Localization of Coronary Artery Disease. Circulation 61:973, 1980.

25. Robinson BF: Relation of Heart Rate and Systolic Blood Pressure to the Onset of Pain in Angina Pectoris. Circulation 35:1073, 1967.

26. Rubio R, Berne RM: Regulation of Coronary Blood Flow. Progr Cardiovasc Dis 18:105, 1975.

27. Schaper W, Remijsen P, Xhonneux R: The size of myocardial infarction after Experimental coronary artery ligation. Z Kreislauff 58:904, 1969.

28. Schaper W, Flameng W, Winkler B, Wüsten B, Türschmann W, Neugebauer G, Carl M, Pasyk S: Quantification of Collateral Resistance in Acute and Chronic Experimental Coronary Occlusion in the Dog. Circul Res 39:371, 1976.

29. Schaper W: Ineffectiveness of physical Training on collateral resistance in chronic coronary artery occlusion in the dog. Circulation 62(Suppl IV):IV–117, 1981.

29a. Schaper W: Influence of Physical Exercise on Coronary Collateral Blood Flow in Chronic Experimental Two-vessel Occlusion. Circulation 65:905, 1982.

30. Simonson E: Evaluation of Cardiac Performance in Exercise. Amer J Cardiol 30:722, 1972.

31. Strauss HW, Harrison K, Langan JK, Lebowitz e, Pitt B: Thallium-201 for Myocardial Imaging. Circulation 51:641, 1975.

32. Thompson PD, Cullinane E, Lazarus B, and Carleton RA: Effect of Exercise Training on the Untrained Limb Exercise Performance of Men with Angina Pectoris. Amer J Cardiol 48:844, 1981.

33. Tubau JF, Chaitman BR, Bourassa MG, Lesperarance J, Dupras G: Importance of Coronary Collateral Circulation in Interpreting Exercise Test Results. Amer J Cardiol 47:27, 1981.

34. Vatner SF, Pagani M: Cardiovascular Adjustments to Exercise: Hemodynamics and Mechanisms. Progr Cardiovasc Dis 19:91, 1976.

35. Verani MS, Hartung GH, Hoepfel-Harris J, Welton DE, Pratt CM, Miller RR: Effects of Exercise Training on Left Ventricular Performance and Myocardial Perfusion in Patients with Coronary artery Disease. Amer J Cardiol 47:797, 1981.

36. Wainwright RJ, Maisey MN, Edwards AC, Sowton E: Functional significance of coronary collateral circulation during dynamic exercise evaluated by Thallium-201 myocardial scintigraphy. Brit Heart J 43:47, 1980.

37. Williams DO, Amsterdam EA, Miller RR, Mason DT: Functional Vessels in Patients With Acute Myocardial Infarction: Relation to Pump Performance, Cardiogenic Shock and Survival. Amer J Cardiol 37:345, 1976.

38. Wolf R, Engel HJ, Hundeshagen H, Lichtlen P: Collateral Myocardial Blood Flow at Rest and After Maximal Arteriolar Dilatation in Patients with Ischemic Heart Disease. In: Coronary Heart Disease. 3rd International Symposium Frankfurt. Edited by Kaltenbach M, Lichtlen P, Balcon R, Bussmann W-D, (Thieme), p 61, 1978.

39. Gottwik M, Schaper W: Do coronary collaterals have protectiv potential? J Cardiovasc Med 7:1272, 1982.

40. Eng C, Patterson RE, Horowitz SF, Halgash DA, Pichard AD, Midwall J, Herman MV, Gorlin R: Coronary Collateral Function During Exercise. Circulation 66:309, 1982.

41. Feldmann RL, Pepine CJ: Evaluation of Coronary Collateral Circulation in Conscious Humans. Amer J Cardiol 53:1233, 1984.

42. Goldberg HL, Goldstein J, Borer JS, Moses JW, Collins MB: Functional Importance of Coronary Collateral Vessels Amer J Cardiol 53:694, 1984.

V. The Role of Psychosocial
Factors in Secondary Prevention

23. Alteration of Type A Behavior and its Effect Upon the Cardiac Recurrence Rate in Post-myocardial Infarction Patients

M. FRIEDMAN, J.J. GILL, C.E. THORESEN and D. ULMER

Abstract

A large group of post-myocardial infarction subjects were randomly selected and enrolled into (1) a group receiving classic cardiologic counseling and (2) a group receiving Type A counseling in addition to the cardiologic counseling.

At the end of three years, reduction in Type A behavior was observed in 43.8 percent of the 592 participants who initially were enrolled to receive both the cardiologic and Type A counseling. The three-year cumulative cardiac recurrence rate was 7.2 percent in participants receiving group cardiologic and Type A behavior counseling and 13 percent in the control participants who received only the group cardiologic counseling. These results suggest that Type A behavior can be significantly modified in a large fraction of post-infarction patients and that such alteration is associated with a significantly reduced rate of cardiac recurrences.

I. The nature of Type A behavior

Dr. Ray H. Rosenman and I announced in 1959, the intimate association of a specific overt behavior pattern with the prevalence [2] and then a few years later, the incidence [23] of clinical coronary heart disease. This behavior pattern which we called Type A behavior, is manifested *overtly* by (1) a sense of time urgency (i.e., impatience) and (2) free-floating hostility (i.e., a tendency to become easily angered or irritated by even the most trivial and inconsequential actions of other persons).

Since the publication of these two articles, dozens of other studies have been published which have confirmed this observed close association of Type A behavior with the prevalence as well as the incidence of clinical coronary heart disease and the interested reader is referred to the reviews of

Jenkins [19] and Price [22] for a description of these articles. Finally, following the confirming results of the Framingham group [18], a review panel on coronary-prone behavior and coronary heart disease convened at the request of the National Heart, Lung and Blood Institute. After reviewing all available epidemiologic, clinical and pathological studies dealing with the possible relationship of Type A behavior to the pathogenesis of coronary heart disease, this panel concluded that this type of behavior was a coronary risk factor fully as important as all other commonly accepted risk factors (e.g., hypertension, hypercholesterolemia and excessive cigarette smoking).

II. The diagnosis of Type A behavior

From the very outset of our studies dealing with Type A behavior, we have emphasized repeatedly [2–5, 14–16, 21] that this disorder *should be diagnosed like any other medical disorder, namely by the clinical detection of characteristic physical signs and the elicitation (by individual questions) of identifying symptoms.* However, an increasing number of non-physician investigators have interested themselves in the possible relationship of Type A behavior to clinical coronary heart disease who unfortunately were not trained in the clinical techniques used for detecting the presence of a medical disorder. Lacking such clinical expertise, these investigators have attempted to diagnose the presence and to assess the severity of Type A behavior in individuals either by having them write out their responses to various pen and pencil and paper tests (i.e., questionnaires)* or to a series of stereotyped questions presented orally to them by non-professional personnel. Indeed a number of recent epidemiological studies, the presence or absence of Type A behavior has been determined in thousands of persons, according to their responses to various series of stereotyped questions (presented either in the form of questionnaires or presented orally by non-professional personnel), without a single one of them ever having been seen, much less *clinically* surveyed by either physicians or possibly qualified paramedical personnel.

The error inherent in this means of diagnosing the presence of Type A behavior quickly becomes apparent when it is realized that no physician would dare to diagnose the presence of any medical disorder (even measles), solely by the written responses of an *unseen* patient to a questionnaire.

This absurdity of singling out Type A behavior as the only disorder in all medicine to be diagnosed by questionnaire becomes even more obvious when it is realized that at least half of all subjects harboring Type A behav-

* At the time of writing this paper, at least 15 different questionnaires 'for the diagnosis' of Type A behavior have been published.

ior are unaware of its identifying stigmata, hence incapable of responding acurately to any questionnaire. Unfortunately too, many cardiologists not knowing the characteristic signs and symptoms of this disorder overlook its presence as they conduct their routine physical exams. Unfortunately sometimes a physical examination carried out too routinely and thoughtlessly can lead to sometimes tragic results.

I have critisized at length this widespread tendency of attempting to detect the presence of Type A behavior without resorting to the usual clinical techniques employed in diagnosing medical disorders because I believe it has created confusion and chaos concerning the role of Type A behavior in the pathogenesis of coronary heart disease.

This confusion of course has hindered attempts to determine the pathophysiology by which Type A behavior may lead to clinical coronary heart disease. It also has hindered attempts to modulate the intensity of Type A behavior because if chaos rules concerning the pathogenetic relevance and also the possible components of Type A behavior, the intent as well as the practicability of treating this disorder diminishes.

On our part however, we have not been hindered in further investigations because from the outset we relied on clinical means of detecting the signs and symptoms of Type A behavior in various individuals. We thus have diagnosed and then selected scores of Type A persons during the past decade upon whom to pursue both laboratory and clinical studies to determine if possible, the pathophysiological processes by which Type A behavior may accelerate the onset of clinical coronary heart disease. Briefly summarized, we have found that most *severely* afflicted Type A subjects long before they exhibit overt coronary heart disease, possess a higher serum cholesterol [6, 7] and a higher fasting and post-prandial plasma triglyceride level than Type B persons [8]. Because of this high serum triglyceride level, sludging of red blood cells occurs in post-prandial Type A but not in Type B subjects [9]. Perhaps most ominous of all, Type A persons secrete more noreprinephrine [10, 11], and ACTH [12]. Finally, the Type A subject secretes more testosterone than this Type B counterpart [26]. On the other hand, the plasma level of growth hormone is significantly lower than that of the Type B person [13].

Many of these findings already have been confirmed by others, notably the elevation of plasma cholesterol in Type A behavior [20, 24, 26], the excess of secretion of norepinephrine [1, 25], ACTH [25] and testosterone [25]. Therefore even at this juncture, it appears quite clear that the conflict against time and other persons (i.e., the core component of Type A behavior) leads to a disarray in the secretion or metabolism of various autonomic and endocrine gland hormones.

Besides studying the possible pathophysiologic effects of Type A behavior, we also began in 1977 a study to determine if Type A behavior could be modified in post-infarction subjects and if it could, would such modification result in significantly less coronary recurrences. If Type A behavior bears a causal relationship to the pathogenesis of Type A behavior, then one might expect its alleviation should have an effect upon either the new occurrence of an infarction in a previously well but Type A person or upon the recurrence of an infarction or cardiac death in a Type A person who already had suffered one or more infarctions.

In this study, we initially recruited for the study, over 1000 persons, 64 years of age or younger, who had one or more infarctions, six or more months earlier. Eight hundred sixteen of these volunteers, while still continuing to be treated by their own physicians also agreed to be randomly selected and enrolled into one of two sections. Section 1 consisted initially of 270 persons who served as controls. They met in groups of ten to receive classic cardiologic advice and instructions from competent cardiologists. Section 2 consisted initially of 546 persons. They too met in groups of ten and in addition to receiving the same cardiologic advice and instructions as section 1 participants, also received Type A behavior counseling. Besides these two randomly enrolled sections, we also followed 150 post-infarction patients as a 'comparison group' in that they were given no counseling of any kind but only re-examined yearly.

At entry, the sociodemographic and the medical findings were essentially the same not only in the two randomly selected but also in the 'comparison group' [14, 15]. The average age of the participants was 53.4 years, height, 69.3 inches, weight 173 pounds. Their average serum cholesterol was 259.6 mg/dl. Approximately 20 percent of the participants had suffered two or more infarctions prior to entry, 55.4 percent had a family history of CHD; 73.8 percent had previously suffered from angina and 25.2 percent had undergone bypass surgery.

All participants were given a videotaped clinical interview for the diagnosis and assessment of their possible present Type A behavior by an independent consultant who was unaware that healthy Type B subjects had been interspersed with the post-infarction subjects. This method of assessing Type A behavior has been fully described in earlier reports [14, 15, 21].

All participants completed a questionnaire designed to obtain their descriptions of the nature and intensity of their sense of time urgency, hostilities, and insecurities. In addition, the spouses and a business associate of the participants receiving Type A counseling (i.e., section 2) also were asked to complete a similar type of questionnaire. These questionnaires are described in earlier reports [15, 21]. All questionnaires were repeated yearly and the videotaped clinical interview was repeated at the end of three years.

All participants also at entry were given a cardiovascular examination including electrocardiogram, blood pressure measurement, urinalysis and the withdrawal of a blood sample for serum cholesterol analysis.

Section 1 groups initially met with their cardiologists biweekly for three months, monthly for three months and then bimonthly. Section 2 groups met monthly in order that they might receive just as much cardiologic counseling as the control group as they also received Type A counseling.

In addition to analyses of the outcome of the two randomized sections, we also conducted an analysis that might provide a more direct test of the relationship between possible change in Type A behavior and cardiac recur- rence. Accordingly, we compared the cardiac recurrence rate for the last two years of the three-year in the study either reported a significant behavior reduction (i.e., more than 1 SD reduction in their questionnaire score at the end of the first year) or failed to report such reduction.

The counseling procedures in both the control and Type A counseled sections consisted of behavioral learning, restructuring of some environ- mental situations and most important of all, cognitive affective learning. These procedures recently have been described in considerable detail [16].

Results

1. The presence of Type A behavior in the participants at entry

Type A behavior was detected at entry in essentially.all post-infarction par- ticipants (98.7%), by employment of the videotaped clinical interview method.

2. Number of patients remaining in the study after three years

A total of 164 control section 1 and 381 Type A counseled section 2 parti- cipants remained at risk in their respective sections for three years. Al- though 97 section 1 and 200 section 2 participants withdrew from the study at the end of three years, 248 of these 'treatment failures' continued to be re-examined yearly. Thus we were able to follow approximately 98 percent of the section 1 and 2 participants for at least three years.

3. Reduction in Type A behavior

As Figure 1 illustrates, a marked reduction in the intensity of Type A behavior as measured by the participants' own questionnaire scores, occur- red in the section 2 participants receiving Type A counseling. Although some reduction also was noted in the section 1 control subjects, it was sig- nificantly less than that observed in section 2 subjects. A similar reduction

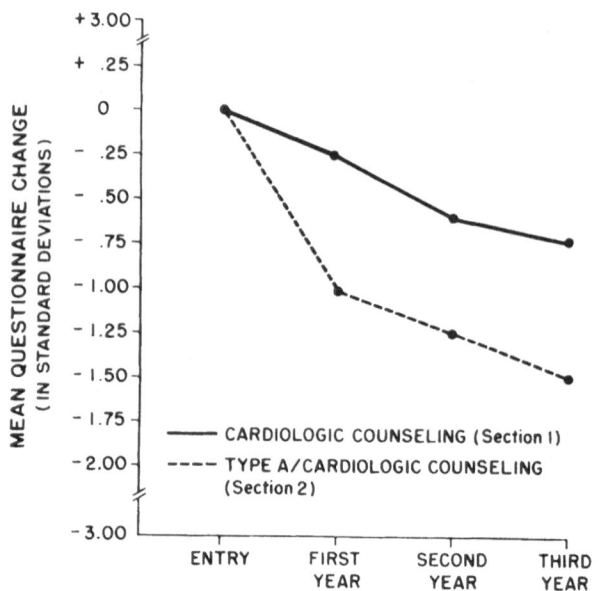

Figure 1. The decremental change observed each year for 3 years in the average Type A behavior questionnaire scores of sections 1 and 2 are depicted. Note that the mean decremental changes in section 1 never equals −1 SD from the initial mean score

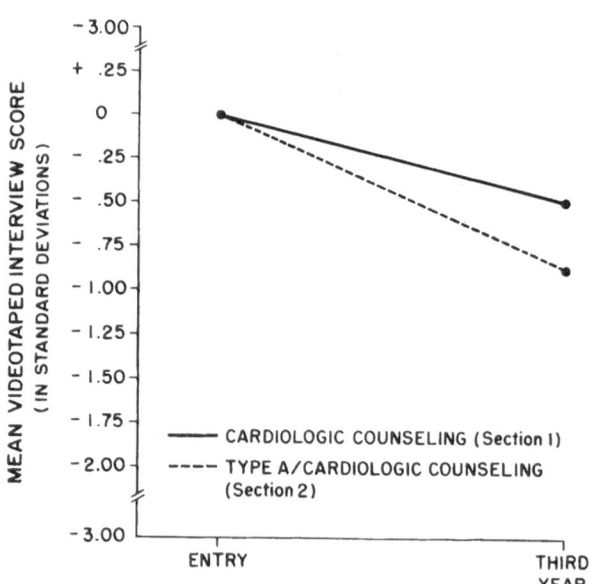

Figure 2. The yearly decremental changes observed in section 2 participants as estimated from the participant's own, his spouse's, and his monitor's questionnaires. Note that each year, although the mean change reported by participants was greater than that observed by the spouses and monitors, these differences were not significantly different

in the Type A behavior of section 2 participants also was observed in the yearly questionnaire scores reported by the spouses and the business associates (i.e., monitors).

Perhaps even more impressive, a very significant reduction in the Type A behavior of section 2 participants at the end of three years also was observed (see Fig. 2) as measured by the videotaped clinical interview score.

4. The recurrence rate in participants exhibiting significant Type A behavioral reduction at the end of their first year

One hundred eighty one participants at the end of the first year of the study exhibited a significant reduction in their Type A behavior pattern. Their coronary recurrence rate (1.7%) during the next two years was one-fourth that (8.6%) of the 326 persons who failed to exhibit a similar reduction in their Type A behavior.

5. The cardiac recurrence rate in section 1, 2 and 3 participants

Employing the 'Intention-to-Treat' principle, the three-year cumulative recurrence rate (7.2%) observed in the Type A counseled participants was significantly lower than the three-year rate (13.2%) observed in section 1 participants or the three-year rate (14.0%) observed in the 'comparison group' participants.

Discussion

The foregoing results indicate four phenomena that we believe are important in the consideration of coronary heart disease.

First, our results demonstrate that in well over 90 percent of successively examined post-infarction subjects, Type A behavior is present. This overwhelmingly intimate association of Type A behavior would have been detected earlier by ourselves and other investigators, if the detection of Type A behavior had been accomplished not by responses to questionnaires or orally presented stereotyped questions but by clinical procedures, – as all other medical disorders also are detected.

Second, the present study demonstrates that Type A behavior can be modified in a sizeable fraction of post-infarction subjects.

Third, when a large group of post-infarction subjects are given cardiologic and Type A counseling, the subsequent cardiac recurrence of the total group is approximately half that of the control group given only the cardiologic component of the counseling.

Fourth, the present data strongly suggest that Type A behavior besides its already demonstrated associative relationship to both the *prevalence* [2] and *incidence* [23] of clinical coronary heart disease, also plays a *causal* role in the early emergence of clinical coronary heart disease.

Acknowledgements

Supported by grants from the National Heart, Lung and Blood Institute (21427), Bank of America, Standard Oil of California, the Kaiser Hospital Foundation, and the Mary Potishman Lard Foundation (Forth Worth, TX).

References

1. Carruthers ME: Agression and Atheroma. Lancet 2:1170, 1969.
2. Friedman M, Rosenman RH: Association of Specific Overt Behavior pattern with Blood and Cardiolvascular Findings. JAMA 169:1286–1296, 1959.
3. Friedman M, Rosenman RH: Type A Behavior Pattern: Its Association with Coronary Heart Disease. Annals Clin Research 3:300–312, 1971.
4. Friedman M: The Modification of Type A Behavior in Post-Infarction Patients. Am Heart J 97:551–560, 1979.
5. Friedman M, Powell LH: The Diagnosis and Quantitative Assessment of Type A Behavior: Introduction and Description of the Videotaped Structured Interview. Integrative Psychiatry 7/8:123–136, 1984.
6. Friedman M, Byers SO, Rosenman RH, Elevitch FR: Coronary-Prone Indiciduals (Type A Behavior Pattern): Some Biochemical Characteristics. JAMA 212:1030–1037, 1970.
7. Friedman M, Rosenman RH, Carroll V: Changes in the Serum Cholesterol and Blood Clotting Time in Men Subjected to Cyclic Variation of Occupational Stress. Circulation 17:852–860, 1958.
8. Friedman M, Rosenman RH, Byers SO: Serum Lipis and Conjunctival Circulation After Fat Ingestion in Men Exhibiting Type A Behavior Pattern. Circulation 29:874–885, 1964.
9. Friedman M, Byers SO, Rosenman RH: Effect of Unsaturated Fats Upon Lipemia and Conjunctival Circulation. JAMA 193:882–886, 1965.
10. Friedman M, St -George S, Byers SO, Rosenman RH: Excretion of Catecholamines, 17-Ketosteroids, 17-Hydroxycorticoids and 5-Hydroxyindole in Men Exhibiting a Particular Pattern (A) Associated with High Incidence of Clinical Coronary Artery Disease. J Clin Invest 39:758–764, 1960.
11. Friedman M, Byers SO, Diamant J, Rosenman RH: Plasma Catecholamine Response of Coronary-Prone Subjects (Type A) to a Specific Challenge. Metabolism 23:205–210, 1975.
12. Friedman M, byers SO, Rosenman RH: Plasma ACTH and Cortisol Concentration of Coronary- Prone Subjects. Proc Soc Exp Biol & Med 140:681–684, 1972.
13. Friedman M, Byers SO, Rosenman RH, Newman R: Coronary-Prone Individuals (Type A Behavior Pattern): Growth Hormone Responses. JAMA 217:929–932, 1971.

14. Friedman M, Thoresen CE, GilGill JJ, Ulmer D, Thimpson L, Powel L, Price V, Elek Sr, Rabin DD, Breall WS, Piaget G, Dixon T, Bourg E, Levy RA, Tasto DL: Feasibility of Altering Type A Behavior Pattern After Myocardial Infarction: Recurrent Coronary Prevention Project Study: Methods, Baseline Results and Preliminary Findings. Circulation 66:83–92, 1982.
15. Friedman M, Thoresen CE, Gill JJ, Posell LH, Ulmer D, Thompson L, Price VA, Rabin DD, Breall WS, Dixon T, Levy RA, Bourg, E: Alteration of Type A Behavior and Reduction in Cardiac Recurrences in Post-Myocardial Infarction Patients. Am Heart J 108:237–248, 1984.
16. Friedman M, Ulmer D: Treating Type A Behavior – And Your Heart. Alfred A. Knopf, Inc., New York. 1984.
17. Grundy SM, Griffin AC: Effects of Periodic Mental Stress on Serum Cholesterol Levels. Circulation 19:496–498, 1959.
18. Haynes SG, Feinleib M, Kannel WB: The Relationship of Psychosocial Factors to Coronary heart Disease in the Framingham Study. III Eight-Year Incidence of Coronary Heart Disease. Am J Epidemiol 111:37–58, 1980.
19. Jenkins CD: Psychologic and Social Precursors of Coronary Disease. New Eng J Med 284:244–255, 1971.
20. Peterson JE, Keith RA, Wilcox AA: Hourly Changes in Serum Cholesterol Concentration: Effects of the Anticipation of Stress. Circulation 25:798–803, 1962.
21. Powell LH, Friedman M, Thoresen CE, Gill JJ, Ulmer DK: Can the Type A Behavior Pattern Be Altered After Myocardial Infarction? A Second Year Report from the Recurrent Coronary Prevention Project. Psychosomatic Medicine 46:293–313, 1984.
22. Price V: Type A Behavior Pattern: A Model for Research and Practice. Academic Press, New York, 1982.
23. Rosenman RH, Friedman M, Straus R, Jenmins CD, Zyzanski SJ, Wurm M: Coronary Heart Disease in the Western Collaborative Group Study: A Follow-Up Experience of $4\frac{1}{2}$ Years. J Chronic Dis 23:173–190, 1970.
24. Wertlake PT, Wilcox AA, Haley MI, Peterson JE: Relationship of Mental and Emotional Stress to Serum Cholesterol Levels. Proc Soc Exp Biol & Med 97:163–165, 1958.
25. Williams RB Jr, Lane JD, Kuhn CM, Meosk W, White AD, Schanberg SM: Type A Behavior and Elevated Physiological and Neuroendocrine Responses to Cognitive Tasks. Science 218:483–485, 1982.
26. Zumoff B, Rosenfeld RS, Friedman M, Byers SO, Rosenman RH, Hellman L: Comparison of Plasma and Urinary Stroids in Men with Type A And Type B Behavior Patterns. Conference Proceedings No. 231, p A12-1. NATO AGARD Conference, London, 1977.

24. A 5-year Controlled Clinical Trial on Psychological Well-being

R. A. M. ERDMAN, H. J. DUIVENVOORDEN and M. KAZEMIER

Abstract

The effects of a cardiac rehabilitation (rehab.) program on psychological functioning, workresumption, smoking-habits and the continued use of gymnastic exercises were studied over a period of 5 years. In 1977, 80 post-myocardial infarct patients (pat.) were randomly allocated to either participation in the rehab. program – duration 6 months – or to encouragement of self-determined home-rehab. Both groups were tested 3 times: before and after 6 months and 5 years later. The psychological questionnaires measured well-being, feelings of disability, feelings of displeasure and social inhibition. Other data were gathered by means of structured interviews. During the last measurement, the rehab. group consisted of 27 pat. and the homegroup of 30 pat. The 5-year follow-up showed that, in comparison to homerehab., participation in the structured rehab. program led to diminished feelings of being disabled, displeasure and social inhibition. Other important results were found: the rehab. program had a favourable effect on workresumption as 56% returned to their activities vs 47% in the homegroup. After 6 months of rehab. 76% of the smokers terminated this habit vs 64% in the home-group. Five years later the percentages were 48 vs 64. After 5 years it appeared that in the rehab. group 41% continued with regular gymnastic exercises vs 30% in the home-group. Also, a significant negative correlation was found between workresumption and smoking-habits. From this study it is concluded that group-rehab. on an out-patient basis is to be preferred over individual efforts. The manner in which such a program is carried out requires further refinement.

Introduction

The aim of cardiac rehabilitation is to achieve as normal as possible somatic and psychologic functioning in cardiac patients. As Croog and coworkers [3] stated: 'As a point of reference we will refer to recovery as 1: achievement of a return to the premorbid state particularly in the physical, psychological, and social spheres and/or 2: achievement of maximal functioning in the social and psychological spheres within the limits of physical capacity'.

However, these aims are general and hence rather vague, and any program that aims to achieve these goals should be evaluated with respect to its effectiveness.

In 1968 Hellerstein [7] reported that after a myocardial infarction his patients derived both physical and psychological benefits from an exercise training program. Nowadays cardiac rehabilitation is widely recommended for two types of psycho-social problems after a myocardial infarction: (a) emotional symptoms and medically unnecessary limitations of activity in early convalescence and (b) the modification of long standing habits and attitudes believed to be riskfactors for further ischemic cardiac disease [8]. Though, it is 'widely recommended' [2, 11] not everybody who is involved in the management of the patient with a myocardial infarction, is convinced of its utility. Predicting the individual outcome of the recovery process after a myocardial infarction is of eminent importance for clinical practice [4]. The purpose of this randomized clinical trial was: to describe over a period of approximately five years the effects of active participation in the Rotterdam cardiac rehabilitation program.

Concretely formulated, the research question was:
Does cardiac rehabilitation have any short-term or long-term beneficial effect on psychological variables and/or behavioural characteristics such as workresumption, regular exercises and smoking habits.

Material and methods

The Rotterdam rehabilitation program is named Capri, which stands for Cardio Pulmonar Research Institute and is an adaptation of the Capri-program from Seattle/U.S.A. [10]. It is an interactional rehabilitation-program consisting of two sessions of two hours training a week in a conventional gymnasium, supervised by a multidisciplinary team including a cardiologist, two physiotherapists, a psychologist, a social worker and a nurse. Each training session consists of a period of warming-up, jogging, gymnastics, volleyball, soccer or hockey and relaxation exercises.

Training is done under cardiologic supervision and resuscitation equipment is available. The entire program takes 6 months. The main goals of the Capri-program are: to restore physical capacity, to reduce fear and anxiety, and to enhance self-esteem [1, 3, 5, 9]. Within the context of this rehabilitation-program we were able to investigate changes in psychic functioning, workresumption, smoking-habits and the taking up of gymnastics as a habit, over a period of approximately 5 years.

During $1\frac{1}{2}$ years 328 cardiac patients were referred to the Capriprogram and of these 80 conformed to the selection criteria of this study. Only male and married patients with a first myocardial infarction which had occurred not longer than 6 months before the first psychological investigation, were considered for the trial. Furthermore, they had to be younger than 65 years and mentally and physically fit to take part in the program. The 80 patients were randomly allocated to either participation in the Capriprogram or to physician encouraged home-rehabilitation. The patients of the home-reha-bilitation (our control-group) received a brochure with guide-lines and advices for physical fitness-training and jogging. All patients received the usual out-patient cardiological care. The drop-out rate was, at the end of a rehabilitation period in both groups 20%. Eight patients quit the Caprigroup earlier than planned: 3 patients died, 2 patients had a re-infarction and 2 had cardiac-interventions and one did not attend. In the Home-group 6 patients were removed from the study since they were no longer motivated to participate in the psychological tests and 2 times the data were incomplete. So each group consisted of 32 patients after 6 months. Five years later both groups were reduced to 27, respectively 30 patients.

In the Capri-group 2 patients died, 2 patients were not longer motivated to participate in the study and from 1 patient the address was lost. In the Home-group 2 patients were eliminated since 1 got a re-infarction and participated in the Capri-program and 1 patient was treated in hospital for cancer. Both groups were examined three times by means of a structured interview and 1 psychological questionnaire, entitled: Heart Patients Psychological Questionnaire [6]. This test measures 4 psychological concepts: WELL-BEING, FEELING OF BEING DISABLED, DISPLEASURE and SOCIAL INHIBITION. The test was validated on a large reference group consisting of 1649 cardiac patients in the Netherlands. The interview gave information about cardiac events, smoking-habits, regular exercise, workresumption and life-events.

Results

The 32 Capri-patients who completed the study, attended on average 75% of the training-sessions offered to them. Both groups were comparable as to the incidence of life-events, age, occupational level and the incidence of cardiac events. At intake, the mean age of all 80 patients was 51 years and ranged from 35 to 60 years. *Smoking-habits.* After six months, within the Capri-group only 28% reported they were smokers versus 47% in the Home-group ($p < 0.01$). Five years later however, the results changed completely; the Capri-group included 52% smokers while in the Home-group 36% reported they were smokers. *Gymnastics.* As could be expected, after 6

236

months in the Capri-group 87% participated in doing sports actively versus only 50% in the Home-group ($p < 0.01$). Five years later, this favourable result is continued. The majority of the Capri-group (67%) has taken up gymnastics as a habit versus 45% in the Home-group. This result, however, was not statistically significant. *Workresumption.* It was striking that in the Capri-group after a follow-up period of 5 years 44% had resumed their work-activities full-time versus only 27% in the Home-group. The greater part of those who resumed their workactivities half-time after 5 years were

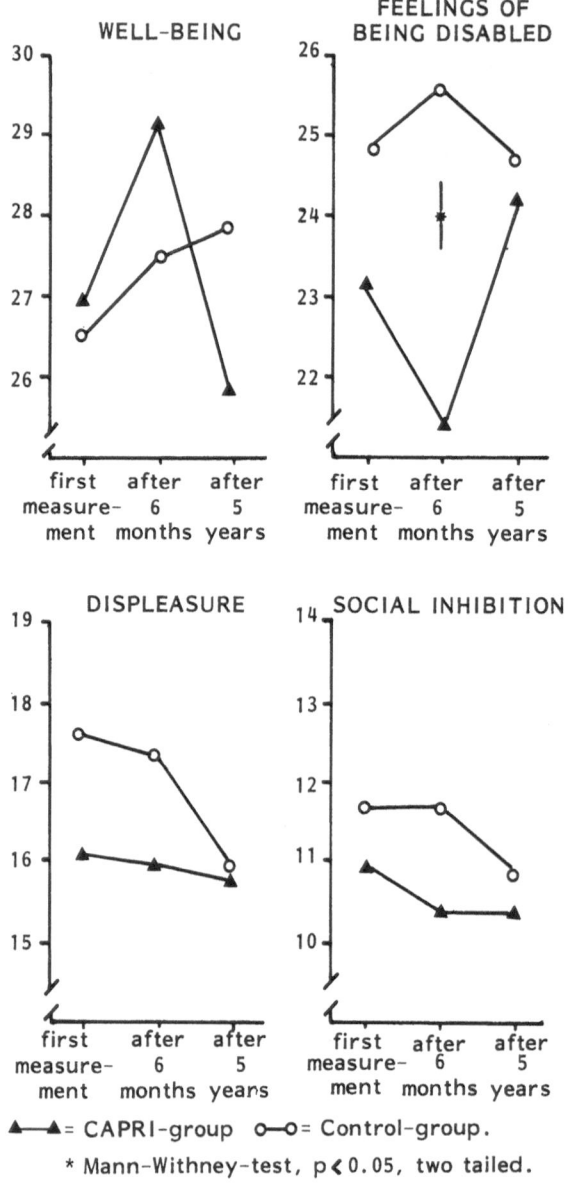

Figure 1. Psychic functioning in CAPRI- and HOME-group.

rehabilitated in the Homegroup: 23% versus 11%. None of these findings were statistically significant. *Psychological measurement.* Figure 1 illustrates the data on the scales of the Heart Patients Psychological Questionnaire. The horizontal axis shows the 3 measurements over about 5 years and on the vertical axis the test-score is represented. Each mark in the graphic represents the mean test-score on the concerning scale. The better the feeling of well-being, the higher the score.

During the second measurement, so when the rehabilitation-program is just finished, the difference in feelings of well-being between the 2 groups is at largest, in favour of the Capri-group. So one can state: Capri has a favourable short-term effect on Well-being, but these findings are reversed five years later. On the other three graphics, the higher score means an unfavourable result. The only statistical significant result is reproduced regarding feelings of being disabled. After 6 months the rehabilitated group feels statistically singificant less disabled than the control-group. After 5 years this result has practically disappeared. This tendency repeats itself on the following two items, concerning displeasure and social inhibition. After 6 months there exists a difference between both groups in favour of the Capri-group, however, these results are not statistically significant. After 5 years these findings have faded away.

Conclusions

1. Participation in the Capri-program has a short-term favourable effect on smoking-habits; this result is abolished 5 years later.
2. After 5 years 67% of the rehabilitated group continued with sporting activities versus only 45% in the Home-group.
3. Participation in the Capri-program has a long-term favourable effect on full-time workresumption.
4. Group-rehabilitation on an out-patient basis enhances feelings of well-being and diminishes feelings of being disabled, displeasure and social inhibition after 6 months. This effect disappeared almost completely after 5 years.

Discussion

Due to the small sample size the results of this study are tentative and as yet not generalizable. Perhaps our patient groups were too small or the attendance-rate within the rehabilitation-group was not sufficient. Another explanation for our results could be that those patients who after 6 months had to leave the rehabilitation-program showed rebound anxiety because cardiological as well as psychological care would decrease in the near future.

238

In further evaluation studies it will be important to answer questions are: For which patients is the rehabilitation-program at issue beneficial and consequently for which patients is the program contra-indicated. The manner in which the Capri-program should be carried out still requires much research and ingenuity.

References

1. Bruce RA, Kusumi F, Bruce EM et al: Cardiovascular and psychological adaptations to prolonged physical training of coronary patients. Cardiology 62:83–84, 1977.
2. Cay EL, Vetter NJ, Philip AE, Dugard P: Psychological status during recovery from an acute heart atack. J Psychosom Res 16:425, 1972.
3. Croog SH, Levine S, Lurie Z: The heart patient and the recovery process. Soc Sci Med 2:111–164, 1968.
4. Diederiks JPM, Sluijs van der H, Weeda HWH, Schobre MG: Predictors of physical acrivity one year after myocardial infarction. Scand J Rehab Med 15:103, 1983.
5. Erdman RAM, Duivenvoorden HJ: Psychological evaluation of a cardiac rehabilitation program: a randomized clinical trial in patients with myocardial infarction. J Card Rehab 10:696–706, 1983.
6. Erdman RAM: M.P.V.H. A Medical Psychological Questionnaire to Assess well-being in cardiac patients (HPPQ). Hart Bull 13:143, 1983.
7. Hellerstein HK: Exercise therapy in recovery disease. Bull N Y Acad Med 44:1028, 1968.
8. Mayou RA: Psychological reactions to myocardial infarction. J R Coll Physicians London 13:103, 1979.
9. Mulcahy R, Hickey N: The rehabilitation of patients with coronary heart disease. Scand J Rehab Med 2:108, 1970.
10. Pyfer HR, Mead WF, Frederick RC et al.: Exercise rehabilitation in coronary heart diseases: community group programs. Arch Phys Med Rehab 342, 1976.
11. Wenger NK: Research related to rehabilitation. Circulation 60:1036, 1979.

25. Psychosomatic Aspects in Secondary Prevention

R. HOPF and J. JORDAN

Abstract

The course of chronic coronary heart disease is dependent among other things on the patient's ability to cope with the concomitant, psychic situation. In patients who can adequately manage the impairment, decrease in vitality, and psychic symptoms seem to be rare. More frequently the patients feel they are heart invalids and just give up or deny their disease and try to go on just as before.

The common depressions, decline in ego, and the diminished value related to their own life makes it necessary not only to follow up cardiologically but also to provide the patient with psychosocial care in interdisciplinary co-operation. Ambulatory heart groups offer the best chances for such intensive care because of the regular, relaxed and trustful contacts between patient and physician.

The first heart group in Frankfurt/M. was founded in autumn, 1974. Because of the great number of patients who gave their written consent for their readiness for participation we were forced to make a selection. Patients with comparable findings were assigned to form pairs. Their assignment to either the heart group (HG) or the control group (CG) was decided by chance. The patients had a systematic follow-up in 1980. And they are still being followed up.

Of the initial 14 patients from each heart and control group, there were 12 of the HG-group and 11 of the CG-group still alive in 1980. Three of the HG-patients did not longer participate in an ambulatory cardiac exercise program then but were still followed up. As could be expected, the risk factors were under better control in HG-patients, their physical ability due to stress-testing had improved. More impressing, however, were the patient's ways of life.

In the HG-group 7 patients were still working versus only 4 in the CG-group. They were more content with their lives and occupations. Most patients' outlook on life had been influenced by their disease and had caused them to focus their attention more on their families. Patients of the HG-group planned their lives more consciously, they showed more self-confidence and were more optimistic regarding the future. On the other hand, depressions and resignations were nearly twice as frequent in the CG-group.

Rehabilitation in ambulatory heart groups provides the opportunity for continuous follow-up and especially individual support in mastering the disease. This chance should not be denied any patient.

Introduction

Sport as therapy for angina pectoris has traditionally been used for some 200 years. Ambulatory cardiac exercise programs have however only reached their current levels of significance since Gottheiner in Israel [2] and Hellstein in the USA [5] could prove that heart patients can sometimes astonishingly improve their physical capabilities through regular, controlled sport activities.

In Germany Hartmann [4] was the first to include patients, who had suffered a myocardial infarction, into an exercise group for disabled persons and to instruct them in an exercise program. Nowadays, there are more than 20,000 heart patients in ambulatory cardiac exercise programs in Germany.

This proves that heart patients urgently desire such a form of personal and intensive care. From the medical point of view, these groups provide ideal opportunities for complete, medical, long-term care. Due to their particular style of work, these groups offer also an opportunity for detailed instruction and patient guidance.

Rehabilitation does not mean merely exercise or training. As early as 1967, the definition of WHO took into consideration that rehabilitation, besides improving physical ability, has to aim at psychosocial adaptation. This means achieving a normal social life for heart patients as far as possible. According to Harbauer [3], psychological, psychiatric and psychotherapeutic knowledge indicates that precisely this group experience can avoid the individual isolation problems and lead him back as part of the social group. Human life can best develop as a member of a protecting group.

We have gathered experience with ambulatory heart groups for ten years now. Right from the beginning, it seemed important for us to study the psychic and social influence of exercise and of group experience on the patients and their families beyond the physical effects which could be measured. Rehabilitation can only be called successful if the patients learn to accept their disease and to cope with problems imposed on them by their diminished physical capability if present [6].

Patients and Methods

In 1974 we wrote to a total of 56 patients with angiographically confirmed coronary heart disease and a physical stress tolerance of at least 75 watts/1.73 m² body-surface from 4 to 6 minutes. The patients were asked whether they were interested in taking part in an ambulatory rehabilitation program regularly. Twenty-eight patients gave their written consent to participate. These patients were grouped in pairs according to their clinical and angiographic findings. (The angiographic findings were classified according to their score for the quantification of coronary sclerosis or left ventricular function, respectively [7]). After that, it was randomly decided who of each patient-pair was assigned to the heart group or the control group. Thus, comparability between both groups was achieved in terms of age, size, body weight, social status as well as physical ability, coronary angiographic findings and left ventricular function. See Table 1 for the data. The heart group (HG) patients met once a week for rehabilitation program during 5½ years, while the control group (CG) had no special maintenance other than routine clinical follow-ups. At the end of these 5½ years both groups were scrutinized with respect to their clinical findings as well as to their psychosocial conditions by questionnaires which had to be anonymously answered [1].

In 1984 another investigation encompassing 26 participants of the rehabilitation program was performed. Some of those patients had taken part in the heart-group for several months, 11, however, for more than 6 years. Some of these patients had been participants in the first study. The patients' ages ranged from 40 to 65 years; the mean was 56 years. At the time of investigation the patients had been ill for an average of 10 years.

Results of the First Study

After 5½ years, 2 HG-patients and 3 CG-patients had died. One HG-patient had left the group too long before to be included into the study. Another 3

Table 1. Heart Group and Control Group

	Heart Group (n = 14)	Control Group (n = 14)
Age (years)	33- 64 (50.1± 6.7)	41- 63 (50.8± 6.3)
Height(cm)	163-186 (174 ± 5.7)	160-180 (171.0± 6.0)
Weight (kg)	65- 85 (75.3± 7.0)	59- 86 (72.6± 9.4)
Minimal work load tolerated (watts/1.73 m²)	75	75
Coronary Score	10- 48 (25.0±10.0)	5- 55 (25.6±12.3)
Ventricle Score	1- 10 (4.1± 2.4)	0- 12 (3.6± 3.2)

patients had left the HG-group due to professional reasons, too great a distance to home and knee joint arthrosis but were taken into consideration in terms of the follow-up. All these 11 patients had a systematic follow-up and all of them fully answered the questionnaires about their psychosocial conditions. The corresponding 11 CG-patients also completed the questionnaires. We were able to follow-up clinically 8 of them.

Clinical Findings

In the HG-patients body weight had a mean increase of 0.9 kg, in the CG-patients 4.5 kg. The blood pressure values showed a systolic decrease of 10 mm Hg and diastolical 9 mm Hg. The control group on the other hand showed a systolic increase of 22 and diastolic 9 mm Hg. Values for cholesterine had slightly increased in the HG-group as well as in the CG-group by a mean of 26 and 20 mg/dl, respectively. Triglycerides were slightly reduced in the HG-group by a mean of 29 mg/dl, whereas in the CG they were increased by 21 mg/dl.

The ergometric investigation showed that HG-group patients could be placed under stress in the mean 138 watts/1.73 m^2 body surface. This means an increase by 20 watts. CG-patients only tolerated stressing up to a mean of 93 watts/1.73 m^2. In other words their physical ability had decreased by 24 watts compared to the previous follow-up. It has to be taken into account that the mean duration of stress took 346 seconds in the HG-group and thus, was longer than in the CG-group with a mean stress tolerance of maximal 311 seconds.

Heart volume had not changed in the heart group (mean 832 and 835 ml/1.73 m^2 body surface) whereas in the CG-group it had slightly increased from 881 to 928 ml/1.73 m^2 body surface (Table 2).

Table 2. Effects of Ambulatory Rehabilitation Program

	Heart Group (n = 11)		Control Group (n = 11)	
	1974	1980	1974	1980
Weight (kg)	73.5± 7	74.4± 5.4	72.6± 9.4	76.6± 8.4
RR sysystolic (mmHg)	138 ± 14	128 ± 19	128 ± 8	150 ± 15
diastolic (mmHg)	86 ± 11	80 ± 6	74 ± 6	85 ± 6
Cholesterol (mg/dl)	244 ± 56	270 ± 65	239 ± 44	259 ± 48
Triglycerides (mg/dl)	151 ± 70	122 ± 60	164 ± 63	185 ± 57
Heart Volume (ml/1.73 m^2)	832 ±178	835 ±131	881 ±201	928 ±232
Work Load (watts/1.73 m^2)	118 ± 34	138 ± 29	117 ± 17	93 ± 15
Tolerated duration of ergometry (sec)	357 ± 9	346 ± 31	340 ± 42	311 ± 55

The Patients' Outlook on Life

The discrepancies concerning the outlook on life were impressive. The patients of both groups were comparable according to education, profession and family status. At the follow-up, only 4 HG-patients vs. 7 CG-patients had retired. Those patients in the HG-group who had not retired worked fewer hours than those of the CG-group (41.4 vs 43.5 hours per week). Most of these patients were satisfied with their occupations and felt they were well able to cope with their tasks (Table 3).

Similar observations were made in their private lives. HG-patients focused their attention more on their families. This became obvious by the increased time the patients spent with their relatives. It was alarming that 2 CG-patients said they felt they were a burden to their families. They felt they had no support in dealing with their problems. For another patient the family was a problem in itself. The HG-patients – in contrast to the CG-patients – based on the feeling that they lived more consiously than thealthy persons of the same age and could take more controlled stress, had set goals which they considered worthwile achieving and considered their lives 'worthwhile'. Three CG-patients but only 1 HG-patient said their basic attitude was depressive (Tables 4, 5).

Dizziness, numbness of the limbs, frequent headaches, weight problems, rapid tiring or sleep disturbances indicated manifest or latent depressions. These symptoms were by far more frequent in the CG-group than in the HG-group. Prior to the start of the program, these symptoms were nearly evenly distributed among both groups (Table 6).

Despite the HG-patients beeing more health-conscious and better informed about their disease they rarely showed a feeling of inferiority compared to the CG-patients. They even reported to have gained in self-respect

Table 3. Effects of Ambulatory Rehabilitation Program

	Heart Group (n = 11)	Control Group (N = 11)
Still Working	7	4
Job is very important	5	4
Fully able to take stress at work	4	1
Mean Weekly working hours	41.4	43.5
Works generally overtime	2	3
Retired	4	7
Content with job/occupation: very	2	1
well	8	4
with restriction	1	6
not at all	0	0

Table 4. Effects of Ambulatory Rehabilitation Program

	Heart Group (n = 11)	Control Group (n = 11)
Outlook on life influenced		
by coronary artery disease: strongly:	7	5
slightly:	1	4
not at all:	3	2
More time for the family:	11	10
Family is a burden:	0	1
I am a burden to the family:	0	2
Recreational activities: family:	10	9
friends:	4	2
single:	2	1
Practising sports regularly: 2 times a week:	11	0
Religion is important:	11	8
Self-confidence: increased:	7	4
same as before:	3	5
decreased:	1	2
Nicotine:	1	1

Table 5. Effects of Ambulatory Rehabilitation Program

	Heart Group (n = 11)	Control Group (n = 11)
'Has Personality Changed?'		
Yes	6	4
No	4	7
Living more conscious than others	10	6
Increase in self-confidence	8	4
Life is future-oriented	9	6

despite their disease, that is to say they lived more consciously and intensely than before, their behaviour towards others having favourably changed. Compared to the CG-patients those of the HG-group reported to be less irritable, to be on good terms with their relatives and to be content with their standard of living despite reduced incomes due to their disease. HG-patients generally showed more drive and, for example in planning their vacations more flexibility. They regularly did some light sport at home once or twice a week. On the whole their activities seemed to be more pleasure-oriented and almost free of anxiety (Table 4).

Table 6. Effects of Ambulatory Rehabilitation Program

Symptoms	Heart Group (n = 11)	Control Group (n = 11)
Angina pectoris	7	8
Depressive	1	3
Rapidly exhausted	7	9
Lack of drive	4	6
Fear to fail	2	3
Puffers from strain	1	6
Discontented	2	4
Irritable	4	7
Numbness of the limbs	4	8
Sleep disturbances	6	5
Too little sleep	4	7

Judging from the frequency of complaints about stomach problems which correlated to regular aspirin usage, their compliance as far as taking the medication was concerned, was obviously favourably influenced.

Results of the Second Study

Twelve of the 26 patients had retired and of the 14 patients still at their jobs only 6 said they worked overtime regularly. On the whole the working patients were quite content with their occupations, although half of them complained of job related nervous stress. Their jobs rated high among all 14 patients, and 11 claimed to be able to take full stress (Table 7).

Despite suffering from their disease on an average for 10 years, all patients reported they felt better now than at the onset of symptoms, even though 10 of them often had cardiac troubles. In only 4 cases did the disease lead to a feeling of inferiority compared to friends and acquaintances.

Half of these patients complained of irritability and 18 were still inclined to swallow private or job-related anger. Half of the patients were convinced

Table 7. 2. Study (Survey based on questionnaires)

Participation of 26 patients in ambulatory cardiac rehabilitation program
Age: 40-65 years, x̄: 56 years
Duration of participation: 3 months till > 6 years

Working:	14/26
Subjectively fully fit, strain is realy felt:	11/26
Working generally overtime:	6/26

that their outlook on life had been changed by their disease and by the support received in the course of the program. They stated in particular that they now lived more consciously. Nearly all the patients said they enjoyed life, only 2 complained of having serious problems. Thus, the results of the first study were essentially confirmed and also supported by the fact that half of the patients spent more time with their families than at the onset of symptoms. Family ties were generally felt to be helpful and extremely important. None of the patients felt they were a burden on their relatives (Table 8).

Discussion

Other studies (Ziegeler, 1982 [14], 1983 [15]; Kerekjarto, 1983 [8]; Maas, 1981 [9]; Wishnie et al., 1971 [2] and Wynn, 1967 [13]) showed that coronary artery disease may cause grave changes within the family relationships. It may be considered proved that the wives of patients with myocardial infarction are confronted with a variety of stress and often feel unable to cope with it. During their husbands' hospitalization they for the most part have to rely on information from the patients. Thus they are not sufficiently able to follow the course of rehabilitation or disease. On the other hand they have to take over an enormous part of the responsibility after the patient has been discharged. As a consequence, communication may be contradictory in many ways (Skelton and Dominian, 1973 [11]). Most wives feel a sense of guilt and try to take good care of the partner and to spare him troubles, very often overdoing it and thus, unconsciously exerting dominance and restraint. This often results in the feeling that their partners show resistance. Repeated attacks of angina pectoris may lead to the feeling of helplessness in the partner who does not know whether to call for the physician or not. The partner also is helpless and does not kwow how to react if

Table 8. 2. Study (Survey based on questionnaires)

Perception of disease (n = 26)	
Duration of disease:	$\bar{x}$: 10 years
Frequent cardiac complaints:	10/26
Condition better than at onset of complaints:	25/26
Frequent decline in ego:	4/26
Help and support by the family:	21/26
Increased irritability:	13/26
Privat/vocational troubles are 'swallowed':	18/26
Fears are *not* always discussed with partner:	13/26

there are changes in the behaviour of the patient e.g. if they recognize the signs of job-related stress or see that the partner acts in a way injurious to his health e.g. smoking, sleep or physical exercise deficit. Often the partners had to make the painful experience that the patients feeling for their family or partners subsided before the onset of disease. Induced by this experience, the partners may unconsciously and subtly make reproaches to or be disappointed by each other. A recent study by the Health Insruance Plan of Greater New York (Rubberman et al., 1984 [10]) points out the importance of emotional stress resulting from direct social relationships of the patients. Emotional isolation and psychic stress within the family may under certain conditions be the very factors which alone can increase infarct mortality rate fourfold.

We studied patients taking part in an ambulatory rehabilitation program or those who were at least interested in them. Thus, we naturally took into consideration only those patients who already were health conscious and interested in taking part in the program. Thus it might have been easier for us to influence their way of living. Naturally it should be our ultimate aim to inform every patient about the disease and the resulting consequences as early as possible, to motivate each to take part in an heart group programs. Therefore it is absolutely necessary to point out to the patient and to make him aware of the importance of rehabilitation and secondary prevention by rehabilitation programs and to induce him to take part in it. This should already be done in the admitting hospital as well as the rehabilitation center. We have made the experience that during the acute phase of their disease the patients can more easily be motivated to take an active part in their therapy. For the future we must not accept that only about 30% of the patients with myocardial infarction can be motivated to take part in heart groups. As our results demonstrate these programs offer manifold ways to help coronary heart patients.

Our study takes into account only a selected group of patients and our results refer to only a small number but painstakingly and systematically examined patients. Nevertheless, our results concur with the experience of others and thus seem to be of general validity.

Our results show that the patients without exception appreciate the offer of information and of help to deal with their problems within the heart group and that they learn to handle their situation emotionally with more frankness. As a result, treatment in heart groups helps to promote the development of constructive attitudes which enable the patient to deal more adequately with himself and his anxieties at home or on the job. One aspect of this positive management is that the patients learn to recognize their disease-related limitations at an early stage, and thus are better prepared to accept this condition. They are able to cope with anxieties and depressive moods instead of having to deny them; and they lead fuller lives which are pleasure-oriented and confident in the future, even though they are fully aware of the risks associated with their disease. We have observed that, while increased devotion to partner or family can be positive in many respects, it may also create new problems in the partner relationship. On the other hand, other studies, as well as our own, have shown that the disease can put a great deal of pressure on partners and relatives. They try to take good care of the patient and take problems off his hands. In the process, they may often repress their own anxieties, wishes, and aggressions, which can lead to chronic emotional strain as well as other problems in the relationship which could be prevented.

Therefore our studies suggest that it would be advisable to bring partners of heart patients, especially those with coronary artery disease, into the therapy situation at an earlier stage. They should be provided with more detailed information and also given the opportunity to participate in the ambulatory cardiac rehabilitation program. In this way, they could share their experiences with the partners of other heart patients. This could also help to facilitate the mechanisms involved in managing the disease and lead to a more open, 'heart-to-heart' communication in the emotional relationship between the partners.

References

1. Görge G: Effekte einer fünfjährigen Betreuung Herzkranker in einer ambulanten Herzgruppe im Vergleich zu einer Kontrollgruppe. Inaugural-Dissertation, Frankfurt, 1982.
2. Gottheiner V: Die Renaissance der Zivilisationskrankheiten und die Wiederherstellung des Herz- und Gefäßleidenden durch maximale körperliche Übung. Die Rehabilitation 3:172–181 and Die Rehabilitation 5:104–116, 1964, 1966.
3. Harbauer H: Psychosoziale Aspekte der Bewegungstherapie. In: Hopf R, Kaltenbach M (eds). Bewegungstherapie für Herzkranke. Urban und Schwarzenberg, München Wien Baltimore, p 165–168, 1981.
4. Hartmann KO: Schorndorfer Modell. In: Hopf R, Kaltenbach M (eds). Bewegungstherapie für Herzkranke. Urban und Schwarzenberg, München Wien Baltimore, p 204–214, 1981.
5. Hellerstein HK, Hornstein ER, Goldberg AN, Dulando AG, Friedman EK, Hirsch EZ, Marik S: The influence of active conditioning upon subjects with coronary artery disease. Can Med Assoc 7 96:901, 1967.
6. Hopf R, Kaltenbach M: Frankfurter Modell. In: Hopf R, Kaltenbach M (eds). Bewegungstherapie für Herskranke. Urban und Schwarzenberg, München Wien Baltimore, p 190–194.
7. Kaltenbach M, Bussmann W-D, Giebeler W: Ziele und zukünftige Entwicklung der Bewegungstherapie für Herzkranke. In: Hopf R, Kaltenbach M (eds). Bewegungstherapie für Herzkranke. Urban und Schwarzenberg, München Wien Baltimore, p 244–250, 1981.
8. Kerekjarto M, von Krasemann EO, Maas G: Wie leben Frührentner nach Herzinfarkt?. Münch Med Wschr 125 34:722–726, 1983.
9. Maas M: Die psychosoziale Lage des Herzinfarkt-Frührentners. Inaugural-Dissertation, Hamburg, 1981.

10. Ruberman W, Weinblatt E, Goldberg J, Chaudhary B: Psychosocial influences on mortality after myocardial infarction. The New England Journal of Medicine 311 9:552 f, 1984.

11. Skelton M, Dominian I: Psychological Stress in wives of patients with myocardial infarction. Br Med J 2:101–103, 1973.

12. Wishnie HA, Wackett TB, Casseu HN: Psychological hazards of convalescence following myocardial infarction. J of the American medical Association 215:1292 f, 1971.

13. Wynn A: Unwarranted emotional distress in men with ischaemic heart disease. Medical Journal of Australia 2:847–851, 1967.

14. Ziegeler G: Individuelle und familiäre Bewältigungsstategien am Beispiel von Herzinfarkt und Diabetes. In: Angermeyer, freyberger (eds) Chronisch Kranke Erwachsene in der Familie, 1982.

15. Ziegeler G: Soll der Lebenspartner in die ambulante Herzgruppe eingezogen werden? In: Halhuber C (ed). Ambulante Herzgruppen – Neue Aspekte 83 Medizin und Information, p 87–92, 1983.

26. Social Isolation and Attitudes Towards Stress: A Behavioral Trap for Patients After Myocardial Infarction

A. EDER, G. CZERWENKA-WENKSTETTEN and
M. NIEDERBERGER

Abstract

Personality traits are known to be risk factors in the occurrence of myocardial infarction and are likely to also influence the success of rehabilitation and secondary prevention. Main elements of these traits are a high level of anxiety and suppressed aggressiveness, and a high need for support of the system of self-esteem through performance and success. These elements form a vicious circle in which social isolation plays an important role.

Methods: We conducted a study in 192 patients after MI and a control group of 67 persons, matched according to socio-demographic criteria. The research instruments were:

1. A questionnaire assessing the patient's attitudes towards vocational stress.

2. The Giessen-Test of personality traits.

3. A time-budget questionnaire, assessing the patient's subjective evaluation of the activities of his daily routine.

Results: Patients with more often than the control group consider vocational stress inevitable and explain this inevitability by their present life situation and professional situation. The Giessen-Test shows MI patients to have a stronger tendency towards avoiding company, suppressing anger, feeling estranged from their social environment, and being more compulsively focused on excelling others than do persons of the control group.

MI patients consider leisure time spent with friends and time spent with the partner less agreeable, time spent with professional work more agreeable than the persons of the control group.

Conclusions: From our results and their interpretation we deduct the necessity for MI patients to gain insight into the vicious circle which systematically induces them to expose themselves to over-charge. We suggest this to be achieved through two parallel therapeutical goals:

1. The enhancement of coping strategies in order to enable the patient to go through the amount of stress necessary for the support of his self-esteem.
2. Encouragement to communication and engagement in social activities in order to open up new resources for emotional support and thereby self-esteem.

This therapeutic approach seems more likely to cause long-term behavioral changes than would mere encouragement of the patient to progressively increase performance or the simple advice to avoid stressful situations.

Introduction

Recent literature on the psychosocial determinants of myocardial infarction (MI) reveals quite clearly that there is a psychological predisposition for the readiness to expose oneself to stress. Conclusions of this type can be drawn even from earlier publications on coronary-prone behaviour patterns (e.g. Friedman, Rosenman, 1960). The syndrome of coronary-prone behaviour pattern, however, seems to be quite resistent to psychotherapy in many cases: According to our hypotheses, this is mainly due to reasons that have to be traced in the psychosocial environment of the patients. In order to obtain further information on a possible vicious circle inducing patients after MI to systematically overloading themselves, we have tried to measure both their readiness to accept stress in their daily lives as well as the readiness to rely on other persons.

Material and methods

We carried out a study with 192 patients after MI – 97 had suffered an infarction within one year prior to the investigation, 95 earlier – and a control group of 67 persons, matched according to socio-demographic criteria.* The research instruments were:
1. A questionnaire assessing the patient's attitudes towards vocational stress, designed by Kemeter and Eder, first described by Eder et al., 1982.
2. The Giessen-Test of personality traits (Beckmann, Richter, 1972).
3. A time-budget questionnaire, assessing the patient's subjective evaluation of the activities of his daily routine (Eder, 1979).

* The study was supported by the Austrian Ministry of Health and Environmental Protection.

Results

1. Attitudes towards vocational stress

The patient's responses to a series of questions dealing with their attitudes towards vocational stress differed significantly from the ones of the control group in the following aspects.

Mere refusal of vocational stress is significantly less frequent in patients after MI than in persons of the control group: 20% of patients with recent infarction and 13% of the patients with earlier infarction, but 28% of the control group agree with the statement: 'I don't have vocational stress and I don't want any'.

On the other hand, patients after infarction agree to a significantly higher extent with statements that define stress as an outside obtrusion that cannot be evaded, which is reflected in the following formulations:

Table 1. Percentage of persons agreeing with the following statements

Vocational stress:	Pat. w recent MI (N = 97)	Pat. w. earlier MI (N = 95)	Controls (N = 67)	Chi Sqr (P<)
I don't have it and I don't want it	20	13	28	05
I don't have it, sometimes that's boring	6	5	8	
I do hace it and I can't help it	31	25	5	.001
I do have it, and I cope with it as well as I can	28	43	31	.001
I do have it and somehow I like it because it keeps me from thinking too much about other things	11	8	6	
I do have it and somehow I like it because I need the feeling of being efficient	37	36	28	
I would be ready to accept it although I don't like it because I need the feeling of being efficient	19	14	8	
I do have it and must endure it because things which I don't do myself just are not done	19	23	9	.003
I must endure it in order to be able to compete with my colleagues	21	21	3	.003
I must endure it in order to get along with my boss	14	16	9	
I·must endure it because that's what they expect from me, given my salary	33	27	9	.002
I must endure it because I need the money	14	18	5	.05
I accept it because otherwise I would be bored	9	12	8	

— 'I do have vocational stress and I cannot help it'
— 'I do have vocational stress and must endure it because things which I don't do myself just are not done'
— I do have vocational stress and must endure it in order to be able to compete with my colleagues'
— I do have vocational stress and must endure it because that's what they expect from me, given my salary'
— 'I do have vocational stress and must endure it because I need the money'.

In the other statements of this part of the questionnaire, stress is being defined as desirable for at least some reason, like: 'I do have vocational stress and somehow I like it because it keeps me from thinking too much about other things'. In these statements, too, patients after MI tend to accept stress more readily than persons of the control group. These results are less marked, however, and statistically not significant.

2. Intimacy with other people

In the items of the Giessen-Test, patients after MI tend to agree with the following items significantly more often than persons of the control group:
— 'I think I tend to suppress anger'
— 'I have the impression that I am very interested in outdoing other people'

Table 2. Percentage of persons agreeing with selected items of the Giessen-Test

Item-Nr		Pat. w. recent MI (N = 97)	Pat. w. earlier MI (N = 96)	Contr. (N = 67)	Chi Sqr (P<)
2	I think I tend to look for company	26	26	51	.002
6	I think I tend to suppress anger	59	45	32	02
7	I think I am very interested in outdoing other pesons	25	25	11	.05
12	I think I tend to avoid close contact with another person	22	21	11	
25	I think I feel emotionally rather distant to other people	20	13	3	.02
39	I find it hard to be really unrestrained	32	31	14	

— 'I tend to avoid close contact with another person'
— 'I feel rather distant to other people'
Patients after MI agree significantly less often with the statement:
— 'I tend to look for company'.

3. Preference of professional work over leisure with family and friends

In a time-budget questionnaire, patients and controls were confronted with a list of activities of daily routine and were asked to state with each activity the amount of time spent with it, and to evaluate whether they considered it rather pleasant, or unpleasant, or neutral.

The proportion or those who considered time spent with professional work pleasant was significant higher in patients after MI than in the control group; the proportion of those who considered time spent with the partner and leisure with friends pleasant was significantly smaller in patients after MI (Table 3).

Conclusions

The positive evaluation of professional work by patients after MI at first sight seems to prove their higher readiness to accept vocational stress as a necessary element of their lives: but they consider stress as being imposed upon them, rather than being a subjective necessity, as can be seen in their responses to statements that try to measure attitudes towards vocational stress.

At the same time, patients after MI seem to be less ready to spend time with their partners and friends, which becomes plausible when we consider that they also feel emotionally distant to other people, as can be seen in the responses to the Giessen-Test.

Table 3. Evaluation of some of the activities of daily routine: Percentage of Persons who rate as pleasant

	Pat. w. recent MI (N = 97)	Pat. w. earlier MI (N = 95)	Controls (N = 67)	Chi Sqr (P<)
Professional work	45	46	33	.05
Time spent with partner	62	68	74	.05
Leisure with friends	59	52	76	.001
Just doing nothing	32	26	49	

These results confirm an idea by G. Czerwenka-Wenkstetten which has been previously presented by the authors (Niederberger et al., 1982), where we tried to design a systematic interaction between attitudinal elements in the lives of patients after MI. Czerwenka calls this interaction a spiral of anxiety and performance: At a certain point in time in the biography of MI patients, a typical social misunderstanding is evoked. It can be triggered by events that date back to childhood, but can also occur throughout professional work. Main elements of this social misunderstanding are:

1. A high amount of vocational stress leaves little room for social activities and thereby probably also reduces the feeling of security that could be transmitted through intimacy with other people. Given the high feeling of professional competence and the low feeling of social competence that seems to be typical for patients after MI, it is a logical reaction for them to try to compensate a loss of emotional security by increased performance.

2. Exaggerated performance sooner or later leads to an exhaustion of physical capacities; at this point in time, the feeling of security and self-esteem is endangered. All energy available is then being spent on increased performance, which leads to further social isolation, thus constituting the beginning of a vicious circle, which in turn often also obstructs psychotherapeutical Intervention.

The decisive importance of the collapse of self-esteem in the process of rehabilitation from MI has been pointed out previously by the authors (Niederberger et al., 1982), as well as by other researchers (Van Der Walk, 1967; Bastians, 1968).

Since performance is a necessary prerequisite for self-esteem in many patients with MI, a reduction of the ability to perform represents a threat to self-esteem. Hence results the ambition of these patients to concentrate all forces on increased performance after an infarction.

The consequences for therapeutic intervention which we deducted from this, focused on showing the patient that social status, affection and self-esteem could be gained through processes that are unrelated to performance. An overt 'therapeutic attack' on the patient's compulsive desire for maximum performance could result in increased anxiety in two ways: trying to help the patient increase performance would expose him to fears of failure; trying to convince him of the unnecessity of performance would endanger his system of self-esteem.

A central element in the therapeutic process is thus the connection between performance and affection. Therapy therefore has to aim at both mechanisms:

1. by enhancing coping mechanisms for stress so that the patient becomes more able to cope with the amount of stress which he considers necessary, and

2. by enhancing the ability to communicate and to engage in social activi-

ties in order to find another support for self-esteem and feelings of security, and thereby reduce his feeling of necessity to perform and to cope with stress.

The long term goal of therapy should be to help the patient to gain insight into and control of the process which systematically induces him to expose himself to vocational overload.

This kind of procedure seems more likely to cause long term behavioral changes than would mere encouragement of the patient to slowly increase performance or the simple advice to avoid stressful situations.

References

1. Bastiaans J: Psychoanalytic investigations on the psychic aspects of acute myocardial infarction. Psychother Psychosom 16, 1968.
2. Beckmann D, Richter HE: Giessen-Test. Bern-Stuffgart-Wien 1975.
3. Eder A: Ein Meßansatz subjektiven Lebensgefüls zum Vergleich von Patienten mit vorwiegend organischer mit solchen mit vorwiegend psychischer Mitbedingtheit. In: Strotzka et al.: Ökonomische Aspekte psychosomatischer und psychosozialer Erkrankungen. Wien Inst f Gesellschaftspolitik 1979.
4. Eder A, Kemeter P, Springer-Kremser M: Cycle disturbances, psychosomatic complaints, and self-image: an analysis of interdependencies between self-perception and psychosomatic disturbances. J Psychosom Obstetrics and Gyn 1:3-4, 1982.
5. Friedman M, Rosenman RH: Overt behavoir patterns in coronary disease. J Amer Med Ass 173:1320-1325, 1960.
6. Niederberger M, Czerwenka-Wenkstetten G, Eder A: Is There Sufficient Appreciation of Vocational Counseling? In: Mathes P, Halhuber MJ (eds): Controversies in Cardiac Rehabilitation. Berlin-Heidelberg-New York, 1982.
7. Van der Valk JM, Groen IJ: Personality structure and conflict situation in patients with myocardial infarctions. J Psychosom Res 11, 1967.

VI. The Role of Reperfusion in Secondary Prevention

27. Effect of Percutaneous Transluminal Coronary Angioplasty

G. KOBER, C. VALLBRACHT, R. HOPF, B. KUNKEL and
M. KALTENBACH

Abstract

Transluminal coronary angioplasty (TCA) has proved to be successful in dilating high-grade stenotic vessel segments. Due to a reduction in the stenosis responsible for angina pectoris and ischemic reactions in the exercise ECG the patients are asymptomatic and can be fully stressed the day after angioplasty provided that complete revascularization has been achieved.

As far as quality of life and rehabilitation are concerned long-term success and restenosis rate which become apparent for example in the frequency of performed bypass graft operations and patients still working are of decisive importance.

Mostly patients can resume work a week after successful angioplasty. Medium-term (3 months) and long-term (12 months after TCA) success can be noninvasively assessed by symptoms and ischemic reactions in the exercise ECG. The hardest criterion is angiographic follow-up. These methods show comparable long-term success of 80 to 85%.

The majority of the patients who had undergone successful TCA were still improved and working at a follow-up 3 to 6 years (mean 3.8 years) later. Only in 6% of the patients bypass graft surgery had been performed in the meantime. Out of those patients in whom dilatation was not successful 50% had undergone surgery and a markedly lower percentage was able to work.

Successful revascularization by TCA shows good long-term results during a follow-up period of till now up to 7 years. Regional restenoses predominantly occur within the first 3 months after TCA. Long-term deterioration is often due to progressive primary disease.

Introduction

Transluminal coronary angioplasty (TCA) has been successfully applied to

262

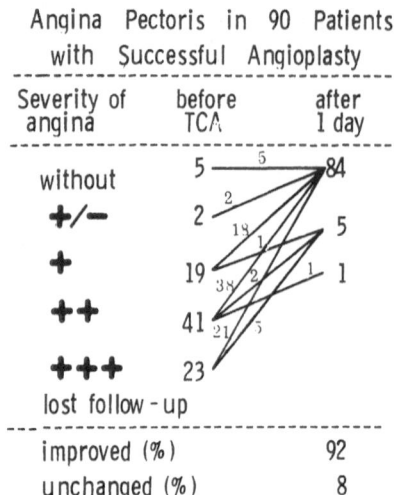

Angina Pectoris in 90 Patients with Successful Angioplasty

Severity of angina	before TCA	after 1 day
without	5	84
+/−	2	5
+	19	1
++	41	
+++	23	
lost follow-up		
improved (%)		92
unchanged (%)		8

Figure 1. Severity of angina pectoris before and after coronary angioplasty (TCA). Angina is graded as uncharacteristic (+/−), slight (+), moderate (++) and severe(+++).

dilate high-grade stenotic coronary vessel segments since its introduction into the treatment of coronary heart disease in 1977. Since October 1977 1040 TCA procedures have been performed in the University Hospital of Frankfurt. Acute success-rate increased from 52% to 91%. In 50 patients (4.8%) emergency bypass operations were necessary, Four patients, three with double-vessel disease and with old myocardial infarctions, died as a consequence of an unsuccessful TCA of a non-infarct-related vessel. This means a fatality rate of 0.4%.

Angioplasty is indicated in patients with clinical symptoms of angina pectoris mostly with ischemic changes in the exercise ECG, the thallium scintigram or the radionuclide ventriculogram. In few patients mostly after a non-transmural infarction several months ago neither angina pectoris nor ischemia could be induced. All patients had high-grade organic coronary artery stenoses which in most cases could be reduced to a hemodynamically ineffective or in a few cases to a minor hemodynamically effective degree.

Methods and results

In a subgroup of 90 patients with successful TCA 83 patients had angina pectoris of varying severity immediately before TCA, 2 had rather uncharacteristic symptoms, 5 had no angina pectoris. In all symptomatic patients angina pectoris was improved after TCA, 84 patients were absolutely symptom- free (Fig. 1).

```
Ischemic  Reaction  in  the  Exercise-ECG
in  90  Patients  with  Successful  TCA
-----------------------------------------------
Severity of        before          after
ischemia            TCA            1 day
-----------------------------------------------
without            8  ⁸           75
+/-                4      ₂         0
+ (<2mm)          37  ³⁵  ₂       14
++ (2-4mm)        29  ¹⁹  ⁹        1
+++ (>4mm)         9      ⁸
at rest            3  ₃
Significant
ischemia          87%            17%
-----------------------------------------------
improved                         83%
unchanged                         3%
∅ or +/-          13%
```

Figure 2. Severity of ischemia in the exercise-electrocardiogram before and after angioplasty. Ischemia is graded as uncharacteristic (+/−), slight (+), moderate (+ +) and severe (+ + +). Three patients had ischemia at rest.

In 78 (87%) of the 90 patients the exercise ECG before TCA definitely showed pathologic changes of different severity. In 4 patients changes were of only borderline degree and in 8 patients there were no pathologic findings. The day after dilatation exercise-ECG was normal in 75 patients, had improved in 10 patients and not changed or slightly deteriorated in 5 patients (Fig. 2).

In all patients coronary angiograms before TCA showed luminal reduction of more than 50%. In 84 percent of the patients percentage stenosis was higher than 75% and in half of the patients it was 90% and more. After dilatation percentage stenosis was reduced to less than 50% in 81% of the patients. None of them had remaining stenosis of 75% or more. Mean stenosis had decreased from 84% to 33% (Table 1).

Table 1. Diameter Stenosis (%) in 90 Patients with Successful TCA

Stenosis	Before TCA (% of patients)	Immediately after (% of Patients)
< 50%	0	81
< 75%	100	19
< 90%	84	0
≥ 90%	49	0
% stenosis ($\bar{x}$)	84%	33%

Table 2. Questionnaires to 243 Patients (1978 to 1981)

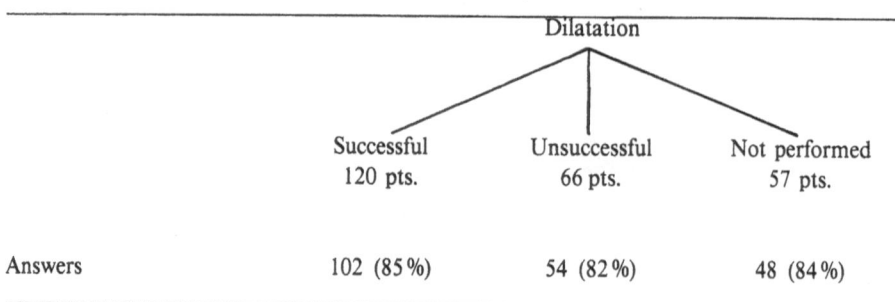

	Successful 120 pts.	Unsuccessful 66 pts.	Not performed 57 pts.
Answers	102 (85%)	54 (82%)	48 (84%)

Thus, acute reduction in percentage stenosis to a hemodynamically inef-fective degree and consequently complete revascularization in cases of fre-quently existing single vessel disease could be achieved by angioplasty in a high percentage of the patients. Even in cases with multiple vessel disease complete revascularization can be achieved. To calculate the functional improvement, exercise tests with maximal work load already can be per-formed the day after TCA. Usually the acute angiographic result was in good accordance to the gain in exercise capacity and disappearance of ischemic reactions.

At follow-ups 3 and 12 months after angioplasty furthermore good results could be confirmed in the majority of the patients. In a big patients group with 439 repeat angiographies the restenosis rate was 17% within a mean follow-up period of 5.6 months.

To obtain information about the long-term-effect of TCA questionnaires were sent to 243 patients who were referred to our hospital between 1978 and 1981 with the question for an indication for TCA. These patients were assigned to the following three groups:
1. 120 patients in whom dilatation had been successful,
2. 66 patients in whom dilatation had been unsuccessful and
3. 57 patients who had been denied TCA because of minor stenoses or too far advanced coronary disease.

Answers were received from 85% of the 120 patients with acutely suc-

Table 3. Dilatation

		Successful (n = 102)	Unsuccessful (n = 54)	Not performed (n = 48)
Dead	Cardiac	1%	3.6%	2.2%
	others	1%	3.6%	
Bypass		5.9%	50%	33%
Symptoms improved		77%	40%	
Working		61%	43%	63%

Repetitive Coronary Angiograms in 22 Patients

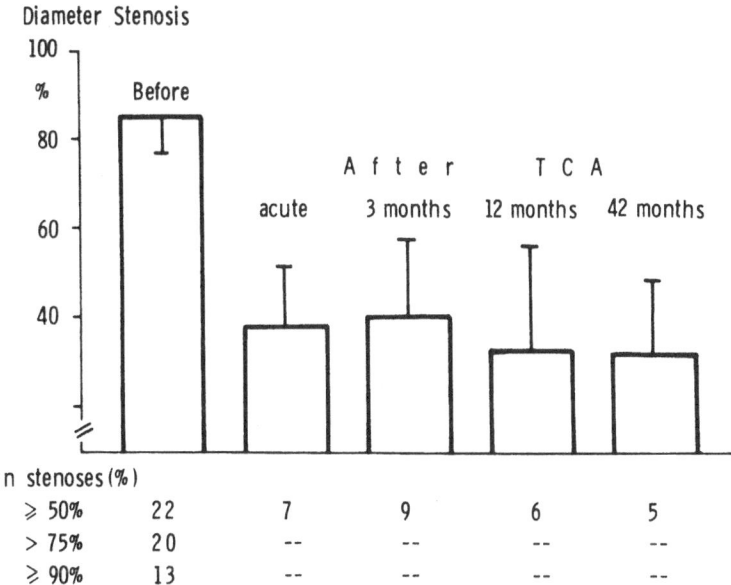

Diameter Stenosis

n stenoses (%)				
≥ 50%	22	7	9	6	5
> 75%	20	--	--	--	--
≥ 90%	13	--	--	--	--

Figure 3. In 22 patients with follow-up angiograms immediately and in the mean 3, 12 and 42 months after angioplasty (TCA) mean residual stenosis of the dilated segment had not changes. Only few stenoses were graded between 50 and 75 %, none was of higher degree.

cessful TCA and from 82 % of the 66 patients with unsuccessful TCA and from 84 % of the 57 patients who had been denied TCA (Table 2).

In the follow-up period of 4-6 years the 3 groups showed relatively low mortality rates (Table 3). It was lowest in the group with successful TCA (2 %). Half of the patients in whom TCA had failed and a third of those who had been denied TCA meanwhile had undergone surgery. In 77 % of the patients who underwent successful TCA clinical findings were still improved compared to 40 % of those with unsuccessful TCA. This information is missing in group 3. A markedly higher percentage of patients in whom

Table 4. Follow-up 4-6 Years after TCA or Bypass-Surgery

Questionnaires (n pts)	TCA 61	Bypass-Surgery 62
Answers	88 %	86 %
Mean Age (years)	53	55
Working	66 %	25 %
Occup. Disability (weeks)		
before	17	25
after	7	38
total	24	64

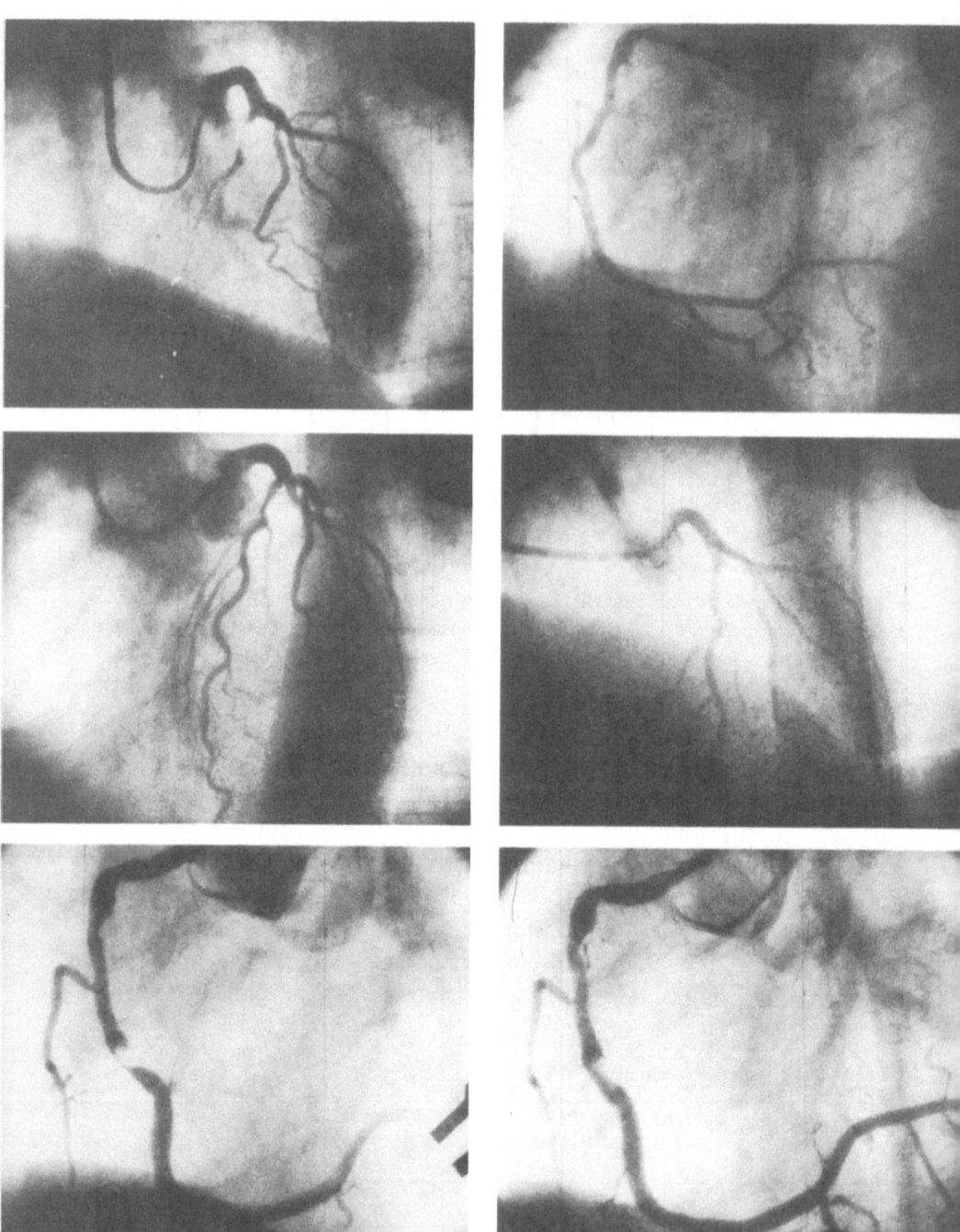

Figure 4a-4f. In 1981 the 54 year old patient showed subtotal proximal LAD-stenosis (4a) and a nearly normal RCA (4b). The good acute TCA-result (4c) could be confirmed after 3 years (4d), but the RCA presented high-grade excentric stenosis (4e), which could be dilated successfully (4 *p* = acute result).

TCA had been successful had returned to work compared to those with unsuccessful TCA.

To quantitate rehabilitational success of TCA a comparison was made between 61 patients with successful TCA and 62 patients who had undergone coronary artery bypass graft surgery (CABG) during the same period (table 4). The number of completed questionnaires and the patients' ages were comparable. 66% of the patients with TCA and 25% of those who had undergone surgery had returned to work. The waiting periods for treatment were nearly equal in both groups. After treatment the period of occupational disability was three times longer in the group with CABG than in the TCA-group. of the patients who underwent TCA 67% had returned to work within 1 to 3 weeks after TCA which never happened after CABG.

Of the 54 patients with successful TCA 22 consented to undergo repeat angiography. This showed good or unchanged regional long-term results in all patients. Before dilatation 20 patients had stenoses of more than 75%. At acute follow-ups and those performed after 3 months and 12 months only few patients had residual stenoses of more than 50% but below 75%. After a mean interval of 42 months following dilatation again only 5 patients had remaining stenoses between 50 and below 75% (Fig. 3) in the dilated coronary segment. In no patient an increase in diameter stenosis of more than 10% had ocurred compared to the study one year after TCA. In 5 patients, however, 4 with primary stenoses in the LAD and 1 in the left circumflex artery, new hemodynamically effective stenoses had developed, 4 in the right coronary artery and 1 in the left circumflex. In the meantime 3 of these patients again had successful dilatation of these new stenoses.

The following figures present the findings in one of these patients (fig. 4a-f). In 1981 the 54 year old patient had subtotal occlusion of the LAD whereas the RCA showed only slight sclerotic changes. The acute result was confirmed by repeat angiography 3 and 12 months later. At repeat angiography 39 months after angioplasty the LAD was still improved but a high-grade excentric stenosis of the right coronary artery was detected and again successfully dilated.

Summary

TCA has proved to be a technique for myocardial revascularization showing not only acute or medium-term but also long-term success over a follow-up period of to date up to 6 years. It reduces or eliminates symptoms, ischemic parameters in the exercise-ECG and stenoses in the angiogram.

In the period between TCA and reinvestigations after 3 and 12 months the majority of patients showed stable angiographic results. Regional restenoses were detected in 17% of the patients within the first year.

Angiographic follow-up studies 3 to 6 years (mean 42 months) after successful angioplasty and still good results after one year showed absence of restenoses in the dilated segments. But progression of the underlying disease led to new stenoses in originally not stenotic vessels in 23% of the patients or in 6.6% of the patients/year.

Taking into consideration the to date still relatively small number of patients no definite differences can be ascertained in terms of mortality and infarctions between those patients successfully treated by TCA and those who had unsuccessful TCA and frequently subsequent bypass surgery. But those patients who underwent successful angioplasty far more frequently had improved clinically and more frequently had returned to work. The periods of occupational disability were markedly shorter after succesful TCA than after CABG.

Angioplasty like bypass-surgery has no influence on the progression of coronary artery disease. Even if long-term success by TCA can be confirmed it must be mentioned that in a considerable percentage of the patients new stenoses develop requiring repeat revascularization.

Consequently it has to be the main aim of treating coronary artery disease to influence the underlying basic disease to prevent progression of coronary sclerosis.

References

1. Grüntzig A, Myler R, Hanna ES, Turina M: Transluminal angioplasty of coronary artery stenosis. Circulation (Abstract) 56:84, 1977.
2. Grüntzig A: Transluminal dilatation of coronary artery stenosis. Lancet 1:263, 1978.
3. Hör G, Maul FD: Beitrag der Myokardszintigraphie in der Therapiekontrolle (Gegenwärtiger Stand und Ausblicke). Z Kardiol 74:65–75, 1985.
4. Kaltenbach M, Kober G, Scherer D: Mechanische Dilatation von Koronaarterienstenosen (Transluminale Angioplastie). Z Kardiol 69:1–10, 1980.
5. Kaltenbach M, Kober G, Scherer D, Vallbracht C: Rezidivhäufigkeit nach erfolgreicher Ballondilatation von Kranzarterienstenosen. Z Kardiol 73(Suppl 2):161–166, 1984.
6. Kober G, Scherer D, Kaltenbach M: Ergebnisse der transluminalen koronaren Angioplastie Med Klin 78:490–496, 1983.
7. Kober G, Lang H, Vallbracht C, Bussmann W-D, Hopf R, Kunkel B, Kaltenbach M: Transluminale koronare Angioplastie 1977–1985 Erfahrungen bei 1000 Eingriffen. Der Radiologe (in press).

28. Single Vessel Stenosis after Acute Myocardial Infarction: Which Patients Should Undergo Percutaneous Transluminal Coronary Angioplasty?

N. DANCHIN, G. ETHEVENOT, M. AMOR, J.-P. GODENIR,
G. KARCHER, M. CUILLIERE, D. AMREIN and F. CHERRIER

Abstract

From April 1980 to December 1983, 33 patients (29 male, 4 female; mean age = 50.3 years) with previous myocardial infarction and one-vessel disease with ⩾ 70% stenosis in the infarct-related vessel, underwent percutaneous transluminal coronary angioplasty (PTCA). Thirteen patients had post-myocardial infarction angina despite medical treatment and 6 had had intracoronary thrombolysis during the acute phase of myocardial infarction. In the remaining 14 patients angiography showed severe proximal stenosis of the infarct-related vessel with a comparatively small akinetic area of the left ventricle and/or exercise Thallium tomoscintigraphy showed a large perfusion defect at maximal exercise, with partial redistribution after exercise, revealing an ischemic zone around the infarcted area.

PTCA was successful in 26 patients (79%) and 3 patients underwent emergency coronary bypass surgery. No further complication occurred.

Among patients with successful PTCA, 2 died during follow-up (mean 18 months), restenosis occurred in 4 of 19 patients who had repeat coronary angiography and all patients with post infarction angina were free of chest pain on follow-up. Exercise Thallium scintigraphy was markedly improved, with complete disappearance of the ischemic area in 6 patients who had a complete radionuclide study before and 3 months after PTCA. In contrast, 3 of the 6 patients with intra coronary thrombolysis had pre-PTCA exercise Thallium tomoscintigraphy with a large defect, stable on redistribution: post PTCA exercise scintigraphy failed to show any improvement.

PTCA is an interesting therapeutic option in patients with previous myocardial infarction single-vessel disease and residual angina. In patients with no residual angina, exercise Thallium tomoscintigraphy seems an interesting method to detect patients with residual ischemia around the infarct area, who are likely to benefit from PTCA; in contrast, PTCA is probably unhelpful in patients with isolated necrosis and no associated ischemia on Thallium tomoscintigraphy.

Introduction

The optimal management of patients with previous myocardial infarction and a single, subtotal stenosis of the infarct-related vessel remains difficult. Surgery is usually considered too aggressive and costly for these patients with single-vessel disease and in whom the area to be by-passed is partially infarcted. Medical treatment, however, cannot prevent re-obstruction of the vessel that may lead to recurrent myocardial infarction. Technically, these subtotal stenoses of infarct-related vessels are often easily amenable to percutaneous transluminal coronary angioplasty (PTCA). The purpose of the present study was to evaluate the role of PTCA in such cases.

Population and methods

From April 1980 to December 1983, 33 patients – 29 males, 4 females; mean age: 50.3 years, range 30 to 64 years – with previous myocardial infarction and single-vessel disease with a 70 % to 95 % proximal stenosis in the infarct-related vessel, underwent PTCA at our institution. During the same time-period, 248 procedures had been performed.

Twenty-five patients had a stenosis of the left anterior descending artery: 24 had had an anterior infarct and one subendocardial infarction. Five patients with an inferior or posterior infarct had a stenosis of the right coronary artery and 3 patients with a previous posterior or lateral infarct had a left circumflex artery stenosis.

Thirteen patients had post-infarction angina despite adequate medical treatment; 6 of them, all with LAD stenosis, had unstable angina.

Six additional patients had undergone intracoronary thrombolysis during the acute stage of myocardial infarction; 3 of them underwent comparative exercise Thallium tomoscintigraphic studies before and 3 months after PTCA.

Lastly, 14 patients with no residual angina had a proximal stenosis of the infarct-related vessel with a comparatively small akinetic area on left ventricular angiography and/or exercise Thallium studies showed the presence of both myocardial necrosis and surrounding ischemia. During the first two years of the study, Thallium planar scintigraphy and, during the last 18 months, Thallium tomoscintigraphy were used routinely for the exercise studies. For Thallium tomoscintigraphy, 32 views of 30 seconds duration each were recorded over 180° with a rotating gamma camera. Tomographic slices oriented in 3 planes according to the long axis of the heart were reconstructed and termed, by comparison with two-dimensional echocardiographic views: short-axis, long-axis, and 4-chamber slices.

Follow-up events were assessed either by an interview and clinical examination of the patient or by a mail or telephone questionnaire. None of the patients were lost to follow-up. The mean duration of follow-up was 18 months (range 6 to 47 months).

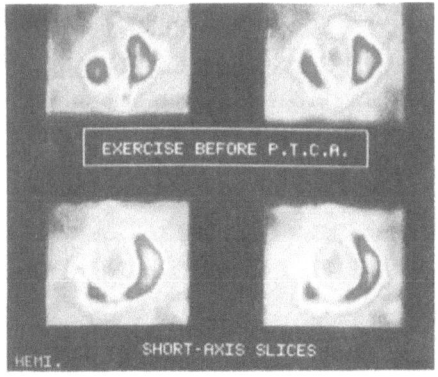

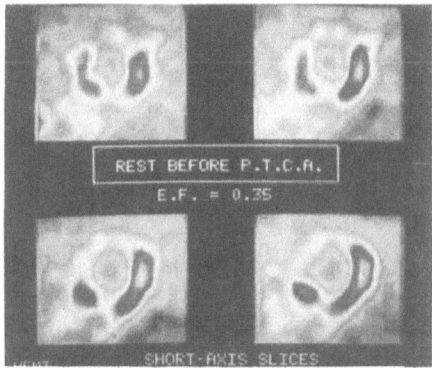

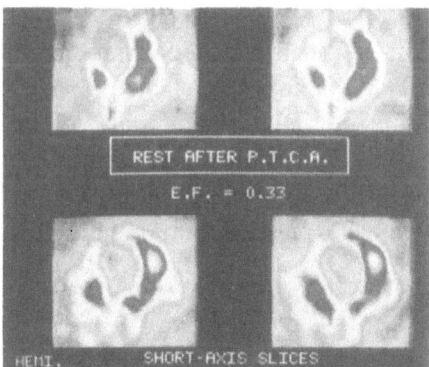

Figure 1. Exercise Thallium tomoscintigraphic studies in a man with previous anterior myocardial infarction. Before PTCA: small defect in the lower septum at basal state (upper left) and large defect of the whole septum during exercise (upper right); ejection fraction decreases from 0.41 at rest to 0.26 during exercise. After PTCA, during exercise: small persisting defect in the lower septum (infarcted area) and complete normalization of the upper septum; ejection fraction: 0.63 during exercise

Results

Primary results

PTCA was initially successful in 26 patients (79%) and 3 patients required emergency aorto-coronary bypass surgery immediately after the procedure. No further complication occured. The primary success rate was related to the vessel involved: 88% for the LAD, 60% (3/5) for the left circumflex artery.

Long Term results

Restenosis occured in 4 out of 19 patients who underwent repeat coronary angiography (21%).

Two patients (6%) died, 6 and 8 months after a successful dilatation of the LAD followed by restenosis; one of these patients, who had had an episode of unstable angina before the first PTCA procedure, died during a second procedure for a recurrent episode of unstable angina.

All 12 other patients with angina before PTCA were totally free of symptoms on follow-up.

All of the patiens with successful PTCA whose Thallium exercise tomoscintigraphy before PTCA showed the association of an area of necrosis (cold spot persisting on redistribution) and of a surrounding ischemic zone (cold spot at peak exercise, disappearing on redistribution) showed considerable improvement on exercise tomoscintigraphy performed 3 months after the procedure: persistance of an infarcted area but disappearance of the ischemic border zone(Fig. 1).

In contrast, 3 patients who had received intracoronary thrombolytic therapy during the acute stage of infarction had pre-PTCA tomoscintigraphic studies showing the sole presence of an infarcted area with no ischemic border zone at maximal exercise (large perfusion defect on exercise, unchanged on redistribution images): post-PTCA exercise tomoscintigraphic studies remained unchanged and ejection fraction did not improve (Fig. 2).

Discussion

Long term prognosis of survivors of acute myocardial infarction with single-vessel disease is good [1, 2] and a conservative therapeutic approach is generally used. Indeed, coronary artery surgery does not seem to improve survival in patients with previous myocardial infarction and single-vessel dis-

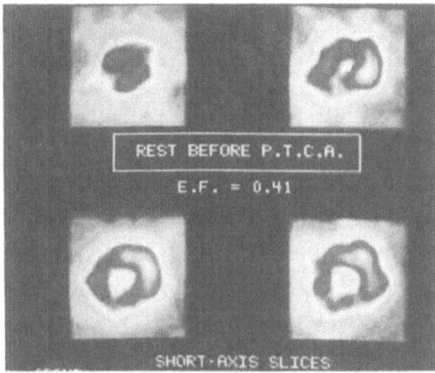

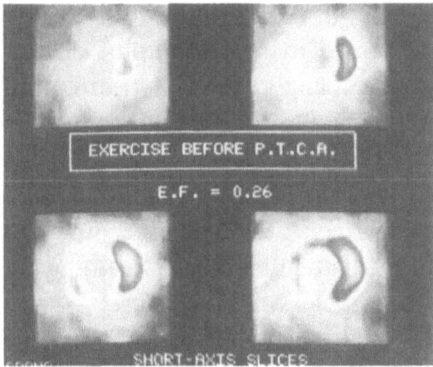

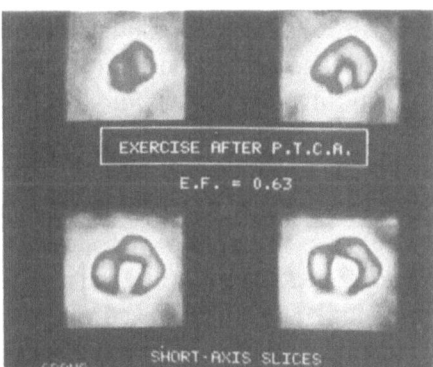

Figure 2. Exercise Thallium tomoscintigraphic studies in a man with previous anterior myocardial infarction treated with intracoronary thrombolytic therapy. Before PTCA: Large defect in the anterior wall and upper septum at rest (upper left), stable during exercise (upper-right). After PTCA, the size of the defect remains unchanged and ejection fraction does not improve.

ease [3, 4]. In a majority of these patients, the infarct-related vessel remains occluded; however, due to spontaneous or therapeutic recanalization, the vessel may be found patent with a high grade stenosis, on subsequent coronary angiography. In these instances, it may be feared that re-occlusion of the vessel lead to re-infarction in the same territory, had some amount of jeopardized myocardium been salvaged by the previous process of recanalization; more aggressive methods of treatment might then prevent recurrent infarction.

Percutaneous transluminal coronary angioplasty is a widely used therapeutic approach in patients with greater than 60% stenosis of a single vessel. Its yields a low but definite operative risk [5, 6], that is markedly increased in patients with previous myocardial infarction when PTCA is performed on one of the non-infarct-related vessels [7, 8]. In our experience, PTCA resulted in the closure of the infarct-related vessel in 3 patients who developed chest pain and electrocardiographic signs of ischemia in the distribution of the occluded vessel; all 3 underwent emergency aorto-coronary bypass surgery and remained free of symptoms on follow-up.

For patients with residual angina after myocardial infarction despite adequate medical treatment, and with a single stenosis on the infarct-related artery, PTCA is an interesting therapeutic option, provided the stenosis is technically suitable. It is less expensive than surgery [9] and the patients may leave hospital a few days after the procedure. After dilatation of the coronary artery, all of our patients became free of symptoms. However, the recurrence rate is comparable with that observed in larger series of patients [10]; restenosis usually occurs within the first few months following the procedure and careful clinical follow-up must be maintained throughout this period. One of our patients died during repeat PTCA for recurrent stenosis of the LAD, which stresses the potential hazards of the procedure that carries a risk slightly inferior to that of coronary artery surgery.

The adequate therapeutic management is more difficult to determine in patients without residual angina. In such patients, detection of silent myocardial ischemia seems an appropriate means to select candidates for PTCA. In our experience, exercise tomoscintigraphic studies enabled to determine the presence and extent of myocardial ischemia during exercise. All patients with a large ischemic border zone surrounding the area of myocardial necrosis improved after successful PTCA, with the complete disappearance of the ischemic zone on exercise, in the absence of antianginal therapy. Similarly, when left ventricular ejection fraction during exercise was studied before and after PTCA in the patients with silent ichemia on effort, its value at peak exercise notably increased after the procedure (Fig. 1). In contrast, patients presenting with isolated myocardial necrosis, without an ischemic border zone during exercise showed no benefit from PTCA. Post-PTCA radionuclide studies showed no reduction of the defect of Thallium uptake and ejection fraction remained unchanged. In these patients, PTCA appeared as a purely 'cosmetic' procedure that failed to improve ventricular function, although the flow in the narrowed coronary artery considerably improved: indeed, the whole myocardial area in the distribution of the narrowed vessel beyond the stenosis appeared to have been destroyed during the previous episode of myocardial infarction. Thus, it is our present opinion that patients with no signs of myocardial ischemia in addition to myocardial necrosis should be treated conservatively. In this regard, contrary to what has sometimes been advocated [11], aggressive therapy following coronary artery recanalization during the acute stage of myocardial infarction should not be considered mandatory in all patients.

Conclusion

Percutaneous transluminal coronary angioplasty can prove a useful method to treat patients with residual angina following myocardial infarction and in whom coronary arteriography shows the presence of a single subtotal stenosis on the infarct-related vessel.

In patients without post-infarction angina, radionuclide exercise studies enable to differentiate between those with or without silent myocardial ischemia during exercise. In the former, PTCA might contribute to preserve left ventricular function and to avoid reinfarction due to reocclusion of the coronary artery, whereas in the latter PTCA is most probably useless.

deel 6 hoofdstuk 28

References

1. Sanz G, Castaner A, Betriv A, Magrina J, Roig E, Coll S, Para JC, Navarro-Lopez F: Determinants of prognosis in survivors of myocardial infarction. A prospective clinical angiographic study. N Engl J Med 306:1065–1070, 1982.
2. Kautner RK, Phillips JH: Coronary angiography post first myocardial infarction in the asymptomatic or mildly symptomatic patient: clinical, angiographic and prospective observations. Cath Cardiovasc Diag 7:1–11, 1981.
3. CASS principal investigators and their associates. A randomized trial of coronary artery bypass surgery: survival data Circulation, 68:939–950, 1983.
4. The Veterans Administration Coronary Artery Bypass Surgery Cooperative Study Group: Eleven-year survival in the Veterans Administration randomized trial of coronary bypass surgery for stable angina. N Engl J Med 311:1333–1339, 1984.
5. Cowley MJ, Forros G, Kelsey SF, Van Raden M, Detre KM: Acute coronary events associated with percutaneous transluminal coronary angioplasty. Am J Cardiol 53:12c–16c, 1984.
6. Dorros G, Cowley MJ, Janke L, Kelsey SF, Mullin SM, Van Raden M: In-hospital mortality rate in the National Heart, Lung and Blood Institute Percutaneous Transluminal Coronary Angioplasty registry. Am J Cardiol 53:17c–21c, 1984.
7. McConahay D, Hartzler G, Rutherford B: Percuteneous transluminal coronary angioplasty: use in management of symptomatic patients with recent myocardial infarction. Circulation 66:II–329, 1982.

8. Murphy DA, Craver JM, Jones EL, King III SB, Curling PE, Douglas JS Jr: Hemodynamic deterioratión after coronary angioplasty in the presence of previous left ventricular infarction. Am J Cardiol 54:448–450, 1984.

9. Jang GC, Block PC, Cowley MJ, Gruentzig AR, Dorros G, Homes DR, Kent KM, Leatherman LL, Myler RK, Sjolander SME, Stertzer SH, Vetrovec, Willis WH Jr, Williams DO: Relative cost of coronary angioplasty and bypass surgery in a onevessel disease model. Am J Cardiol 53:52c–55c, 1984.

10. Holmes DR Jr, Vlietstra RE, Smith HC, Vetrovec GW, Kent KM, Cowley MJ, Faxon DP, Gruentzig AR, Kelsey SF, Detre KM, Van Raden MJ, Mock MB: Restenosis after percutaneous transluminal coronary angioplasty (PTCA): a report from the PTCA. Registry of the National Heart, Lung and Blood Institute. Am J Cardiol 53:77c–81c, 1984.

11. Walker WE, Smalling RW, Fuentes F, Lance Gould K, Johnson WE, Reduto LA, Sterling RP, Weiland AP, Wynn MM: Role of coronary artery bypass surgery after intracoronary streptokinase infusion for myocardial infarction. Am Heart J 107:826–829, 1984.

29. The Role of Coronary Bypass Surgery in Rehabilitation

E. VARNAUSKAS

Abstract

Although the results of the three major prospective randomized trials may appear contradictory, they rather complement each other.

Coronary bypass surgery improves survival in high risk but not in low risk patients defined by non-invasive (resting ECG, exercise ECG, history of peripheral disease, age) and invasive predictors (extent and location of coronary artery narrowings).

Coronary bypass surgery does not prevent from myocardial infarction, but it protecs from dying (in most cases from myocardial infarction).

Coronary bypass surgery dramatically relieves angina and improves exercise tolerance in most patients. This improvement of comport of life does not produce long-lasting effect on the rate of retirement. The intensity and duration of angina pectoris prior to coronary bypass surgery has a significant effect on the rate of retirement at five year follow-up.

Recurrence of chest pain and development of new myocardial infarction cannot be entirely explained by gradual graft closure; progress of coronary arteriosclerosis in native vessels should be considered as a major contributory factor.

Introduction

This presentation is based on a review of two major prospective randomised trials: The European Coronary Surgery Study (767 patients recruited 1973-74) [1-4] and CASS (780 patients recruited 1975-79) [5-7]. The reports of these studies include the data on survival as well as on the quality of life, while the third major trial VA Study (686 patients recruited 1972-74) [8] has mainly reported survival results.

Prospective randomised studies are generally accepted as having fewer sources of error and bias than non-randomised studies. However, it should be kept in mind that even with proper randomisation misleading results can emerge. Unintentional deviation from the protocol rules after randomisation can also upset the outcome of the study. Thus, the results of every study be it randomised or non-randomised should be carefully and critically evaluated.

CASS was not designed to check the results of the European Study just as the European Study was not designed to check the results of the VA Study. Thus, by definition the results of these studies cannot be expected to agree with each other. However, there is no doubt that the results on quality of life are very similar in the European Study and CASS.

Angina pectoris whether mild or moderate is dramatically relieved or improved in the vast majority of patients by the policy of early surgery as compared with conventional treatment in which surgery is reserved to the patients who develop angina pectoris refractory to medical therapy. Early surgery is also significantly superior to the conventional medical treatment in improving exercise performance and reducing the need of antianginal drugs such as beta-blockers or nitrates.

These differences in the results on the quality of life between the two treatments gradually diminish with time but are still significant at five year follow-up.

In spite of marked improvement of symptoms and functional status the rate of retirement from work is not significantly altered by the early surgery as compared to the conventional therapy. The results of the European Study show that annual retirement gradually increased from 21% at entry to 43% at five years in both treatment groups with a possibly significant difference between the groups at one year. Class III angina at entry and duration of angina of two years or more prior to the admission in the study were predictive of significantly increased rate of retirement in both treatment groups at five years ($p = 0.0015$ and $p = 0.047$, respectively); there was no significant difference between the two treatment groups.

There was no significant difference in the occurrence of non-fatal infarction between the two treatments in both studies. Apparently early surgery was unable to protect the myocardium from infarction.

In spite of these numerous similarities in the results on the comfort of life and myocardial infarction, the two studies differ from each other in terms of the results on survival.

Results and discussion

The European Study convincingly demonstrates that early surgery significantly improves five and eight year survival as compared with the conven-

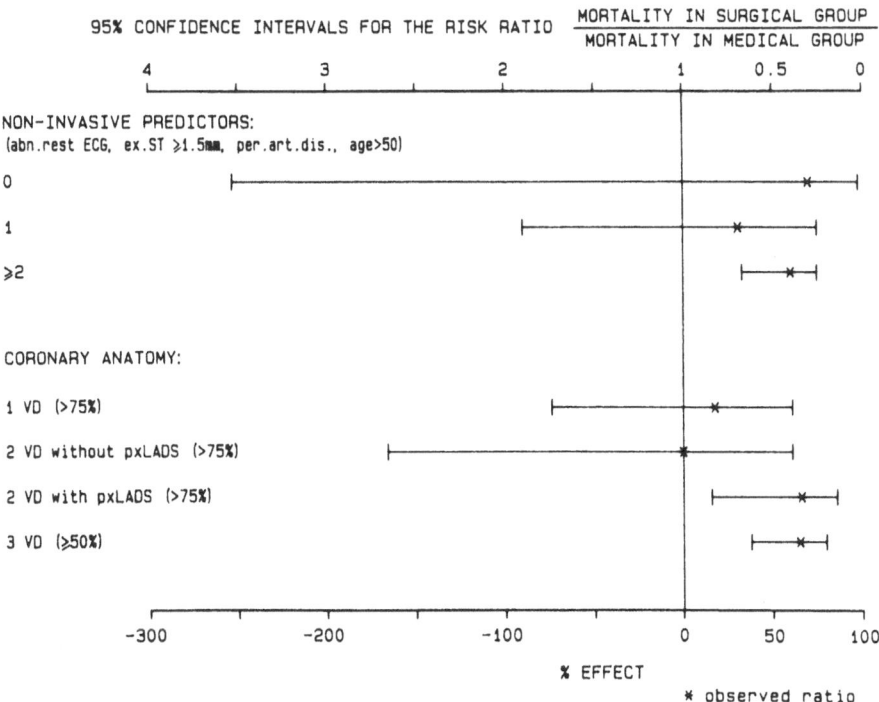

Figure 1. Efficacy of early surgery on survival in different cathegories of patients defined by prognostic predictors.

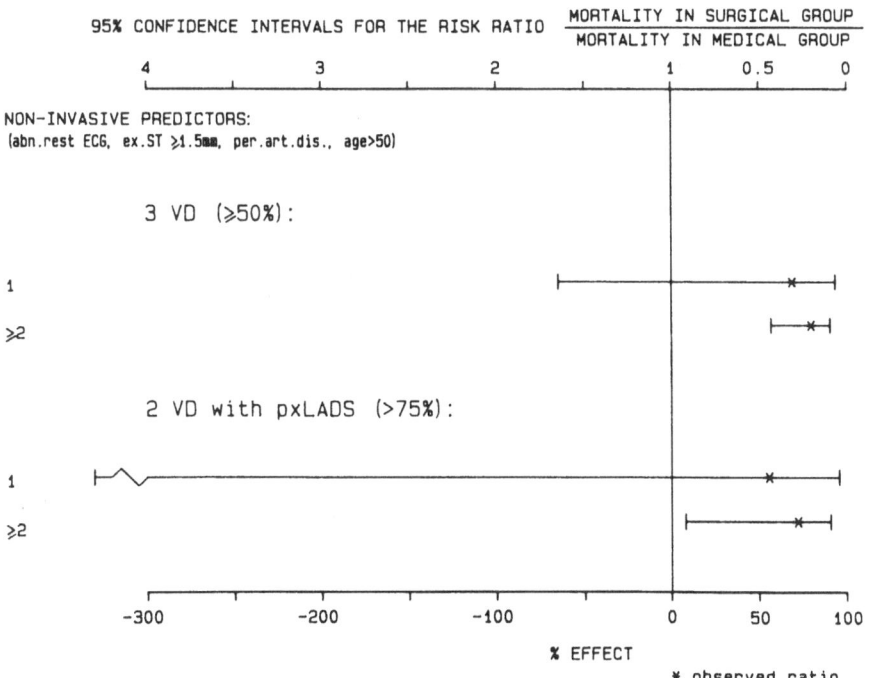

Figure 2. Efficacy of early surgery on survival in patients with 3-vessel disease and 2-vessel disease and the influence of prognostic predictors.

tional therapy. This survival improvement is dependent on the extent of coronary disease and which is even more important on the non-invasive prognostic predictors. These non-invasive predictors are electrocardiographic abnormalities (Q-wave, ST-segment shift and T-wave inversion) reflecting myocardial ischaemia [9, 10]; peripheral arterial disease diagnosed by history and physical examination which reportedly is associated with significantly shortened life expectancy [1]; and age. The efficiency of early surgery to improve mortality in relation to various prognostic predictors is shown in Fig. 1. The benefit of surgery increases with increasing number of predictors. Conversely, absence or presence of only one of these predictors suggest insignificant result of surgery even in patients with 3-vessel disease, Fig. 2. The difference in survival in favour of surgery is also seen in patients with 2-vessel disease defined by 75% or more stenosis in whom one of the diseased vessels is the proximal segment of the left anterior descending artery and who also have two or more prognostic predictors. Early surgery does not alter the prognosis in patients with single vessel disease.

Variables related to left ventricular function (ejection fraction, segmental wall abnormalities and left ventricular end-diastolic pressure) were not predictive of survival nor the outcome of coronary bypass surgery because patients with ejection fraction of less than 50% were not included in the study.

Although reflecting myocardial ischaemia, angina pectoris is not an independent predictor of survival or of the outcome of coronary bypass surgery.

Unlike the European Study, CASS was unable to show significant differences in survival between the two treatment groups. The major difference in the survival results between the European Study and CASS appears to be the excellent survival rate observed in CASS medical patients. An explanation that this finding might be due to variations in medical therapy or differences in angina pectoris could be considered, provided that the prevalence of prognostic characteristics in the two populations is the same. Unfortunately the available evidence suggests that there are substantial differences in the prevalence of prognostic factors between the two study populations and in the subsets of medical patients who received surgery. 20% of CASS patients were included because they had relatively recent myocardial infarction but had no angina suggesting no residual myocardial ischaemia. Considerably larger proportion of the European patients had electrocardiographic signs of ischaemia at rest and particularly during exercise. Although more detailed studies are needed to clarify the differences in risk factors between the two studies, it is reasonable to conclude that the two study populations deviate from each other so much that the survival results of the study should be expected to be different. Thus, the two studies do not contradict each other but rather complement each other.

The results of the European Study clearly suggest that non-invasive prognostic predictors ought to be of great help in selective appropriate patients for coronary angiography and prophylactic surgery. Postponing bypass surgery until development of angina pectoris refractory to medical treatment is associated with significantly increased risk of premature death. On the other hand, surgery should not be performed too early because of great risk for repeat operation which is associated with increased operative mortality.

A rehabilitation program which does not include the possibility of prophylactic coronary bypass surgery cannot be considered comprehensive and complete.

References

1. European Coronary Surgery Study Group: Coronary bypass surgery in stable angina pectoris: survival at two years. Lancet I:889, 1979.
2. European Coronary Surgery Study Group: Prospective randomized study of coronary artery bypass surgery in stable angina pectoris. Second interim report. Lancet II:491, 1980.
3. European Coronary Surgery Study Group: Prospective randomized study of coronary artery bypass surgery in stable angina pectoris: a progress report on survival. Circulation 65(suppl. II):67, 1982.
4. European Coronary Surgery Study Group: Long-term results of prospective randomized study of coronary artery bypass surgery in stable angina pectoris. Lancet II:1173, 1982.
5. CASS Principal Investigators and Their Associates: Coronary artery surgery study (Cass): A randomized trial of coronary artery bypass surgery. Quality of life in patients randomly assigned to treatment groups. Circulation 68:951, 1983.
6. CASS Principal investigators and their associates: Coronary artery surgery study (CASS): a randomized trial of coronary artery bypass surgery. Survival data. Circulation 68:939, 1983.
7. CASS Principal investigators and their associates: Myocardial infarction and mortality in the coronary artery surgery study (CASS) randomized trial. N Engl J Med 310:750, 1984.
8. Takaro T, Hultgren HN, Detre KM, Peduzzi P: The Veterans Administration Cooperative Study of Stable Angina: current status. Circulation 65(suppl II):60, 1982.
9. McNeer JF, Margolis JR, Lee KL et al.: The role of the exercise test in the evaluation of patients for ischemic heart disease. Circulation 57:64, 1978.
10. Gohlke H, Samek L, Betz P, Roskamm H: Exercise testing provides additional prognostic information in angiographically defined subgroups of patients with coronary artery disease. Circulation 68:979, 1983.
11. Hughson WG, Mann JI, Tibbs DJ et al.: Intermittent claudication: factors determining outcome. Br Med J 1:1377, 1978.

30. Social Fate after Aorto-Coronary Bypass Surgery

J. GEHRING, W. KOENIG, N. WRANA and P. MATHES

Abstract

Between January 1980 and December 1983 the medical and social status of 423 patients (pts.) who were considered candidates for aortocoronary bypass surgery (ACBS) was assessed by a questionnaire, mean 16 months after coronary angiography. 54 pts. had refused surgery, 15 pts. were reoperated, 23 pts. had angioplasty and 7 pts. had died on the waiting list. After exclusion of these 117 pts. 306 pts. remained, who form the basis of this report.

53 pts. (17%) had retired before surgery, 4 pts. (1.3%) had died perioperatively and 19 pts. were on sick-leave less than three months. Of those pts. who were still employed preoperatively 102 (44.3%) went back to work, 85 (37%) had retired and 42 (18%) were on sick-leave longer than three months.

Significant differences were noted between the 102 working and the 85 retired pts. as far as medical and social factors are concerned. Of the medical factors postoperative freedom of symptoms ($p < 0.0001$), postoperative exercise tolerance ($p < 0.0001$) and completeness of revascularisation ($p < 0.05$) seemed to have influence on return to work. Of the social factors age ($p < 0.0001$), type of occupation ($p < 0.0002$), duration of preoperative absence from work ($p < 0.001$) and heavy manual work ($p < 0.05$) showed significant differences between the groups.

Since duration of preoperative absence from work is the only preoperative factor that can be modified, strategies for improving the return-to-work-rate should aim at shortening of waiting times for coronary angiography and ACBS.

Introduction

Aortocoronary bypass surgery (ACBS) is a well accepted and effective surgical procedure for the treatment of medically intractable angina pectoris and – in certain subgroups – shall improve the prognosis of patients with coronary artery disease [6, 19]. Although many studies have demonstrated improved quality of life of those patients, most authors were not able to find a net increase in resumption of work [1, 2, 11, 12, 14, 16, 17]. While studies from the United States and Canada show a return-to-work-rate of 60% to 90%, West German studies conducted between 1974 and 1983 revealed a rate of 20%–57% [3–5, 9, 10, 13, 18]. The reason for this difference may be attributed to more extensive disease in operated patients in this country and/or to differences in the systems of social security.

The role of economy and unemployment rate has often been stressed to explain these results. Convincing data, however, do not exist for the Federal Republic of Germany, since most relevant studies were completed before 1975 when the unemployment rate was very low. A study from the United States showed an inverse relationship between the economical situation and the resumption of work of blue collar workers [7]. These results, however, are not contradictory, since they have to be regarded on the background of a different social system.

The purpose of our study was to evaluate the influence of social and medical factors determined pre- and postoperatively on the rate of return to work after bypass surgery.

Patients and methods

Between January 1980 and December 1983 447 patients, who had undergone coronary angiography at our institution were considered as candidates for ACBS. 16 months after coronary angiography a questonnaire was sent to these patients to assess their medical and social status. The response rate was 95%.

Fifty-four patients had refused surgery because of their family physician's advise or their own decision (Fig. 1). Twenty-three patients were referred for percutaneous transluminal angioplasty. 346 patients were on the waiting list for ACBS; the mortality rate was 2.1%. For further evaluation we excluded 53 patients who had retired already preoperatively for cardiac reasons or age and 15 patients who underwent reoperation. The remaining 306 patients who had undergone ACBS consisted of 282 males and 24 females with a mean age of 53.4 years. All had stopped working because of cardiac reasons (myocardial infarction in 78.2%). 58.7% were blue collar workers (BCW), 13.2% were white collar workers (WCW) and 11.2% were professionals (P). Preoperative angiography showed single vessel disease in 9.6%, double vessel disease in 34.3%, triple vessel disease in 48.5% and left main stem stenosis in 7.6%. Mean ejection fraction was 62%. Mean duration of preoperative absence from work 6.8 ± 5.8 months, mean waiting time for ACBS was

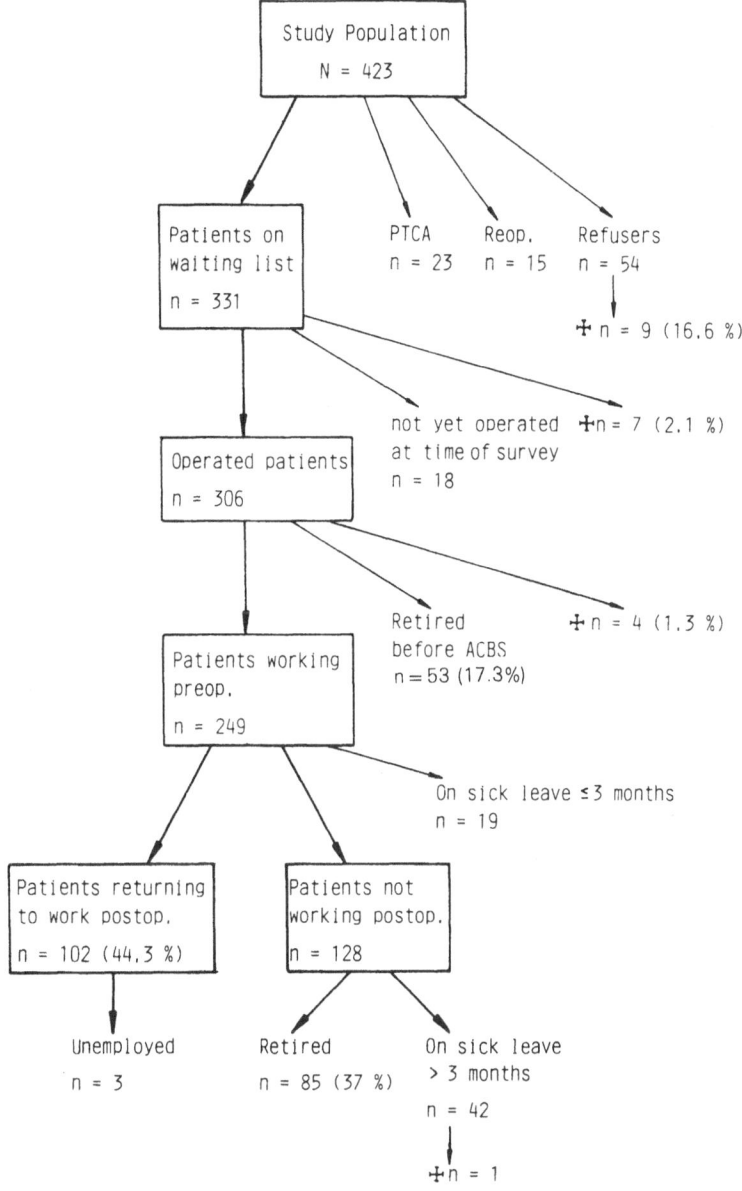

Figure 1. Medical and social fate of 423 candidates for aortocoronary bypass surgery.

3.7±2.9 months. Patients were referred for surgery to 10 different surgical centers in Germany and other European countries. A mean of 2.6±1.1 grafts were implanted, perioperative mortality rate was 1.3%, perioperative infarction was seen in 7.6%. In 3.4% ACBS plus aneurysmectomy were performed. Completeness of revascularisation was assumed, if all significantly stenosed vessels to the non-infarcted myocardium had received a bypass.

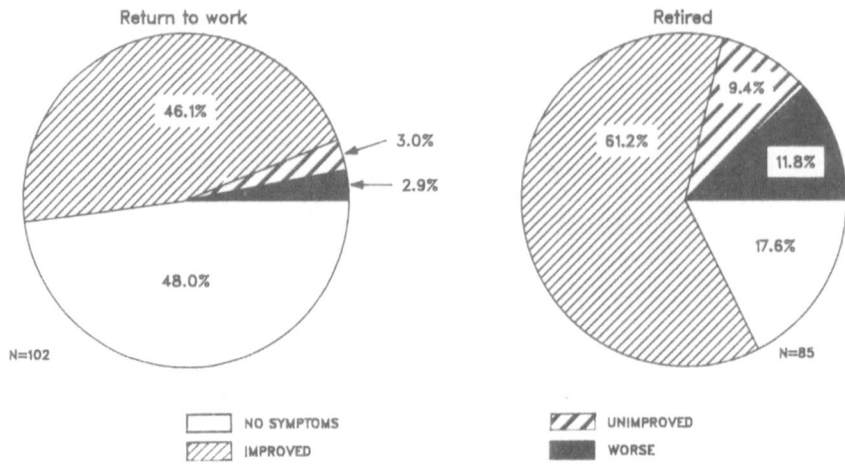

Figure 2. Postoperative cardiac symptoms of patients returning to work and of postoperatively retired patients.

Chi^2 tests and unpaired t-tests were used for comparison between groups. A *p*-value of less than 0.05 indicated a statistically significant difference. Means are presented with a standard deviation.

Results

Role of medical factors

At the time of the survey (mean one year postoperatively) 44.3% of the operated patients had returned to work, three patients had lost their job. Of the patients not working postoperatively, 85 (47%) had retired, 42 were on sick leave longer than three months.

One year after surgery 29.3% were free of cardiac symptoms, 54.4% felt improved, 8.5% unimproved and 7.2% worse than before surgery. There were significant differences between the patients working postoperatively and the ones who had received a pension as far as symptoms are concernd (Fig. 2). While 48% of the working patients were free of symptoms, only 17.6% of the retired ones had no symptoms. It should be noted, that the latter group did not return to work although they had obtained complete relief of symptoms.

Postoperative exercise tolerance turned out to be another medical factor with probable influence on resumption of work (Fig. 3). Patients with an exercise capacity of equal or less than 50 watts did return to work in only 23%, whereas patients, who achieved more than 100 watts during bicycle

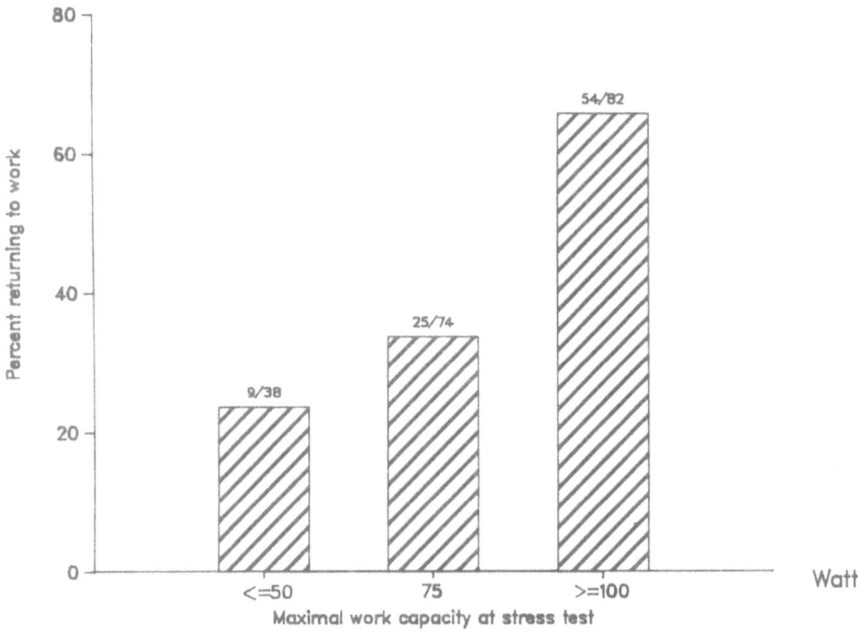

Figure 3. Return-to-work-rate in relation to the result of early postoperative stress test.

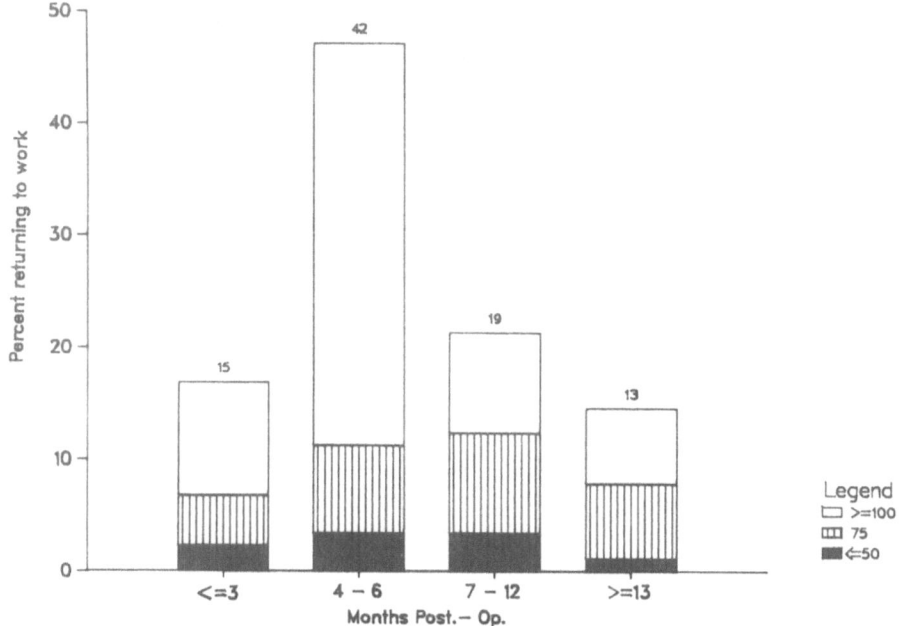

Figure 4. Duration of sick-leave in relation to the exercise tolerance 3–6 weeks after ACBS.

ergometry returned to work in 66%. Postoperative functional capacity also seemed to be related to the duration of the postoperative sick-leave period (Fig. 4). Most patients of the group with the highest exercise capacity returned to work during the 4th and 6th month, while patients reaching their limit at 75 watts showed a much more delayed resumption of work.

Completeness of revascularisation seems to be another factor with influence on resumption of work (Table 1). Other medical factors such as extent of coronary artery disease, preoperative infarction rate, preoperative ejection fraction, perioperative infarction rate, postoperative angina pectoris on stress test did not differ significantly, although there were some differences in the perioperative infarction rate and the stress-induced occurrence of postoperative angina (Table 2).

Role of non-medical factors

Of major importance were non medical factors, all being discernible already before ACBS (Table 3). Age, occupation and duration of preoperative absence from work did have a major influence on resumption of work. Looking separately at the group of blue collar workers, white collar workers

Table 1.

Variable	Working n = 102	Retired n = 85	Univ. test P
Postop. free of symptoms	48%	17.6%	$chi^2 < 0.0001$
Postop. exercise tolerance	94.9 ± 26.4 W	76.4 ± 23.5	$t < 0.0001$
Complete revascularis.	84.2n%	71.1%	$chi^2 < 0.05$

Table 2.

Variable	Working n = 102	Retired n = 85	Univ. test P
Coronary artery disease	1: 4.9% 2:37.3% 3:47.1% 4:10.8%	1: 8.2% 2:30.6% 3:54.1% 4: 7.1%	n.s.
Periop. infarction	4.9%	10.6%	n.s.
Postop. angina at stress test	13.5%	23.9%	n.s.
Preop. myocardial infarction	80.4%	78.8%	n.s.
Ejection fraction	62.8 ± 12.3%	61.1 ± 12.7%	n.s.

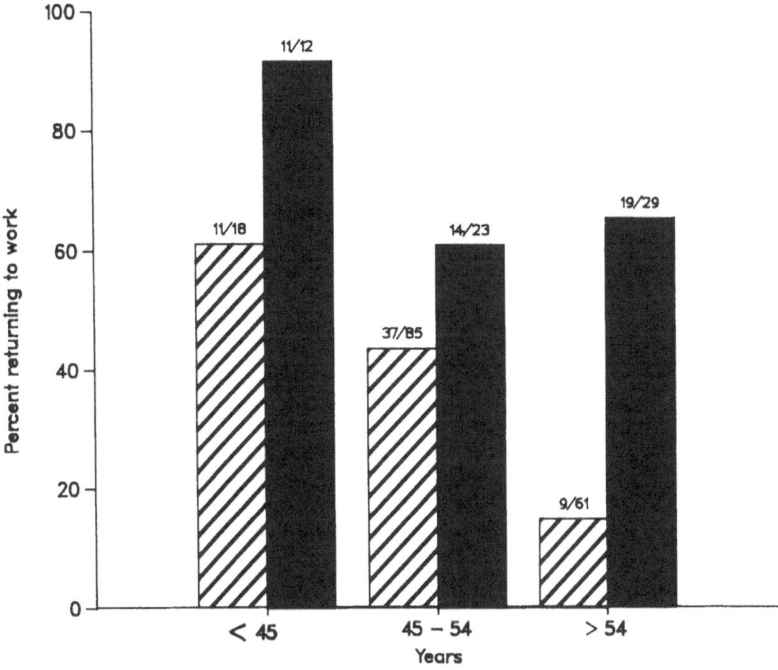

Figure 5. Return to work rate in relation to age and occupation.

and professionals age did have a considerably different influence on resumption of work. While there was a steep decline of the return-to-work-rate in blue collar workers by age, for the group of white collar workers and professionals age did not have a similar impact on return-to-work-rate beyond the age of 54 years (Fig. 5).

Discussion

Resumption of work after ACBS is influenced by medical, non-medical as well as pre- and postoperatively discernible factors. The literature reveals

Table 3.

Variable	Working n = 102	Retired n = 85	Univ. test P
Age (yrs.)	50.5 ± 7.1	54.7 ± 5.1	< 0.0001
Occupation (BCW; %)	55.9	82.4	< 0.0002
Duration of preop. absence from work (Mo)	5.0 ± 3.8	7.1 ± 4.5	< 0.001
Heavy manual work (%)	29.4	44.7	< 0.05

some controversial results as far as the influence of medical factors is concerned. Most authors give high priority of the postoperative relief of cardiac symptoms [1, 2, 8, 13, 14, 16, 17]; this holds true also for our study. Another important factor in our study seems to be the postoperative exercise capacity. While some authors came to similiar conclusions [9], others found no influence of this factor on resumption of work [4]. As a result of our study we consider the result of the postoperative stress test an important predictor of resumption of work. It is, however, not only influenced by the quality and completeness of revascularisation but also by the degree of general physical conditioning.

The role of completeness of revascularisation on resumption of work is another controversial subject in the literature. While some authors found no positive influence of this factor [3, 10, 13, 16], in our study and in those of others [2, 9] a higher percentage of patients with complete revascularisation was seen amongst those who resumed work after ACBS. However, since not all patients did have a postoperative coronary angiogram, the patency rate and the degree of revascularisation could not be determined in our study. Yet on the basis of the surgical reports we could decide wether complete revascularisation was attempted.

As far as the other medical factors are concerned, such as severity of coronary heart disease, preoperative left ventricular funciton, pre- and perioperative myocardial infarction rate there are conflicting results reported in the literature [1–3, 9, 14, 16]. In general those factors do not appear to be of any major influence on resumption of work.

Our study confirms the previously reported results in that resumption of work after ACBS is predominantly influenced by age, type of occupation and duration of preoperative absence from work [8, 10, 11, 18]. These factors allowed a prediction in 80%–90% of patients who were to return to work postoperatively [15, 17]. Since only the duration of preoperative absence from work can be modified, this factor should receive great attention. Presently the time-lag between the first manifestation of coronary heart disease and its diagnosis by coronary angiography, is too large in the Federal Republic of Germany. This holds true for the waiting time for ACBS as well. Besides shortening of the duration of preoperative disability, intensive vocational counseling in the frame work of a comprehensive rehabilitation program should be initiated already preoperatively for those patients and be resumed after surgery as early as possible.

References

1. Anderson AJ, Barboriak JJ, Hoffmann RG, Mullen DS: Retention or resumption of employment after aorto-coronary bypass operations. Jama 243:543, 1980.

2. Barnes GK, Ray MJ, Obermann A, Kouchoukos NT: Changes in working status of patients following coronary bypass surgery. Jama 238:1259, 1977.

3. Benesch L, Neuhaus KL, Rivas-Martin J, Loogen F: Clinical results and return to work after coronary heart surgery. In: Roskamm H, Schmutziger M (eds). Coronary heart surgery. Springer, Berlin, Heidelberg, New York, 1979.

4. Blümchen G, Scharf-Bonhofen E, Brandt D, van den Berg C, Bierk G: Clinical results and social implications in patients after coronary bypass surgery. In: Roskamm H, Schmutziger M (eds). Coronary heart surgery. Springer, Berlin, Heidelberg, New York, 1979.

5. Blümchen G, Barthel W, van den Bergh C, Bierk G, Brandt D, Scharf-Bonhofen E, Reidemeister JC: Soziales Schicksal bei operierten und konservativ behandelten Koronar- und Aneurysmapatienten. Z Kardiol 69:632, 1980.

6. Coronary Artery Surgery Study (CASS): A randomized trial of coronary artery bypass surgery. Quality of life in patients randomly assigned to treatment groups. Circulation 68:951, 1983.

7. Crosby JK: Return to work after coronary artery bypass surgery. Int. Symposium on Return to Work after ACBS, Rotenburg/Fulda, 1984.

8. Danchin N, David P, Robert P, Boutassa MG: Employment following aortocoronary bypass surgery in young patients. Cardiology 69:52, 1982.

9. Gohlke H, Gohlke-Bärwolf CH, Schnellbacher K, Heidecker K, Samek L, Görnandt L, Stürzenhofecker P, Roskamm H: Long-term effects of aortocoronary bypass surgery on exercise-tolerance and vocational rehabilitation. In Controversies in Cardiac Rehabilitation. Mathes P, Halhuber MJ (eds). Springer, Berlin, Heidelberg, New York, p 71, 1982.

10. Gregori AN, Hetzer R, Schwarz B, Mayer B, Buser K, Lichtlen P, Borst HG: Veränderungen der Lebensqualität nach Koronarrevaskularisation. Z Kardiol 72:12, 1983.

11. Hammermeister KE, DeRouen TA, English MT, Dodge HT: Effect of surgical versus medical therapy on return to work in patients with coronary artery disease. Amer J Cardiol 44:105, 1979.

12. Johnson WD, Kayser KL, Pedraza PM, Shore RT: Employment patterns in males before and after myocardial revascularisation surgery. Circulation 65:1086, 1982.

13. Lichtlen P, Liese W, Leitz K, Borst HG: Postoperative Klinik nach aortokoronarem Venenbypass in Relation zum Ausmaß der Revaskularisation. Z Kardiol 67:83, 1978.

14. Oberman A, Wayne JB, Kouchoukos NT, Charles ED, Russel RO, Rodgers WJ: Employment status after coronary artery bypass surgery. Circulation 65:115 (suppl. II), 1982.

15. Sergeant P, Suy R, Flameng W, Lesaffre E: Reemployment after coronary surgery in a country in severe economic crisis. Int. Symposium on Return to Work after ACBS, Rotenburg/Fulda, 1984.

16. Smith HC, Hammes LN, Gupta S, Vlietstra RE, Elveback L: Employment status after coronary artery bypass surgery. Circulation 65:120 (suppl II), 1982.

17. Stanton BA et al.: Predictors of employment status after cardiac surgery. Jama 249:907, 1983.

18. Walter P, Thies B, Gerhardt U: Wie viele Patienten nehmen nach einer Koronaroperation ihre Arbeit wieder auf? Med Klin 78:276, 1983.

19. Varnauskas E et al.: Long-term results of prospective randomized study of coronary artery bypass surgery in stable angina pectoris. Lancet 1173, 1982.

31. Clinical and Occupational Status of Patients with Coronary Artery Disease (CAD) who Underwent Aorto Coronary Bypass Surgery (ACBS)

M. WELSCH, G. BERGMANN, H. C. MEHMEL, W. SAGGAU and W. SCHMITZ

Abstract

To assess the postoperative clinical and occupational status of patients with CAD who underwent ACBS we analyzed the data of 267 patients (90% male) with an average age of 48 years with a range of 30 to 55 years at the time of surgery; all of these patients had been working up to this event.

The clinical data include information obtained from pre- and post-operative coronary arteriography and left ventriculography; also included is information from the surgery procedure and prior as well as postoperative symptoms. The demographic data contained information concerning the occupational status before and after surgery, reason for failure of resumption of work and patient satisfaction with the outcome of the operation; this information was collected using a standardized questionnaire on the last reexamination an average period of 25 (range 9 to 36) months after surgery. The symptomatic relief and rehabilitation was determined for each patient at the same time.

On average 3.3 months after ACBS 53% of all patients went back to work, 47% didn't take up a professional activity within the follow up period.

The 145 'workers' after ACBS with an average age of 46.3 years were significantly younger than the 112 'non workers' with 49.5 years ($p < 0.001$).

The lack of physical stress at work showed a highly significant influence on resumption of work. Whereas out of 85 white collar workers (59 employees, 18 employers and 8 civil servants) 82% continued working after ACBS, out of 182 blue collar workers only 39% resumed their professional activity ($p < 0.001$).

Based on the comparable initial degree (3.4 versus 3.5) the extent of the angina symptomatic after ACBS averaged 1.2 ± 0.5 in the 'worker' and

1.5 ± 0.8 in the 'non worker' group, and thus the difference was significant at the 1% level.

The participation in a rehabilitation program with 91 patients in the 'worker' and 48 patients in the 'non worker' group was significantly different at the 1% level.

Whereas preoperatively both groups showed a similar value of left ventricular ejection fraction (57.6% against 56.5%), the postoperative value with $61.3 \pm 5.6\%$ in the 'worker' and $57.4 \pm 8.3\%$ in the 'non worker' group was significantly different at the 5% level.

We conclude that the strategy for improving resumption of work is to decrease the considerable waiting time for preoperative diagnosis and surgery; and with five objective predictive factors, it is possible to discern patients with the lowest resumption of work prognosis and to submit them to an individualized postoperative rehabilitation program.

Introduction

Within the last 17 years aorto-coronary bypass surgery (ACBS) as an essential basic principle of therapy for atherosclerotic coronary artery disease (CAD) has gained an important standing. Venous aorto-coronary bypass graft (ACBG) for eliminating relevant coronary artery stenosis was introduced by Rene Favaloro in 1967 [6].

In most of the cases vena saphena magna has been used for ACBS and the complete revascularisation has become the main object at ACBS [14].

The aims of ACBS consist in improvement of life expectancy and quality of life. Life expectancy of surgically treated patients is approaching that of the average population. The prognosis of patients with multiple vessel disease and main stem stenosis undoubtedly has improved [5, 11–13, 15, 16].

The improvement of the quality of life by drastic reduction of anginal complaints has been achieved in 85 to 90% of the patients, while complete removal of angina pectoris can be registered in 60 to 75% of all patients [13, 17]. It is true that based on the progress of the primary disease, the extent of the symptomatic recovery gradually decreases on a scale of 3 to 4% per year [9], but in the majority of the patients at least stops for some years. The symptomatical improvement normally allows a professional rehabilitation [1, 2, 4, 7, 8, 16, 17, 19].

In view of these positive results of ACBS regarding symptoms and signs as well as prognosis of CAD for all involved in health care, the proportion of patients resuming work after ACBS in Western Germany and the resulting social and economical effect is disappointing [9, 17].

While according to relevant studies, the probability of professional reintegration in Western Germany ranges between 20 to 57% in the USA 63 to

80% resume work postoperatively, without essential differences with respect to the result of an operation, individual exercise tolerance and professional demand [1, 2, 4, 7, 9, 10, 16, 17, 19].

Patients and Methods

To assess the postoperative clinical and occupational status of patients with CAD who underwent ACBS we analyzed the data of 327 patients (90% male) with an average age of 47.9 ± 5.5 years with a range of 30 to 55 years, at the time of surgery; all of these patients had been working up to this event.

The average severity of preoperative angina pectoris judged by the criteria of the Canadian Cardiovascular Society was 3.5 ± 0.6 with a range of 1 to 4.

Further preoperative clinical and demographical characteristics are shown in Table 1 to 3.

These patients were taken from a total number fo 521 patients who underwent ACBS between April 1981 and May 1983 at the Department of Cardiac Surgery at the University Clinic of Heidelberg.

The data of the Federal Agency for Statistics shows that the average frequency of early retirement in Germany 1982 was: at the age of 58 years

Table 1.

No of patients	327	
Age (years)	47.9 ± 5.5	(30–55)
Sex ♂	294	(90%)
♀	33	(10%)

Table 2.

Myocardial infarction	195	(59.5%)
— anterior localisation	105	
— posterior localisation	90	
Coronary artery disease	2.2 ± 0.8	(1–3)
— single-CAD	8.2	(24.8%)
— double-CAD	89	(29.7%)
— triple-CAD	147	(45.5%)
— left main included in 1–3-CAD	60	(18,2%)
Ejection fraction (%)	54.1 ± 9.0	(23–68)

296

Table 3.

Severity of angina pectoris (CCS-criteria I-IV)	3.5±0.6 (1–4)
Period of time (months)	
— Symptoms → C. Catheter	16.1±23.4 (0–99)
— C.Catheter → Surgery	4.0±2.8 (0–15)

17.5%, for the 59 year olds 21.5% Furthermore the Agency comes to the conclusion that 25% of all males had prematurely left employment before reaching the age of 60.

Considering the criteria for taking up patients in this study, these facts led us the decision to determine the upper age limit to 55 years at time of surgery. Preoperative retirement or application for this and second disease influencing the capability to work were further exclusion criteria from this study.

The surgical procedure was performed with aid of pulsatile cardiopulmonary bypass at moderate whole systemic hypothermia (25–28 °C). The cardiac arrest was induced by continuous aortic cross-clamping with profound topical cardiac cooling (10–15 °C) and infusion of cardiplegic Bretschneider solution (4 °C).

To be direct myocardial revascularisation vena saphena magna grafts were used exclusively. The proximal anastomoses were performed with a

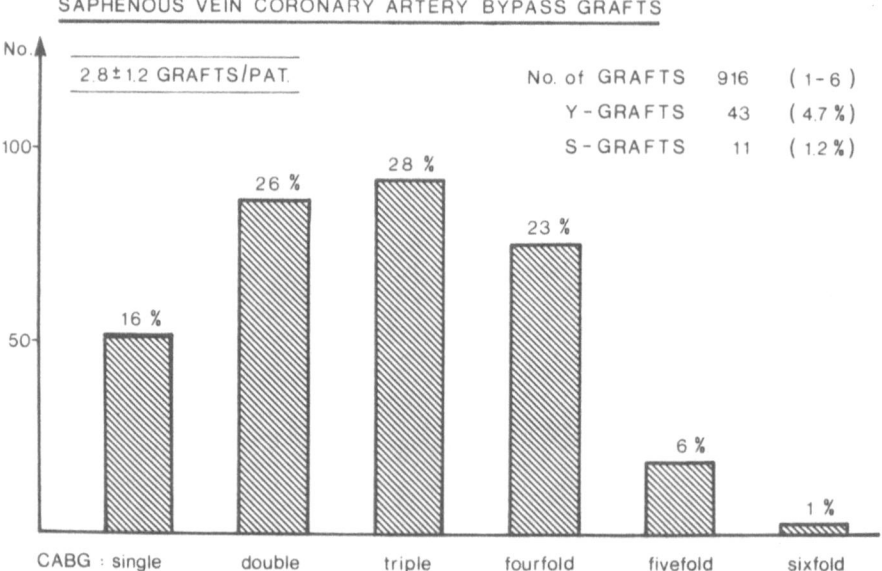

Figure 1. Frequency and extent of the inserted coronary artery bypass grafts (Cabg). [18]

partial occlusion clamp after completion of distal anastomoses. Figure 1 despicts frequency and extent of the inserted grafts.

Coronarographic restudy was done in each patient to the Sones or Judkins technique in the Heartcatheter Laboratory of the Department of Cardiology, on average 1.6 ± 0.5 (range 1 to 3) months after ACBS to determine early graft patency.

The second angiographic study reports were reviewed to obtain the following parameters:

1. Number of diseased vessels with a stenosis of cross-sectional diameter greater than 50%.
2. Condition of inserted grafts.
3. Measurement of biplan left ventricular ejection fraction.

Besides using the patency rate to assess revascularisation, a graduation for angiographic qualitive determination of revascularisation developed by Roskamm et al. [13] was modified respectively by one further grade.

The severity of angina pectoris was classified through the criteria of the Canadian Cardiovascular Society [3]. The clinical data include information obtained from pre- and postoperative selective coronary arteriography and left ventriculography in 30° right anterior oblique and 60° left anterior oblique projection with a cineradiographic film; also included is information from the surgery procedure and prior as well as postoperative symptomatic. The demographic and relevant historical facts contained information concerning the work status before and after surgery, reason for failure to return to work and patients satisfaction with the outcome of the operation; this information as collected by the same person using a standardized questionary on the last reexamination in an average period of 22 ± 16.9 months with a range of 9 to 34 months after surgery. The symptomatic relief and rehabilitation was determined for each patient at the same time.

A computerized data base containing the mentioned clinical and demographic information for each of the 327 patients was constructed and analyzed via the HADES basis and SAS statistic system of the University Calculating Centre. All data was then correlated with the patients postoperative work status.

Results

Patency Rate

At the re-coronary angiography, on average 1.8 months after ACBS, out of 916 inserted grafts 840 were open. The corresponding early mean patency rate was 91.7%. With a patency rate of 96%, 303 grafts were connected with the left anterior descending artery (LAD); 184 grafts to the diagonalis artery

298

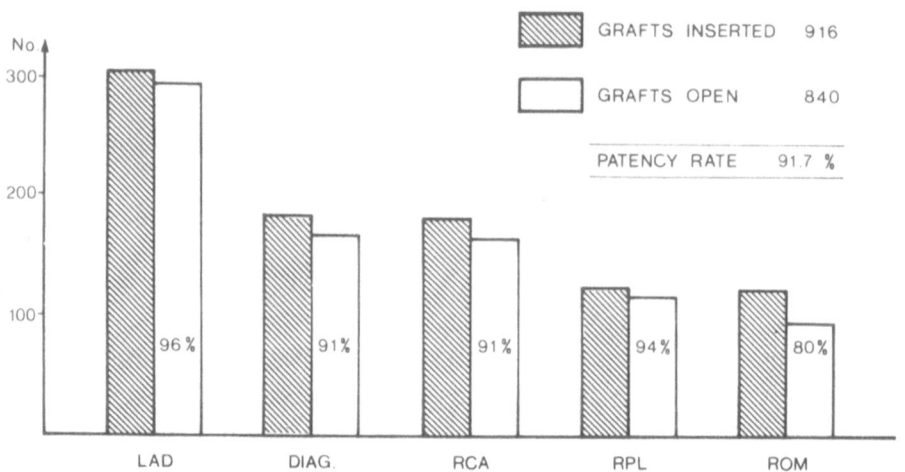

Figure 2. Localisation of the inserted grafts an the corresponding patency rate (symbols see text) [18].

(DIAG) and 182 grafts to the right coronary artery (RCA), each with a patency rate of 91%. The patency rate of 125 grafts to the posterior lateral artery (RPL) was 94%. The lowest patency rate was found in 122 grafts to the obtuse marginal artery (ROM) with 80% (Fig. 2).

Grade of Revascularisation

A differentiated analysis of the operative results is possible with the division of the angiographic data into five grades of revascularisation. This graduation takes into consideration the extent of stenosis, the angiographic condition of the grafts and the different value of the varying vascular regions.

A complete revascularisation – all vessels with a significant stenosis (greater than 50 per cent) were provided with an open graft – was achieved in 62,8% of all cases. An incomplete revascularisation – all main branches with a significant stenosis were provided with an open graft – was found in 10.7% of the patients. In 15.8% we observed a sufficient revascularisation – all main branches with a significant stenosis were provided with an open graft but at least one graft had a significant stenosis. While an insufficient revascularisation was registered in 9.9% – all main branches with a significant stenosis were provided but at least one graft was occluded. In three patients the revascularisation was miscarried – all grafts were occluded. As shown in Table 4.

Table 4.

		Localisation- stenosis > 50%	Condition of inserted grafts	n	%
I	complete:	all vessels	open	205	(62.8)
II	incomplete:	main branches	open	35	(10.7)
III	sufficient:	main branches	with signif. stenosis	52	(15.8)
IV	insufficient:	main branches	at least one occluded	32	(9.9)
V	miscarried:	all vessels	occluded	3	(0.8)

Angina pectoris and Left-Ventricular Function

The angina pectoris symptoms were classified according to the criteria of the Canadian Cardiovascular Society. The initial mean degree of 3.5 ± 0.6 improved impressively to 1.4 ± 0.3 at the last reexamination 9 to 34 (mean 22) months after surgery ($p<0.001$).

Before aortocoronary bypass surgery the left ventricular ejection fraction was $54.1\pm9.0\%$ and increased postoperatively to $59.1\pm7.6\%$ ($p<0.005$).

The grading of left ventricular regional wall motion (in seven segments) showed postoperatively a striking improvement. Segmental hypocinetic wall motion normalized postoperatively in 86.3% (Fig. 3).

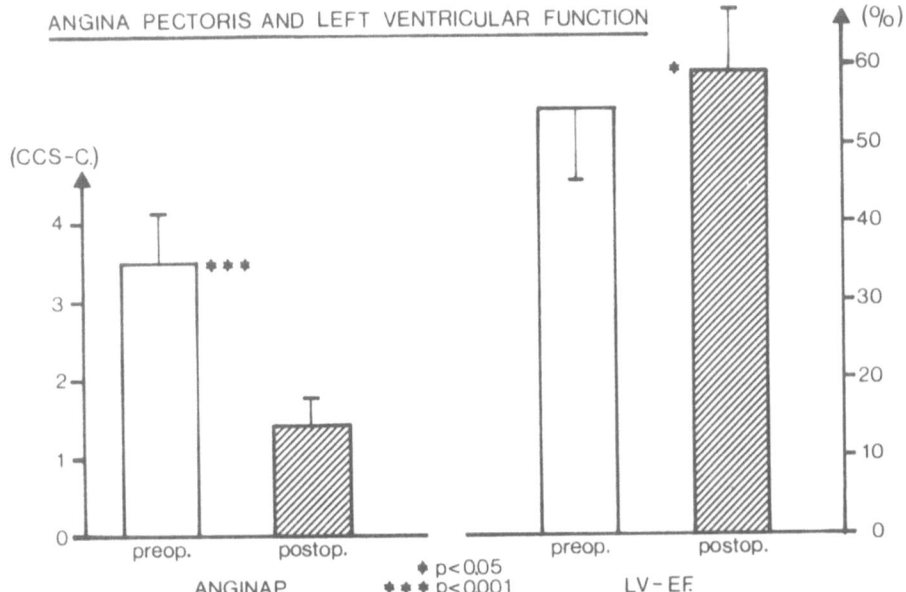

Figure 3. Angina pectoris and left ventricular function pre- and postoperatively (n = 327).

Status of Employment

According to the social and economic status, resumption of work after ACBS shows a quite different proportion: Of the blue-collar workers 39% went back to work, whereas 88.9% of the employees resumed their professional activity. 75% of the employers carried on their business, among the civil servants 50% retired.

With a comparable mean age in all groups the difference between blue-collar worker and employees in relation to resumption of work is highly significant at the 0.1% level. On average 3.3 months after ACBS 52,9% of all patients went back to work (Table 5).

In contrast to the patients resuming work, 47.1% didn't take up a professional activity within the follow up period of 22 ± 16.9 months ranging from 9 to 34 months.

Factors without visible Influence

Relevant factors without visible influence on resumption of work are the extent of CAD with an identical average vascular involvement of 2.2 ± 0.8 and a similar frequency of prior myocardial infarction with 35 in the 'WORKER' and 37 in the 'NON WORKER' group. In both groups the

Table 5.

	No./total pat.	%	Mean age
Status of employment			
– blue collar	87/222 ***	(39.0)	46.0 ± 5.2
– employees	64/ 72	(88.9)	47.0 ± 6.7
– employers	17/ 23	(75.0)	45.9 ± 5.5
– civil servants	5/ 10	(50.0)	46.5 ± 2.1
	173/327	(52.9)	46.4 ± 5.7

*** $p < 0.001$.

Table 6.

	'Worker' 173/327 (52.9%)	'Non worker' 154/327 (47.1%)
Coronary artery disease	2.2 ± 0.8	2.2 ± 0.8
Myocardial infarcion	96	99

Table 7.

	'Worker'	'Non worker'
Grafts	2.8 ± 1.1	2.8 ± 1.2
Patency rate	93.7 ± 0.2	91.6 ± 0.2
Revascul grade	1.8 ± 1.1	1.7 ± 1.1

Table 8.

	'Worker'	'Non worker'
Period of time (month)		
— Symptoms → C. Catheter	15.4 ± 24.3	16.8 ± 22.7
— C. Catheter → Surgery	4.0 ± 3.1	3.9 ± 2.5
Participation in coronary-training group	15	6

number of inserted grafts per patient with 2.8 ± 1.1 compared with 2.8 ± 1.2 is nearly identical. The grade of revascularisation with 1.8 ± 1.1 in the 'WORKER' group versus 1.7 ± 1.1 in the 'NON WORKER' group is comparable. The mean patency rate with $92.7\pm0.15\%$ and $91.6\pm0.17\%$ is not essentially different. As to the period of time between the first symptoms and coronary angiography with 15.4 ± 24.3 contrasted to 16.8 ± 22.7 months there was no visible influence on resumption of work. The 'waiting time' between coronary angiography and ACBS with 4.0 ± 3.1 months in the 'WORKER' group versus 3.9 ± 2.5 months in the 'NON WORKER' group was also without visible influence and relatively short in both groups. The participation in outpatient coronary training groups with 15 against 6 of our 327 patients was amazingly low (Table 6 to 8).

Factors with significant Influence

Some influencing factors with varying statistical significance could be found.

The 173 worker after ACBS with an average age of 46.3 ± 5.7 years, were significantly younger than the 154 non-workers with 49 ± 4.7 years ($p<0.001$). As to the rate of resumption of work the lack of physical stress at work showed a high significant influence. Whereas out of 105 withe-collar workers (72 employees, 23 employers and 10 civil servants) 82.1% continued working after ACBS, out of 222 blue-collar workers only 39% resumed their professional activity ($p<0.001$). Based on the comparable initial degree (3.4 ± 0.7 versus 3.5 ± 0.3), the extent of the angina symptomatic after ACBS averaged 1.2 ± 0.5 in the 'WORKER' and 1.5 ± 0.8 in the 'NON WORKER' group, and thus the difference was significant at the 1% level.

The participation in the rehabilitation programme with 108 patients in the 'WORKER' – and 61 patients in the 'NON WORKER' group was significantly different at the 1% level. Whereas preoperatively both groups showed a similar value of left ventricular ejection fraction with 54.6% against 53.8%, the mean postoperative value with 60.1 ± 5.3% in the 'WORKER' – and with 57.4 ± 8.5% in the 'NON WORKER' group was significantly different at the 5% level (Table 9).

Discussion and Conclusion

The aim of ACBS consists in improving life expectancy and quality of life [4, 5, 11–13, 15]. The improvement in quality of life by drastic reduction or complete removal of angina pectoris was achieved in a large proportion of patients [7, 13, 16, 17]. The symptomatical improvement normally allows a professional rehabilitation [7, 16]. A study comparing medical and surgical treatment of CAD found no difference between the two for patients returning to work [10]. Despite comparable surgery results with respect to the grade of myocardial revascularisation, individual exercise tolerance and professional demand, many studies show that the extent of resumption of work in other countries is significantly higher than in Western Germany [1, 2, 7–10, 16, 17, 19]. Visible differences are based on a different social system with reduced chances of calculating the pension, on a significantly shorter morbidity – pre- and postoperatively – and on a considerably shorter waiting time for preoperative filtering diagnosis as well as ACBS.

The variables which influenced the postoperative resumption of professional activity after ACBS were, in order of importance (Fig. 4): age, type of physical activity in preoperative occupation, anginal class, participation in rehabilitation programme and left ventricular function.

Table 9.

	'Worker'	'Non worker'
Age	46.3 ± 5.7	49.7 ± 4.7 ***
White/blue collar	86/87	19/135 ***
Angina pectoris	1.2 ± 0.5	1.5 ± 0.8 **
Ejection fraction	60.1 ± 5.3	57.4 ± 8.5 *
Participation in rehabilitation	108	61 **

*** $p < 0.001$ ** $p < 0.01$ * $p < 0.05$

CONCLUSION

CONTRIBUTING FACTORS TO RESUMPTION OF WORK AFTER

CORONARY ARTERY BYPASS SURGERY :

YOUNGER AGE

LACK OF PHYSICAL STRESS AT WORK

RELIEF OF ANGINA PECTORIS

GOOD OR IMPROVED LEFT VENTRICULAR FUNCTION

PARTICIPATION IN REHABILITATION PROGRAMME

We conclude that a strategy for improving resumption of work is to decrease the considerable waiting time for preoperative filtering diagnosis and surgery; and with five objective predictive factors, it is possible to discern patients with the lowest resumption of work prognosis and to submit them to an individualized postoperative rehabilitation programme.

References

1. Anderson AJ, Barborjak JJ, Hoffmann RG, Mullen DC: Retention or resumption of employment after aortocoronary bypass operations. J Am Med Ass 243:543, 1980.
2. Benesch L, Neuhaus KL, Rivas-Martin J, Loogen F: Clinical results and return to work after coronary heart surgery. In: Roskamm H, Schmuziger M (eds). Coronary heart surgery, Springer: Berlin, Heidelberg New York, 1979.
3. Campeau L: Grading of angina pectoris, Circulation 54:522, 1976.
4. Denolin H: Rehabilitation bei Herzkranken. In: Krayenbühl HP, Kübler W (eds). Kardiologie in Klinik und Praxis, Georg Thieme: Stuttgart, New York, p 71–71.10, 1981.
5. Detre K, Peduzzi P, Murphy M, Hultgren H, Thomson J, Obermann A, Takaro T: Effect of bypass surgery on survival in patients in low- and high-risk subgroups delineated by the use of simple clinical variables. Circulation 63:1329–1338, 1981.
6. Favaloro RG: Saphenous vein graft in the surgical treatment of coronary artery disease. Operative technique. J thorac cardiovasc surg 58:178, 1969.
7. Gehring J, Koenig W, Wrana N, Mathes P: Aortocoronare Bypass-Operation: Welche Faktoren beeinflussen die Arbeitswiederaufnahme, Herz und Gefäße 4:205–223, 1984.
8. Gohlke H, Gohlke-Bärwolf Chr, Samek L, Stürzenhofecker P, Schmuziger M, Roskamm H: Verbesserte anginafreie Arbeitstoleranz bis zu 6 Jahren nach der Bypass-Operation in Abhängigkeit vom Revaskularisationsgrad. Schweiz med Wschr 112:1616–1618, 1980.

304

9. Hacker RW, Torka M, v d Emde J: Revaskularisation des Myokards durch aortocoronaren Bypass, Dt. Ärzteblatt 47:23–28, 1982.
10. Hammermeister KE, de Rouen TA, English MT, Dodge HT: Effect of surgical versus Medical Therapy on Return to Work in patients with Coronary Artery Disease. Amer J Cardiol 44:105, 1979.
11. Lichtlen PR: Natural history of coronary artery disease based on coronary angiography. Cleveland Clin Quart 45:153, 1978.
12. Mathur VS, Hall RJ, Gracia E, de Castro CM, Cooley DA: Prolonging life with coronary bypass surgery in patients with three-vesseldisease. Circulation 62(suppl I):90–98, 1980.
13. Roskamm H, Schmuziger M et al.: Bestimmt die Vollständigkeit der Revaskularisation die funktionelle Verbesserung und die Überlebensdaten koronaroperierter Patienten? Z Kardiol 70:590–599, 1981.
14. Schmuziger M: Herzchirurgie. In: Roskamm H, Reindell H (eds).Herzkrankheiten. Springer: Berlin, Heidelberg, New York, p 802, 1980.
15. Suter B, Hirzel HO, Fischer M, Turina M, Senning A, Krayenbühl HP: Bringt die aortocoronare Bypass-Operation einen Nutzen bei Patienten mit fortgeschrittener Koronarsklerose und schlechter Ventrikelfunktion? Schweiz med Wschr 112:1688–1694, 1982.
16. Symmes JC, Lenkei SCM, Bermann ND: Influence of aortocoronary bypass surgery on employment. Canad med Ass J 118:268–270, 1978.
17. Walter P, Thies B, Gerhardt U: Wie viele Patienten nehmen nach einer Koronaroperation ihre Arbeit wieder auf? Med Klin 78:276–280, 1983.
18. Welsch M et al.: Factors contributing to resumption of work after Aortocoronary Bypass Surgery. In: Walter PJ (ed). Return to Work after Coronary Bypass Surgery (in press). Springer: Berlin, Heidelberg, New York, 1984.
19. Wenger NK: Coronary Bypass Surgery as a Rehabilitative Procedure. Adv Cardiol 31:80–85, 1982.

32. Which Factors do Influence the Rate of Employment after Surgical and Medical Treatment in Patients with Coronary Heart Disease?

J. JEHLE, P. GROSSMANN, L. KAMPA, M. KLOKE and F. LOOGEN

Abstract

The status of employment was examined in a total of 353 patients with coronary artery disease. The diagnosis was established in the year 1976. In 204 patients an operation was performed (group op), 149 patients were treated medically (group nop). According to their profession the patients were assigned to labourers, office workers and professionals.

In group op 26 patients and in group nop 33 patients died during the observation time. In 49 patients of group nop a complete analysis was not possible because no further informations were available. There were no significant differences in the status of employment between the patients of the two groups.

The results showed that 44% in group op and 50% in group nop returned to work without significant differences in these two groups. Labourers showed the lowest, professionals the highest rate of reemployment irrespective of the kind of treatment. The extent of coronary artery disease influenced the prognosis of medically treated patients and therefore the status of employment of the surviving patients. The degree of revascularization did not influence the status of reemployment in the surgically treated group. Left ventricular function did not significantly influence the rate of employment in the operated patients, too. The same effect was seen in the non-operation group, when only the surviving patients were observed. In all groups patients who did not work and received pension were older than the other patients. No significant differences were found concerning angina pectoris of the patients who returned to work and who did not. But the patients of group nop had minor symptoms on the average.

In summary the results show that about 50% of the patients returned to work. Coronary artery surgery does not influence this rate significantly. The rate of reemployment in this study is not influenced by therapeutic measures – either surgical or medical – but by the status and profession of the patients as well as by the degree of angina pectoris 'postoperatively'.

306

Introduction

Bypass surgery reduces angina pectoris in most of the patients with coronary artery disease. Although the exercise capacity improved in nearly all patients after surgical intervention the return to work differs in various countries. In the United States studies have shown that about 60–90% of all patients return to work, whereas in Western Germany the rate is less than 50% [1–3]. There are only few studies on the return to work among patients with medical treatment [4].

The aim of this retrospective study was to find out which factors do influence the rate of employment after surgical and medical treatment, respectively.

The operation group consisted of 204 patients, 21 of them were women (group op). The mean age was 52 years, ranging from 25 to 71 years. In this group 26 patients died, 9 early postoperatively. In all patients a coronary bypass procedure was performed. The medically treated group consisted of 149 patients, 12 women (group n-op). The mean age was 50 years, ranging from 29 to 67 years. In this group 33 patients died during the observation period. In 49 patients a complete analysis of all data was not possible mainly because no further information was available. In most of the patients treated medically there was no indication for surgery because of minor symptoms. The indication for surgery was given in 31 patients. In 26 cases the patients refused operation, in 5 cases the surgeons.

The observation time lasted from 1976 to 1983, that means all patients of

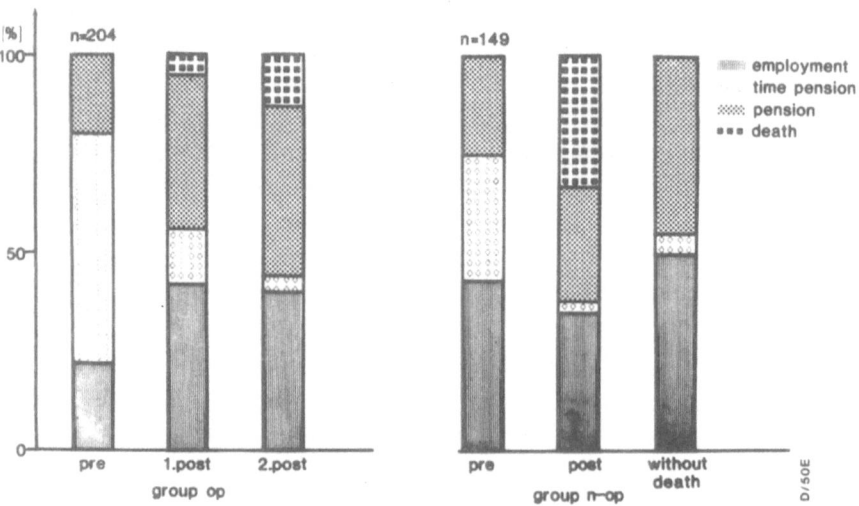

Figure 1. The employment status in the operation (op) and non-operation (n-op) group before and after surgery and diagnostic angiography, respectively. Properatively most patients were receiving time pension, postoperatively 44% were working. Before and after medical treatment (group n-op) about 50% returned to work

the operation group were operated in 1976. The 1. postoperative examination took place 9 months, the 2. examination 6–7 years after surgery. In all patients treated medically the exact diagnosis was established by angiography performed in 1976, too.

The status of the patients in both groups before surgery and before the diagnostic procedure showed no significant differences between the patients with and without surgery:
37 and 45% were labourers, that means skilled or unskilled blue collar workers,
50 and 43% were office workers (white collar workers) and
13 and 12% were professionals.
Figure 1 shows the employment status of the operation and non-operation group. The patients were divided into four groups: employment, time pension, pension, and death ('Time pension' implies that a final decision concerning the employment status of these patients had not yet been made before the operation).

In the operation group most patients (58%) received time pension, 22% were working and 20% received a pension. The rate of employment increased at the 1. examination in comparison to the preoperative rate and remained nearly unchanged up to the 2. examination (40%). The number of patients receiving time pension decreased, most of them received pension, so that the pensioneers increased from 20 to 40% postoperatively.

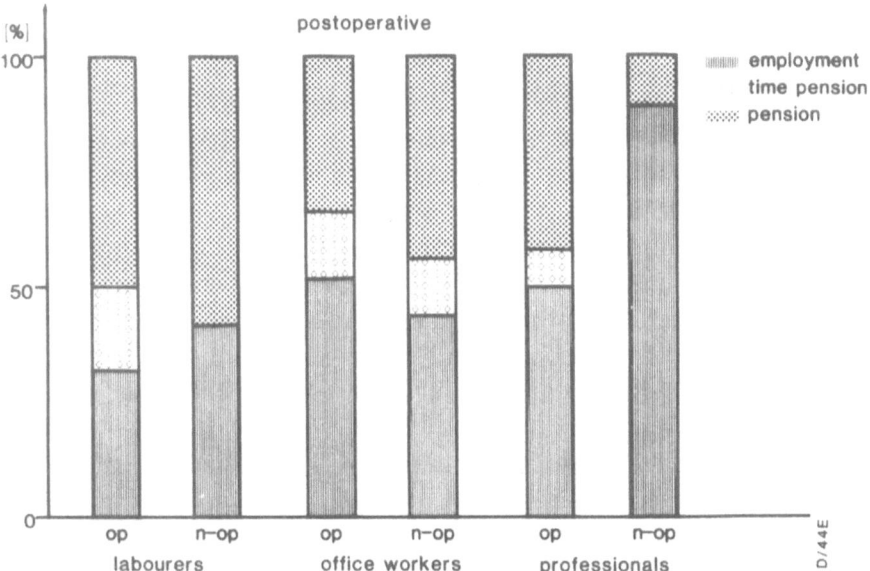

Figure 2. The employment status after treatment of laboures, office workers and professionals in the operation (op) and non-operation (n-op) group. In both groups most of the labourers received pension, whereas most of the professionals were working

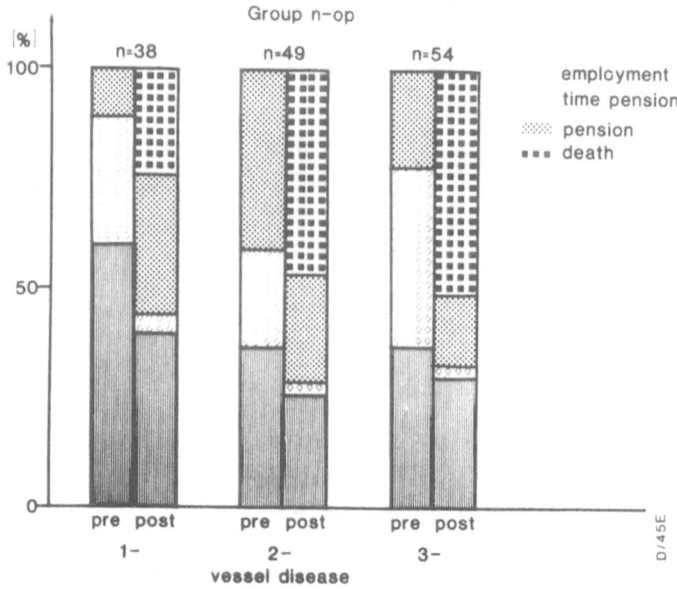

Figure 3. Influence of the extent of coronary artery disease on the employment status in the non-operation (n-op) group. About 50% of the patients with 2- and 3-vessel disease died during the observation period. Concerning only the surviving patients there is no difference in the rate of employment

In the medically treated group more patients were working at the time when the diagnosis was established (43%). This rate did not change significantly after 7 years, even when the deceased patients were excluded. Similar results were found in patients receiving pension. In both groups no patient receiving pension prior to treatment returned to work later on.

The postoperative status of employment of the three professional groups without the deceased patients – labourers, office workers, professionals – are shown in Figure 2.

More than 50% of the labourers received a pension in both groups. Only 32% of the labourers operated and 42% of those treated medically were working. Among the office workers the rate of employment was higher postoperatively, 52 and 44% respectively. No significant differences were found in the two groups (surgically or medically treated). 50% of the professionals were working postoperatively, whereas 89% of those medically treated were still working. Because of the small number of patients (26 patients in the group n-op) there was no significant difference.

These results show that about 50% of all patients – 44% in the operation group and 50% in the non-operation group returned to work without any differences in the surgical and medically treated groups. Labourers showed the lowest and professionals the highest rate of employment irrespective of the kind of treatment.

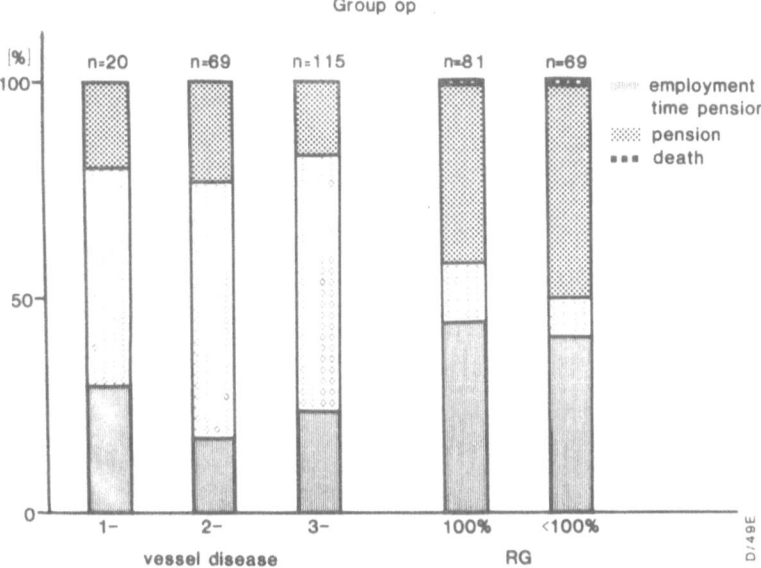

Figure 4. Influence of the extent of coronary artery disease and the degree of revascularization on the employment status in the operation (op) group. Extent of coronary artery disease and degree of revascularization did not influence the rate of reemployment in the surgically treated patients

Which factors do influence the rate of employment in these two groups? One factor may be the extent of coronary artery disease. In Figure 3 the employment status in the non-operation group is depicted in correlation to 1-, 2- and 3-vessel disease.

The rate of employment was highest in patients with 1-vessel disease. About 50% of the patients with 2- and 3-vessel disease died during the observation period. Regarding only the surviving patients there was no difference in the rate of employment between the two examinations, i.d. before and 7 years after heart catheterization.

In the operation group (Fig. 4) there is no difference of working and non working patients among the patients with 1-, 2- and 3-vessel disease. Postoperatively 150 patients were reexamined by angiography. We divided these patients into two groups: complete (100%) and incomplete (< 100%) revascularization. There was no significant difference concerning the employment status of both groups.

From these results we conclude that the extent of coronary artery disease influences the prognosis of medically treated patients, therefore the employment status of these patients. In the surgically treated patients the prognosis was improved. The degree of revascularization did not influence the employment status in these patients.

310

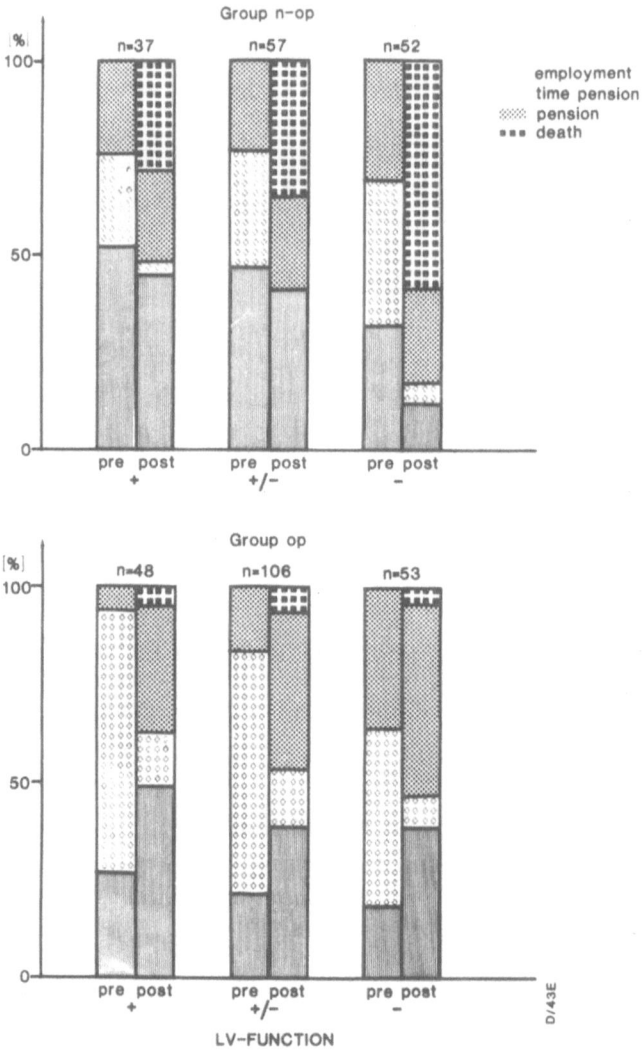

Figure 5. Influence of left ventricular function on the employment status in the operation (op) and non-operation (n-op) group. (+ good, +/− slightly impaired, −/− severely impaired). In group n-op there was a distinct correlation between left ventricular function and survival. In group op no differences were found

The influence of left ventricular function on the employment status is depicted in Figure 5. The left ventricular function is described as good, slightly or severely impaired. In the non-operation group there seemed to be a correlation between the left ventricular function and the return to work. More patients with a good or slightly impaired function returned to work than in the third group. But regarding only the surviving patients there were no differences between the two examinations in the single groups.

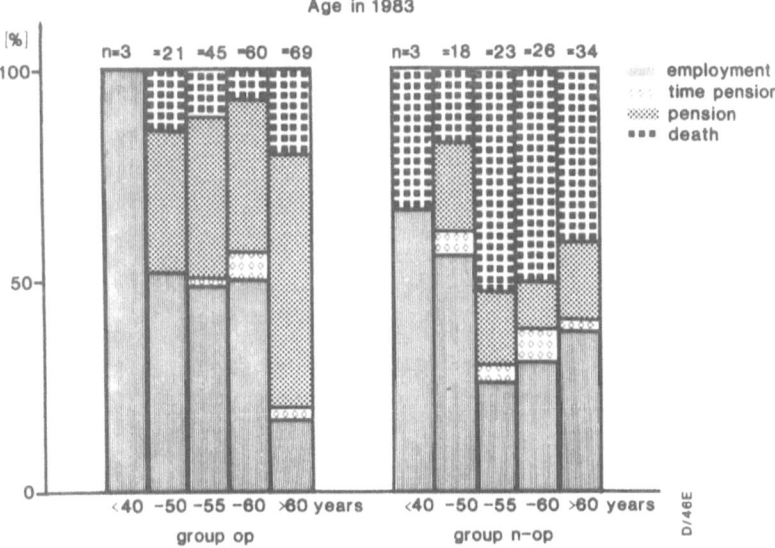

Figure 6. Influence of age on the employment status in the operation (op) and non-operation (n-op) group. In group op about 50% of all patients younger than 60 years were working. In group n-op less patients were working because of the high mortality rate in patients older than 50 years

In the operation group less patients were working before operation than in the non-operation group irrespective of left ventricular function. After surgery about the same percentage of patients returned to work as in the non-operation group. The mortality rate was not significantly different in the three groups of various left ventricular function and much less than in the non-operation group.

These results show that the left ventricular function did not significantly influence the rate of employment in the operated patients. The same effect was seen in the non-operational group. But in this group the survival rate was influenced by left ventricular function.

One important factor for employment after treatment may be the age of the patient. Figure 6 shows the patients of both groups subdivided into groups of different ages. The age considered was that in the year of the last examination in 1983. In the operation group about 50% of the patients younger than 60 years were working. Most patients older than 60 years were receiving a pension. In the non-operation group similar results seemed to be evident. But the lower rate of employment in patients older than 50 years was simulated by the high mortality rate in these age group. Neglecting the deseased patients more than 50% of the older patients returned to work until 1983. The relatively high rate of employment in the older patients is caused by the large number of professionals, whereas in the group of labourers only younger patients returned to work.

312

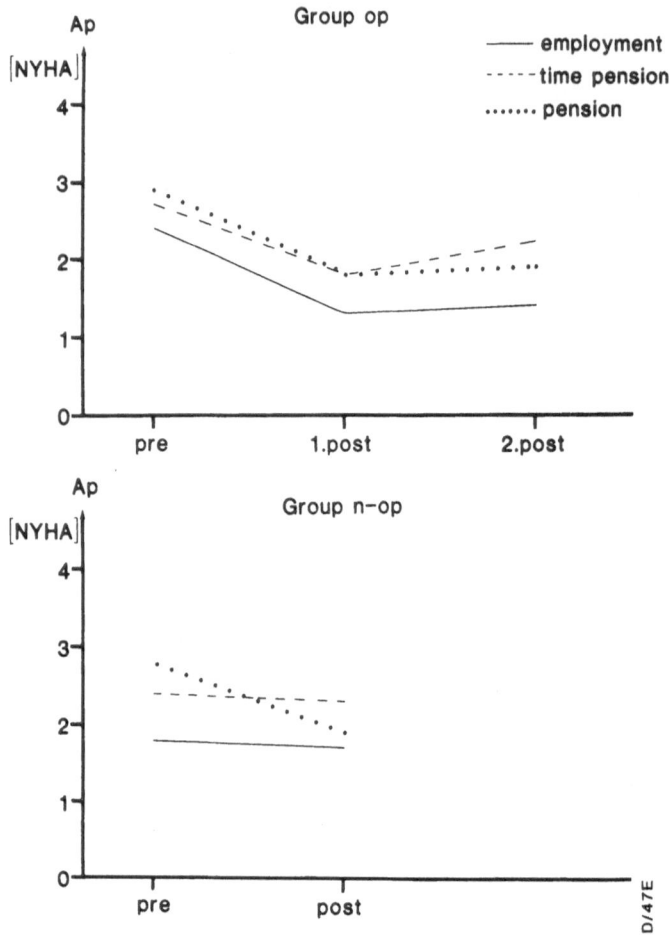

Figure 7. Influence of the degree of angina pectoris on the employment status in the operation (op) and non-operation (n-op) group. Patients with less angina were working in both groups with no significant differences prior and after treatment

The complaints of the patients is another factor which may influence the return to work. In Figure 7 the degree of angina pectoris was correlated to the employment status. In the operation group a significant improvement was seen in all patients. Patients working had less angina than the other ones. This difference was evident pre- and postoperatively, however. In the non-operation group angina did not change on the average. The marked decrease in angina in the group of patients receiving pension was simulated by the fact that in this group more patients with severe angina died and only patients with less angina survived. Besides these changes it is evident that patients in the nonoperation group, especially of the working patients, generally had less angina before heart catheterization than the operated patients preoperatively.

The results of this study show:

1. The mortality rate was significantly higher in patients without surgery.

2. There was no difference in the rate of employment in the surgically and medically treated group.

3. Not the therapeutic measure but the profession and the employment status (pension, 'time pension', working) prior to treatment and the degree of angina pectoris influence the rate of employment.

References

1. Benesch L, Neuhaus KL, Rivas-Martin J, Loogen F: Clinical Results and Return to Work After Coronary Heart Surgery. In: Roskamm H, Schmuziger M (eds). Coronary heart surgery. Springer, Berlin, Heidelberg, New York, 1979.

2. Blümchen G, Scharf-Bornhofen E, Brandt D, van den Bergh C, Bierck G: Clinical Results and Social Implications in Patients After Coronary Bypass Surgery. In: Roskamm H, Schmuziger M (eds). Coronary heart surgery. Springer, Berlin, Heidelberg, New York, 1979.

3. Gehring J, Koenig W, Wrana N, Mathes P: Aortokoronare Bypass-Operation Welche Faktoren beeinflussen die Arbeitswiederaufnahme Herz + Gefäße 4:205, 1984.

4. Hammermeister KE, DeRouen TA, English MT, Dodge HT: Effect of Surgical Versus Medical Therapy on Return to Work in Patients With Coronary Artery Disease. Am J Cardiol 44:105, 1979.

33. Late Results of Reperfusion with Intracoronary Streptokinase

P. G. HUGENHOLTZ, M. L. SIMOONS, P. W. SERRUYS, P. J. DE FEYTER, M. VAN DEN BRAND and P. FIORETTI

Abstract

The reasons for attempting to salvage myocardium threatened by ischemia during temporary or permanent occlusion of one of the nutrient arteries, such as after coronary thrombosis, is based on the observation that the major determinant of survival and the main reason for complications after recovery is the extent to which myocardium has been lost through infarction. Approaches proven to be of relevance under human clinical circumstances, fall into three groups: attempts to reduce the use of oxygen through pharmacological means when oxygen supply is jeopardized, attempts at restoring the blood supply and oxygen delivery at an early stage by manipulations on the coronary arteries and interventions aimed at reducing the damage of cardiac cells after onset of ischemia or during reperfusion. Endpoints considered to be proof of improved left ventricular performance will be: wall motion studies, ejection fraction measurements and reduction in death rate and other serious cardiovascular complications.

Studies involving beta blockers, calcium antagonists, prostaglandines and other pharmacological agents will be contrasted with results obtained from intracoronary thrombolysis through streptokinase and related products. In addition, results will be reported of vasodilator drugs such as nitrates and sodium nitroprusside. Although final proof from prospective randomized studies, one of which is carried out in our Institute and the Netherlands Interuniversitary Cardiological Institute, with intracoronary streptokinase with 302 patients, will not be available at the time of this presentation, arguments will be provided which indicate that the second major approach i.e. restoration of blood supply at an early stage, preferably supported by pharmacological therapy with beta blockade and calcium antagonists, is to be preferred; inasmuch as current data indicate improved function and in certain subsets, improved life expectancy.

Introduction

The feasibility of rapid dissolution of intracoronary thrombi by semiselective or selective infusion of thrombolytic substances has been demonstrated in experimental series (Boucek and Murphy, 1960; Bolton et al., 1961; Chazorv et al., 1976). However, the concept of limiting infarct size as a contribution to the aims of secondary prevention by early re-establishment of anterograde flow, was not introduced into clinical practice until 1978 by Rentrop et al., 1978, 1979. Since then we have witnessed an explosion in the number of patients with acute ischemic cardiac disorders who have been treated by intracoronary streptokinase infusion. Whereas a review of the recent literature leaves no doubt that intracoronary lysis of the thrombus with streptokinase can re-establish blood flow through the acutely occluded coronary artery in approximately 80 % of the cases (Rentrop et al., 1981; Hugenholtz and Rentrop, 1982; Serruys et al., 1982), this fact alone does not necessarily indicate that such a form of treatment is beneficial to the patient in terms of reduced reinfarction and mortality. In fact, the wide-spread dissemination of the new technique appears to be premature since its benefits and risks have not yet been adequately investigated (Bresnahan et al., 1974; Smith et al., 1974; Reimer et al., 1977; Schaper et al., 1979; Ganz et al., 1981), while experimental evidence is not uniformly encouraging.

Neither is it clear after 13 major international trials with intravenous streptokinase, in well over 15,000 patients (European Working Party 1971, European Cooperative Studygroup 1979), that by this means a definite reduction in mortality or reinfarction rate can be achieved. Even today a major trial, in progress in Germany, had to extent the number of individuals included to > 2000 in an effort to achieve statistical significance (Voehringer et al., 1984). Recent data, by Ganz and Lew, 1984, claiming a high successrate of over 90 % are very difficult to interpret as to their relevance in daily practice given the highly restrictive admission criteria (limiting the interval between symptoms and active treatment to one hour) the soft endpoints and the non randomized design which introduced strong selection bias in their patients.

The purpose of this paper is to detail the course of events in the first year of follow up of 302 patients with acute infarction, randomly assigned to intracoronary thrombolysis with streptokinase or to conventional treatment. These data are relevant in terms of their potential significance for secondary prevention. The data form part of an ongoing trial and have to be seen as an interim opinion (Simoons et al., 1984).

Methods and Materials

A flow chart of the protocol employed in the ongoing study of the Nether-

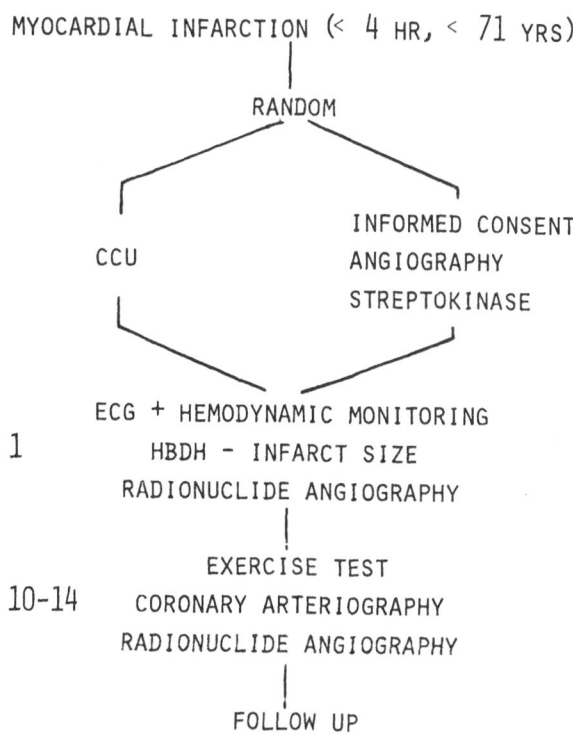

Figure 1. Flowchart of patients included in the randomized trial on intracoronary streptokinase versus conventional therapy in the CCU. (see text).

lands Interuniversitary Institute is presented in Figure 1. Patients randomised to the active treatment were asked for informed consent, prior to the cardiac catheterisation which had a diagnostic as well a therapeutic component. Patients who refused consent, were treated according to the same conventional treatment protocol as was given to the control individuals.

Conventional treatment was that which was indicated by the hemodynamic status of the patient. It was attempted to keep heart rates between 60 and 90 beats per minute, systolic blood pressure between 100 and 140 mm Hg, while signs of left ventricular failure, were treated accordingly (Simoons et al., 1982).

All patients were treated with full dose heparin, followed by coumadin until hospital discharge. After hospital discharge coumadin was continued only in those patients who had signs of intra ventricular thrombus, valvular incompetence or large ventricles with poor contraction.

Patients assigned to the active treatment were initially treated with nitroglycerine i.v. in a dose which reduces systolic blood pressure to 100–140 mm Hg. They were also given lidocaine 2 mg/min and intravenous heparine, 5000 E, in addition to 250 mg acetyl-salicylicacid and 100 mg prednisolone.

Coronary angiography was performed with the Judkins technique. If the artery appeared occluded, streptokinase was given at a rate of 4000 U/min until all visible intracoronary clots had disappeared or the lumen was reasonably patent. The maximum was usually 250,000 U. Upon completion of the desobstruction, complete left and right coronary arteriography was performed and, when the clinical condition permitted this, left ventriculography was carried out in the RAO-projection. In 27 patients angioplasty was carried out in the same setting.

Further details of other laboratory procedures can be found in earlier publications from our institution. All patients were followed at the outpatient clinic for at least one year after admission. The incidence of recurrent myocardial infarction, angina pectoris, heart failure and the need for bypass surgery or PTCA, as well as prescribed medication were recorded and form the substance of this report.

Results

The data were analysed from 302 patients, who prior to 1.1.1984 were allocated to conventional treatment in 150 and to active treatment in 152 instances. Recanalisation was achieved in 88 out of 111 occluded arteries, while 25 arteries were found to be patent at the time of the initial cardiac catheterisation. Sixteen patients refused when informed consent was asked or were found to have major contraindications after randomisation (Table 1). Whilst there were no differences observed in the classification based on hemodynamic data, measured in the coronary care unit between the two groups, pericarditis occurred less frequent in the treated group, 6 individuals versus 23 in the control group.

Severe heart failure or shock occurred in 20 instances of the controlgroup and in 8 actively treated patients. Ventricular fibrillation occurred in 31 instances in the controlgroup, 20 in the actively treated group, none of these differences are statistically significant.

Table 1. Results at 10 month follow up after randomisation

	Controls	Treated	Refused	Angiography $\circ \to \circ$	$\bullet \to \bullet$	$\bullet \to \circ$
Patients	150	152	16	25	23	88
Deaths	22	17	4	–	7	6
Reinfarction	9	20	7	3	1	14

When analyzed according to the 'intention to treat principle', there also appeared to be no difference in mortality at the 3 month follow up (18 deaths in the controls, 14 deaths in the streptokinase group) nor at a median of the 10 month follow up (22 deaths in the controls and 17 in the streptokinase group).

At the tenth month there were 9 reinfarctions in the control group and 20 in the thrombolysis group. Coronary artery bypass grafting, and or PTCA was performed in 29 patients out of the control group versus 30 in the group treated with streptokinase.

In the subgroup of patients who refused streptokinase therapy after randomisation and in those in whom recanalisation failed, complications were worse than in those in whom recanalisation was achieved, inasmuch as 4 of the 16 patients who had refused after randomisation died in addition to 7 out of 23 patients in whom recanalization was unsuccessful. On the other hand, there was only one death among the 27 patients in whom balloondilatation was carried out immediately after successful recanalisation. This subset also had the best functional improvement (Fig. 2). Results of hemodynamic studies are provided in Table 2.

Discussion

Rapid relief of chest pain after reperfusion, a change in arrhythmias or reduction of ST segment abnormalities and shifts in the released cardiac enzymes, reported by Rentrop et al., 1981; Ganz et al., 1981; Rutsch et al.,

Table 2. Evidence for preserved left ventricular function after intracoronary thrombolysis in a subset in whom complete catheterization data were available

Mean ± SD	Ia	Ib	IIa	IIb	IIIa	IIIb
EDV (ml/m^2)	81±20	99±27*	75±23	100±26*	86±17	97±27
ESV (ml/m^2)	39±15	55±27*	35±16	56±26	41±14	55±29
EF (%)	54±11	46±14*	56±11	45±14	53±11	46±14

$$* \ p < 0.005$$

Group Ia = 59 patients with intracoronary streptokinase therapy
Group Ib = 63 patients with conventional therapy
Group IIa = 27 patients with inferior infarction and streptokinase therapy
Group IIb = 31 patients with inferior infarction and conventional therapy
Group IIIa = 33 patients with anterior infarction and intracoronary streptokinase
Group IIIb = 32 patients with anterior infarction and conventional therapy

SUCCESSFUL PTCR VS PTCR+PTCA VS UNSUCCESSFUL PTCR
CHRONIC STAGE
ANTERIOR INFARCTION

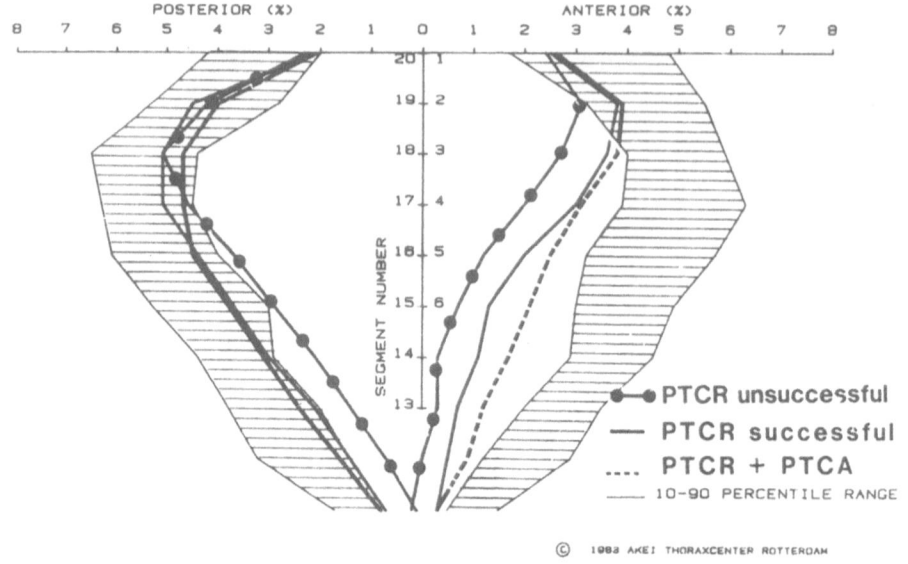

Figure 2. Regional cardiac wall motion in 20 segments of the left ventricle. After thrombolytic therapy (PTCR) and PTCA, the improvement in left ventriculat function is best. (personal comunication by P.W. Serruys, 1984)

1981 and Fioretti et al., 1982 may indicate relief of ischemia or acceleration of the evolution of infarction. All these signs, however, are 'soft' endpoints which may be explained by other mechanisms. They offer only very partial evidence of benefit. Better to interpret are the effects of reperfusion upon left ventricular function. These have been assessed in several studies, some of which allow definite conclusions, since ejection fractions improved significantly. Tutsch et al., 1981 and Merx et al., 1981, in their most recent collection series of 174 patients, reported that for a subset of 68 patients in whom early recanalization of the completely obstructed vessel could be achieved, ejection fraction, determined by contrast angiography, rose slightly but significantly from $52 \pm 13\%$ before intervention to $58 \pm 13\%$ immediately after intracoronary streptokinase infusion. Our randomized study showed that while by isotope studies no significant immediate differences could be demonstrated in ejection fraction between both groups, from the second week onwards angiographic data demonstrated much improved left ventricular function (Simoons et al., 1982; Hooghoudt et al., 1982). In fact, the ejection fraction in the actively treated group was 54% versus 46% in the control group (Table 2), a difference which is statistically significant. Also enddiastolic and endsystolic volumes were normal, in contrast to 'untreated' patients. As changes in left ventricular function immediately after the acute intervention are difficult to assess because of other interrelated factors such as early reduction in compliance (stiff left ventricle), blood viscosity, absence of collaterals, additional drug therapy such as nitrates, etc., the two week data gain further significance as to the extent of recovery. Also, as indicated by the experimental data of Ross et al., 1975 and by the observations of Serruys et al., 1980 from our unit following open heart surgery, complete recovery of function of a reperfused ischemic zone may take up to six weeks, so that further improvement could have been seen had we restudied the patients later.

Serruys et al., 1982 and Hooghoudt et al., 1982 analysed moment-to-moment changes of function in various segments of the left ventrice wall by means of a computer program, which divides the left ventricular in 20 segments. They found significant functional improvement in those segments perfused by a permanently recanalized vessel, while no changes were noted in those segments supplied by (re)occluded vessels (Fig. 2). This would explain the increase in function shown in Table 2. In some successfully treated patients, however, the amelioration in left ventricular global function appeared to be also due to improvement in the function of non-infarcted segments. This may be related to the perfusion of collateral vessels which were not functioning prior to reperfusion or to improvement in marginal areas or to a permanent compensation (beginning hypertrophy?) by non-infarcted areas. Even so, our data confirm that at least a large part of the improvement in global left ventricular function, seen by most authors after streptokinase infusion, must be due to the salvage of previously non-functioning, but viable cardiac cells. It strongly suggests that even up to several hours after the onset of occlusion a concept of the 'stunned' but viable myocardium (Braunwald and Kloner, 1982) is a proper one and that early reperfusion is an essential component for secondary prevention.

Recently, Schofer et al., 1984 attempted to measure the extent of myocardial necrosis immediately after coronary thrombolysis by means of intracoronary injection of technetium-99m pyrophosphate. They found, 20 to 30 minutes after thrombolysis, localized accumulation of the indicator, a finding not seen in patients conventionally treated after myocardial infarction, since their scintigrams became only positive 12 to 36 hours after the onset of symptoms. Since this accumulation of radio-active labelled pyrophosphate, depends not only on the presence of myocardial necrosis, but also on the restoration of a certain amount of bloodflow through the area, the data indicate that after intracoronary thrombolysis, flow can be reestablished, even to the area of necrosis itself. This method may therefore provide a better means to assess the extent of loss of myocardium. Even though not yet confirmed by other authors, this method is potentially much more accurate than the various measurements in the ECG, such as the extent of R-wave preservation or Q-wave reduction or ST-segment mapping which all have been recommended as indicators of the extent of necrosis. However, we believe they are very 'soft' endpoints, and very difficult to accept as final proof, since so many other factors may influence their outcome. The only parameter that may relate to the extent of necrosis is the reduction of the amount of a-HBDH released in the blood stream, indicating a smaller over-all infarct size in the treated group compared to the controls as shown by Simoons et al., 1984. By far the most convincing evidence that intracoron-ary streptokinase indeed has a major beneficial influence on interim out-come would have been a reduction in the rate of reinfarction, a lesser need for subsequent procedures or a lower mortality. In the current trial, interim data analysis on the 'intention to treat principle' shows that in patients recanalized within the first 4 hours after onset of symptoms, mortality was slightly but not significantly lower at 10 months follow up, when compared to those who are treated conventionally. However, if one removes the sub-group of patients who refused angiography and those in whom recanaliza-tion failed, in whom mortality is high, and contrasts this with only 1 late death out of the 27 patients in whom the recanalization with balloon angio-plasty was successful, the therapy would appear much more promising. This kind of interpretation of the data, obviously not allowable under the 'inten-tion to treat principle', but often applied in the interpretation of open trials without randomisation indicates that successful therapy, when accepted, where applicable and provided it is done early, may lead to a marked reduction in mortality and reinfarction rate, presumably one of the aims of good secondary prevention.

Since the aim of this symposium is to indicate the optimal approach of secondary prevention in the patient with acute myocardial infarction, this mode of therapy must be compared with others which portend similar ben-efits. Of these, clearly the intravenous use of thrombolytic agents must be seriously considered and the recent data reported by Ganz et al., 1984 attest to a similar beneficial action.

One alternate approach is the immediate or early administration of beta-blocking agents. The recent trials with metoprolol do provide clear evidence that a beneficial effect can be expected on enzyme release and ECG signs, the magnitude of which is, however, not overwhelming. No reduction in mortality has been reported. On the other hand, a significant reduction in mortality figures in the first year after onset of therapy with beta blockade in the other of 25% was achieved for a relatively restricted number of patients with acute myocardial infarction who met both the exclusion and the inclu-sion criteria of the BHAT, the metoprolol and timolol trials (Hjalmarson et al., 1983, Int. Collaborative Studygroup, 1984), when treated within the first 2 weeks after onset of infarction. When one looks carefully at these criteria at best 25% of the population offered to the recent beta blocker trials could in fact be included. If a similar kind of selection were to be applied to the ongoing intracoronary streptokinase trial, for example by looking only at those who entered very early (< 2 hours) and who were given intracoronary streptokinase and angioplasty with balloon dilatation in the same setting, preferably after prior intravenous streptokinase, a totally different image would emerge.

The difficulty with the exclusion criteria and the disappointing results from the recent trial with early intravenous and oral administration of metoprolol in patients with acute myocardial infarction (MIAMI for short, 1984), in which for mortality no significant difference in favour of beta-blockade administered within 24 hours after onset of infarction could be demonstrated would lead one to believe that perhaps aspirine may offer the greatest protective influence. It certainly would be the cheapest drug of all, it has the least number of exclusion criteria and the recent data from Lewis et al., 1983 would indicate that a marked reduction in one year mortality can be achieved. Unfortunately their data apply to patients with unstable angina, who certainly are not identical to those with acute myocardial infarction.

It has been the purpose of this paper to report on the current status of intracoronary streptokinase in acute myocardial infarction, as one method to effect secondary prevention. Since ours is but one of the three large scale randomized trials with i.c. streptokinase currently in progress in the world (Rentrop 1984 in New York and Kennedy et al., 1983 in Washington State conducted others), it is reassuring but disappointing that neither has indicated great benefits in terms of reduction of mortality.

Since the greatest efficacy of the therapy was achieved in that subset of patients in our trial in whom after successful thrombolysis a PTCA procedure could be carried out, it is very likely that the optimal restoration of bloodflow early after a myocardial infarction remains the route to strive for rather than to await the protective results of beta-blockade or aspirin treatment after occlusion. Meyer et al., 1984, will argue this point forcibly. In fact this is the observation reported by De Wood et al., 1980, 1983 in which it is advocated to use coronary artery bypass grafting in all patients who, within 4 or 6 hours after the onset of symptoms, can reach the operating table. Although their data were not obtained in a randomized fashion and have not yet been confirmed by an on-going trial in the United States, the attraction in this hypothesis is that corresponds to ours advocating early i.v. and i.c. streptokinase in selected cases. Both agree that it means early restoration of blood supply perhaps by a combination of techniques, as advocated by Mathey et al., 1981, and Yasuno et al., 1984, deserves further systematic study.

In summary, this indicates that several benefits can be derived from intracoronary streptokinase even when assessed on an 'intention to treat' basis. Subset analysis confirms the views of those who subscribe to the notion that early reperfusion of ischemic. cardiac tissue is the only efficacious therapy available today but a systematic study of this is lacking thus far.

References

1. Bolton HE, Tapia FA, Cabral H, Riera R, Mazel MS: Removal of Acute Coronary Thrombus with Fibrinolysis – In Vivo Experiment. JAMA 175:307–310, 1961.
2. Boucek RJ, Murphy WP jr: Segmental perfusion of the coronary arteries with fibrinolysis in man following a myocardial infarction. Am J Cardiol 6:525–533, 1960.
3. Braunwald E, Kloner RA: The stunned myocardium: Reduction of CK and CK-MB indexes of infarct size by intravenous nitroglycerine. Circulation 63, 3:615–622, 1982.
4. Bresnahan GF, Roberts R, Shell WE, Ross J Jr, Sobel BE: Deleterious effects due to hemorrhage after myocardial reperfusion. Am J Cardiol 33:82–86, 1974.
5. Chazov EL, Mateeva LS, Mazaev AV, Sargin KE, Sadovshaya M, Ruda Y: Intracoronary administration of fibrinolysis in acute myocardial infarction. Ter Arkh 48(4):8, 1976.
6. Collen D: Coronary Thrombolysis with Tissue-type plasminogen activator (t-PA) in acute myocardial infarction. Proceedings Conference: Improvement of Myocardial Perfusion, Mainz, abstract pp 6, 1984.
7. European Cooperative Study Group for streptokinase treatment in acute myocardial infarction: streptokinase in acute myocardial infarction. N Engl J Med 301:797–802, 1979.
8. European Working Party: Streptokinase in recent myocardial infarction: A controlled multicenter trial. Br Med J 3:325–331, 1971.
9. Fioretti P, Simoons ML, Serruys PW, Brand M vd, Fels Ph, Hugenholtz PG: Clinical Course after attempted thrombolysis in Myocardial Infarction. Results of pilot studies and preliminary data from a randomized trial. Eur Heart J 3:422–432, 1982.
10. Ganz W, Buchbinder N, Marcus H, Mondkar A, Maddahi J, Charuzi Y, O'Connor L, Shell W, Fischbein MC, Kass R, Miyamoto A, Swan HJC: Intracoronary thrombolysis in evolving myocardial infarction. Am Heart J 101:4–13, 1981.
11. Ganz W, Geft I, Shah PK et al.: Intravenous streptokinase in evolving acute myocardial infarction. Cedars-Sinai Med Center Los Angeles, Ca USA, Am J Cardiol 53:1505–1516, 1984.
12. Ganz W, Lew AS: Can early Reperfusion salvage myocardium? Proceedings Conference: Improvement of Myocardial Perfusion, Mainz, abstract pp 14, 1984.
13. Ganz W, Ninomiya K, Hashida J, Fishbein MD, Buchbinder N, Marcus H, Mondkar A, Maddahi J, Shah PK, Berman D, Charuzi Y, Geft I, Shell W, Swan HJC: Intracoronary trombolysis in acute myocardial infarction: experimental background and clinical experience. Am Heart J 102:1145–1149, 1981.
14. Hjalmarson A, Herlitz J, Holmberg S, Rijden L, Swedberg K, Vedin A, Waagstein F, Waldenstroem A, Waldenstroem J, Wedel H, Wilhelmsen L, Wilhelmssom C: The Göteborg metoprolol trial. Effects on mortality and morbidity in acute myocardial infarction. Circulation 67:6, 2, 126–132, 1983.
15. Hooghoudt TEH, Serruys PW, Reiber JHC, Slager CJ, Brand van den M, Hugenholtz PG: The effect of recanalization of the occluded coronary artery in acute myocardial infarction on left ventricular function. Eur Heart J 3:416–421, 1982.
16. Hugenholtz PG, Rentrop P: Thrombolytic therapy for acute myocardial infarction: quo vadis? Eur Heart J 3:395–403, 1982.

17. Hugenholtz PG, Simoons ML: Thrombolytic Therapy for Acute Myocardial Infarction. Hammersmith Cardiology Workshop Series, Raven Press 1:175–184, 1984.

18. Kennedy JW, Ritchie JL, Davis KB, Fritz JK: Western Washington Randomized Trial of Intracoronary Streptokinase in Acute Myocardial Infarction. N Engl J Med 309:1477–1482, 1983.

19. Lewis HJ jr, Davis JW, Archibald DG, Steinke WE, Smitherman TC, Doherty JE, Schaper HW, LeWinter MM, Linares E, Pouset JM, Sabharwal SC, Chesler E, DeMots H: Protective effects of aspirin against acute myocardial infarction and death in men with unstable angina. Results of a Veteran Administration Cooperative Study. N Engl J Med 309, 7:396–403, 1983.

20. Merx W, Dorr R, Rentrop P, Blanke H, Karsch KR, Mathey DG, Kremer P, Rutsch W, Schmutzler H: Evaluation of the effectiveness of intracoronary streptokinase infusion in acute myocardial infarction: Postprocedure management and hospital course in 204 patients. Am Heart J 102:1181–1187, 1981.

21. Meyer J: Elsewhere in these proceedings.

22. Miami Trial: Personal communication, detailed report to appear in the Lancet, 1984.

23. Reimer KA, Lowe JE, Rasmussen MM, Jennings RB: The wavefront phenomenon of ischemic cell death. I. Myocardial infarct size vs duration of coronary artery occlusion in dogs. Circulation 56:786–794, 1977.

24. Rentrop P: Personal Communication, 1984.

25. Rentrop P, Blanke H, Karsch KR, Kaiser H, Kostering H, Leitz K: Selective intracoronary thrombolysis in acute myocarcial infarction and unstable angina pectoris. Circulation 63:307–317, 1981.

26. Rentrop P, Blanke H, Kostering K, Karsch KR: Acute myocardial infarction: Intracoronary application of nitroglycerine and streptokinase in combination with transluminal recanalization. Clin Cardiol 5:354, 1979.

27. Rentrop P, De Vivie, ER, Karsch KR, Kreuzer H: Acute coronary occlusion with impending infarction as an angiographic complication relieved by a guide wire recanalization. Clin Cardiol:101–107, 1978.

28. Ross J, Theroux P, Sasayma S, McKown C, Franklin D: Late recovery of cardiac function after coronary artery reperfusion (abstr). Circulation, 51 supp II:21, 1975.

29. Rutsch W, Schartl M, Mathey D, Kuck K, Merx W, Dorr R, Rentrop P, Blanke H: Percutaneous transluminal coronary recanalization: Procedure, results, and acute complications. Am Heart J 102:1178–1180, 1981.

30. Schaper W, Frenzel H, Hart W, Winkler B: Experimental coronary artery occlusion. II. Spatial and temporal evolution of infarcts in dog heart. Basic Res Cardiol 74:233–239, 1979.

31. Schofer J, Strizler P, Montz R, Mathey DG: Assessment of myocardial necrosis immediately after intracoronary thrombolysis by intracoronary injection of Technetium-99m pyrophosphate. Eur Heart J 5:617–621, 1984.

32. Schwartz F, Hofman M, Schuler G, von Olshausen K, Zimmerman R, Kubler W: Thrombolysis in acute myocardial infarction: effect of intravenous followed by intracoronary streptokinase application on estimates of infarct size. Am J Cardiol 53:1505–1510, 1984.

33. Serruys PW, Brand M van den , Hooghoudt TEH, Simoons ML, Fioretti P, Ruiter J, Fels PhW, Hugenholtz PG: Coronary recanalization in acute myocardial infarction. Eur Heart J 3:404–415, 1982

34. Serruys PW, Brower RW, Katen HJ ten, Meester GT: Recovery from circulatory depression after coronary artery bypass surgery. Eur Surg Res 12:369–382, 1980.

35. Simoons ML, Balakumaran K, Serruys PW, Brand M vd, Fioretti P, Hugenholtz PG: The effect of intracoronary thrombolysis with streptokinase on myocardial thallium redistribution and global and regional left ventricular function. Eur Heart J 3:433–440, 1982.

36. Simoons Ml, Neef de KJ, Serruys PW, Fioretti P, Brand van den M: Recanalization on acute myocardial infarction on intracoronary infusion of streptokinase. Interim results of a randomized trial. Proceedings of a Symposium New techniques in Cardiology, Amsterdam, (Editor: V. Manger Cats) pp 25–35, 1984.

37. Smith GT, Soeter JR, Haston HH, McNamara JJ: Coronary reperfusion in primates. Serial electrocardiographic and histologic assessmant. J Clin Invest 54:1420–1427, 1974.

38. The International Collaborative Study Group: Reduction of infarct size with the early use of timolol in acute myocardial infarction. N Engl J Med 310:9–15, 1984.

39. Vöhringer HF, Linderer TH, Schröder R: Intravenöse Streptokinase Behandlung beim Acuten Myokardinfarct: Langzeitverlauf. Zeitschr für Kardiol 73:45, 1984.

40. Wood de MA, Spores J, Notske R, Mouser LT, Burroughs R, Golden MS, Lang HT: Prevalence of total coronary occlusion during the early hours of transmural myocardial infarction. N Engl J Med 303:897–902, 1980.

41. Yasuno M, Saito Y, Ishida M, Suzuki K, Endo S, Takahasi M: Effects of percutaneous transluminal coronary angioplasty: intracoronary thrombolysis with urokinase in acute myocardial infarction. Am J Cardiol 53:1217–1220.

34. Percutaneous Transluminal Coronary Angioplasty after Thrombolysis to Prevent Reinfarction

J. MEYER, R. ERBEL, T. POP, G. SCHREINER, B. HENKEL, K. HENRICHS, H. J. RUPPRECHT and H. KOPP

Abstract

After successful intracoronary and intravenous thrombolysis in acute myocardial infarction in about 90% of all cases a more than 60% organic stenosis of the diseased vessel can be found. This stenosis may impede coronary blood flow and be the reason for recurrent angina in the rehabilitation phase. Despite the consequent anticoagulation with heparin and coumadine rethrombosis at the same site may occur. We therefore perform the intracoronary transluminal angioplasty of such stenoses immediately after successful thrombolysis within the same cath-lab session to prevent reinfarction.

In a prospective, controlled, randomized study group I patients with successful thrombolysis and group II patients with successful thrombolysis with PTCA are controlled with respect to infarction rate, reocclusion rate, mortality, and myocardial infarction.

Patients of both groups did not differ in age, distribution of sex and diseased vessel, time elapsed between symptoms and start of intracoronary lysis, time to maximum of CPK-curve.

In group I 36 patients are restudied after four weeks. Five out of 32 recanalized vessels showed a reocclusion. In group II dilatation was achieved in 60% (1 occlusion). Out of the successfully dilated patients only 5% had a reocclusion, while 5/14 patients (36%) with unsuccessful dilatation had a reocclusion.

In group I the survival rate was 40/48 patients (83%) compared to 45/51 patients (88%) in group II. The reinfarction rate during the hospital phase was seven patients in group I and two patients in group II with a cardiac mortality of seven patients group I and two patients group II. There was one noncardiac death in group I and four in group II.

While ejection fraction and analysis of segmental wall motion are not different between both groups, postextrasystolic potentiation showed improved contraction patterns in group II.

Introduction

PTCA following successful thrombolysis can be performed with a low complication rate. It seems to lower in-hospital reinfarction and mortality rate, while myocardial function seems not to be improved.

After successful reopening of an occluded coronary artery either by intravenous or by intracoronary application of thrombolytic agents or by the use of tissue-type plasminogen activators the long-term results are depending on the permanent patency of the diseased vessel. The patency rate is depending on a strict anticoagulation regime in the acute as well as in the chronic phase. On the other hand the regularly underlying coronary stenoses may be the cristallization point of another thrombus formation. In a randomized prospective study we treated 99 consecutive, unselected patients with acute transmural myocardial infarction by either streptokinase alone or by streptokinase plus sequential intracoronary balloon angioplasty (PTCA).

Patients and methods

Technique of thrombolysis

Thrombolysis could be started in all 99 patients within the first six hours after the onset of the first symptoms of an acute myocardial infarction. The randomization of all patients was defined prior to the begin of the study.

The patients were given 1 g acethylsalicylic acid, 250 mg of prednisone and 5000 IU of heparin intravenously together with a loading dose of 250,000 IU streptokinase intravenously within 20 min. After selective coronary angiography of both coronary vessels an initial bolus of 50,000 IU of streptokinase was injected via a special infusion catheter directly infront of the occluding thrombus. This catheter was advanced through a Judkins 8F-catheter. A continuous infusion of 4000 IU/min of streptokinase was given until the vessel was reopened and 30 min thereafter to dissolve the remaining clot material.

After the cath-lab procedure all patients were monitored hemodynamically and electrocardiographically on the CCU. The heparinization started six hours later (infusion rate 800–1200 IU/h) for three days followed by an overlapping of coumadine, until the control study at the fourth week.

Patient selection and pretreatment interval

The study population consisted of 99 patients (Table 1) in group I 48 patients were treated by streptokinase alone. In group II 51 patients were

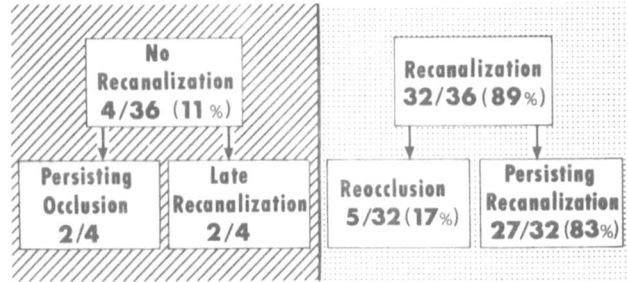

Figure 1. Patency rate of the coronary arteries between the acute phase and the end of the hospital period of four weeks, group I, lysis without dilatation

Table 1. Randomized group. Thrombolysis with/without dilatation

	Without Dilatation n = 48	With Dilatation n = 51	
♂ ♀	42/6	45/6	n.s.
Age	56.3±11.6 y	56.4±9.9 y	n.s.
≥ 70 y	9	8	n.s.
Diseased Vessels	24	LAD = 22	n.s.
	19	RCA = 24	n.s.
	5	CX = 5	n.s.
Time Symptoms → i.c.Lysis	202±74 min	204±63 min	n.s.
Max. CPK	1345±1039 IU	1165±911 IU	n.s.

treated by streptokinase and immediately after reopening of the vessel also with the PTCA of the remaining stenosis. Both groups did not differ with respect to age, sex distribution, infarct localization, time between onset of symptoms and begin of the intracoronary lysis as well as maximum of CPK. There was no age limit. In group I nine patients and in group II eight patients were more than 70 years old.

Results at the end of the hospital phase

In group I of thrombolysis without PTCA 36 patients were controlled after four weeks (Fig. 1). In four of them (11 %) no recanalization was initially reached. In two of them the occlusion persisted while the other showed a late spontaneous recanalization.

In the group of primary recanalization by thrombolysis five out of 32 patients (17 %) had a spontaneous reocclusion of the infarct related vessel

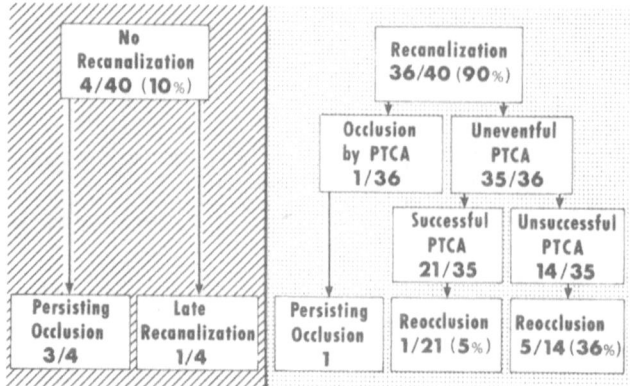

Figure 2. Patency rate of the coronary arteries between the acute phase and the end of the hospital period of four weeks, group II, lysis with dilatation

during the hospital phase, while 27 (83%) demonstrated a persistent recanalization.

In group II 40 patients were controlled angiographically after four weeks (Fig. 2). In four out of 40 controlled patients (10%) no recanalization of the infarct related vessel was reached by thrombolysis. In three of them the vessel occlusion persisted after four weeks. In one patient a late spontaneous recanalization had occurred.

In all 36 patients with successful recanalization (group II) PTCA was attempted. In one patient a reocclusion was caused by the balloon. This artificial occlusion could not be reversed either by catheter maneuvers or by additional streptokinase application.

In 35 out of 36 patients the PTCA procedure was without complications. It was successful in 21 (60%) of them. One of these 21 patients (5%) showed a late reocclusion at the end of the hospital phase. In the group of an

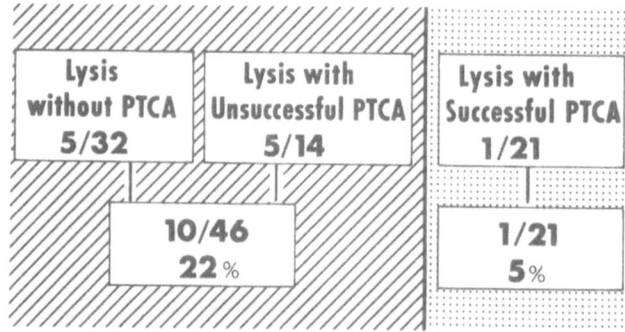

Figure 3. Patency rate of coronary arteries, lysis with successful dilatation vs. lysis without and with unsuccessful dilatation

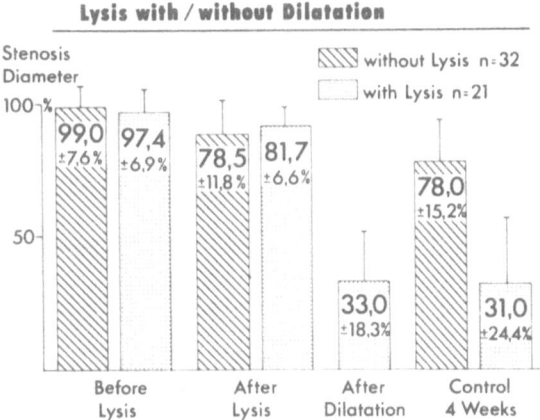

Figure 4. Degree of coronary stenosis (luminal diameter) of patients with and without dilatation before thrombolysis, after successful lysis as well as at the control study after four weeks

unsuccessful PTCA procedure in five out of 14 patients (36%) the vessel was occluded at the control study.

If the patients with lysis alone and those with an unsuccessful PTCA attempt were combined (Fig. 3) the reocclusion was quite high. Ten out of 46 patients (22%) showed occluded vessels. In the group of 21 patients with lysis and successful dilatation only one patient had a late reocclusion (5%).

Degree of vessel obstruction

In group I 32 pts. were controlled angiographically after four weeks (Fig. 4). Before thrombolysis the vessel obstruction was $99,0 \pm 7.6\%$. After thrombolysis a resting stenosis of $78.5 \pm 11.8\%$ luminal diameter remained. At the control study after four weeks the average stenosis had not changed significantly $(78.0 \pm 15.2\%)$.

In group II the initial stenosis before lysis was $97.4 \pm 6.9\%$. Immediately after thrombolysis the resting stenosis was calculated by $81.7 \pm 6.6\%$. After successful dilatation a resting stenosis of $33.0 \pm 18.3\%$ was seen. At the control study the remaining stenosis was $31.9 \pm 24.4\%$. The difference between group I and group II after four weeks was highly significant $(p < 0.0001)$.

Left ventricular function

In 24 pts. of group I and in 10 pts. of group II left ventricular ejection fraction was measured by using extrasystole-free angiograms (Fig. 5). In

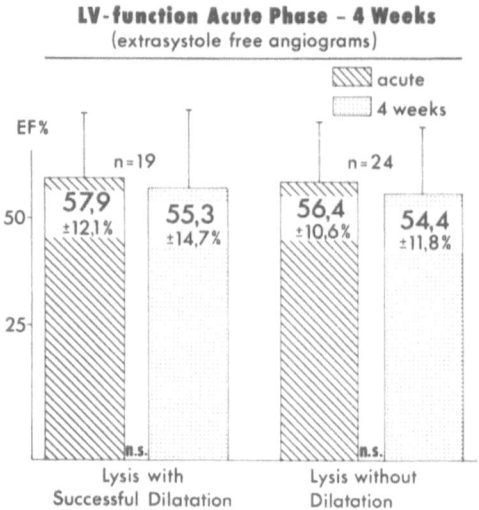

Figure 5. Development of ejection fraction between the acute phase and the control study

both groups there were no significant differences between the acute phase and the control study after four weeks. There were also no differences between group I and group II in the acute phase and at the time of the control study. In a group of 30 pts. at the control study after four weeks the postextrasystolic potentiation was analyzed by two-dimensional echacardiography (Fig. 6). The coupling interval of the extrastimuli was 400 msec. The postextrasystolic potentiation was measured as a difference of the ejection fraction (delta-EF). With this parameter in the group of lysis with successful dilatation a significant better contraction was found compared to the group of lysis without successful dilatation ($p < 0.05$) and lysis without dilatation

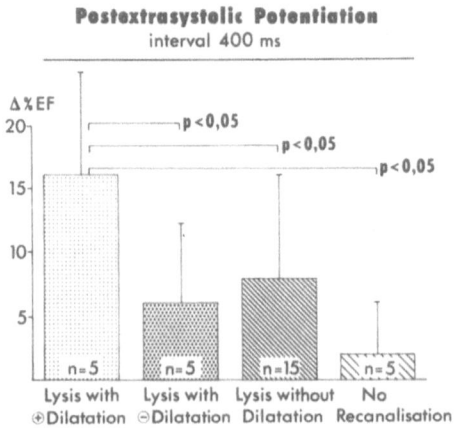

Figure 6. Differences of delta-EF in the postextrasystolic beat (coupling interval 400 ms)

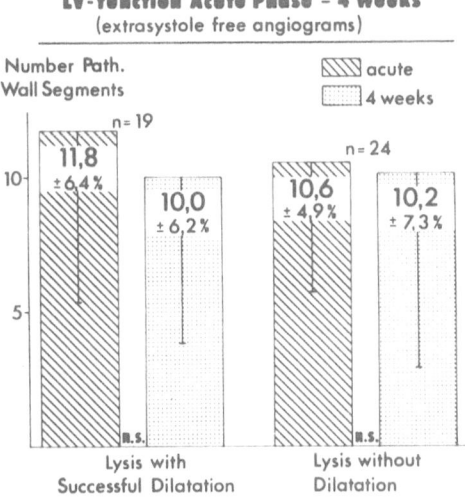

Figure 7. Number of pathological wall segments in the acute phase and at the control study. Postextrastolic beat, coupling interval 400 ms

($p < 0.05$). In patients without recanalization by thrombolysis there were no changes of the wall motion. The infarcted area was replaced by definite scar.

In 43 patients the number of pathological wall segments in the acute phase was compared to that at the time of the control study (Fig. 7). There were slightly less pathological wall motions in the group of lysis with successful dilatation (10.0 ± 6.2 vs $11.8 \pm 6.4 \%$). These differences, however, were not significant. In the group of lysis without dilatation there were no differences. This parameter was not able to show any advantage of either procedure.

In group I 40 out of 48 patients survived (83 %) (Table 2). There were seven reinfarctions, seven cardiac and one non-cardiac death. In group II 45

Table 2. Clinical course during hospital phase

	Lysis without Dilatation n = 48	Lysis with Dilatation n = 51
Survivors	40 (83 %)	45 (88 %)
Reinfarctions	7	2
Cardiac Deaths	7	2
Non-cardiac Deaths	1	4
Control Studies	36 (75 %)	40 (78 %)
Denied Controls	4 (8 %)	5 (10 %)

out of 51 patients survived (88 %). There were two reinfarctions, two cardiac and four non-cardiac deaths.

In group I we were able to perform a control study in 36 patients (75 %), while four patients denied this control study. In group II the numbers were 40 patients for the control and five for the refusers.

The reason for the lethal outcome of both groups are listed in Table 3 and 4. In group I there was a higher rate of cardiac deaths. In group II three patients died from shock lung. Only two patients died from cardiac reasons. There were no significant differences regarding the interval between the onset of infarction and the time of death. The mean age of the non-survivors in both groups was relatively high compared to the average age of the whole group.

At the post-mortem-study in group I only three out of eight patients showed an open vessel compared to four out of six in group II. In two patients no autopsy was performed.

Table 3. Data of non-survivors, lysis without dilatation

Cause of death	Day of infarction	Age	Diseased vessel	Vessel status
Sudden Death	13	58	LAD	Fresh Thrombus
Reinfarction	2	46	RCA	Reocclusion
Reinfarction	2	54	LAD	Reocclusion
Reinfarction	17	55	RCA	Reocclusion
Ventric.Rupture	2	57	RCA	Open
Card. Shock	in tabula	71	LAD	Occluded
Reperfus. Arrhythmia	in tabula	60	RCA	Open
Pneumonia	22	68	LAD	Open

Table 4. Data of non-survivors, lysis with dilatation

Cause of death	Day of infarction	Age	Diseased vessel	Vessel status
Asystole	in tabula	76	RCA	open
Shock Lung	7	69	LAD	open
Card. Shock	2	60	LAD	?
Shock Lung	13	70	LAD	open
Cerebral Bleeding	1	71	LAD	?
Shock Lung	9	54	LAD	open

Discussion

After successful intravenous and intracoronary thrombolysis of an acute myocardial infarction a highgrade coronary stenosis of at least 60% can be found at the site of the previous occlusion in the majority of cases [1–4]. These obstructions may be flow-limiting and by this impede a reperfusion of still viable myocardium [5–7].

On the other hand such a stenotic area may be the site of another thrombus formation within the near future [8]. Thus, we have the opinion that the immediate elimination of the underlying stenosis by either subsequent angioplasty or by early bypass surgery seems to be reasonable [9–17]. If, however, such a treatment is useful it should not be postponed by several days or weeks in order to observe the clinical symptoms and to analyze the definite viability of the myocardium. The limited perfusion during the waiting period may lead to a reocclusion in the meantime.

Our series of 99 patients with acute transmural myocardial infarctions was equally randomized into two groups. Both groups were not significantly different with respect to age, sex distribution, infarct location, and time until recanalization.

At the end of the thrombolytic phase the reperfusion rate was similar in both groups. In group II we attempted PTCA in all patients, despite in some of the older ones highgrade, calcified and irregular stenoses were found. In a regular PTCA procedure because of stable or unstable angina these patients might not have been selected for the procedure. Since we did not attempt a PTCA procedure in the same strict manner as we regularly do in patients with angina pectoris the successrate of 60% was comparatively low.

PTCA in the acute infarction phase bears the same risk of an artificial occlusion of the coronary vessel as in-patients with angina pectoris. In our series one artificial occlusion occurred. This is in the same range as in our series of 424 patients with stable and unstable angina, treated since 1978 (1.9%). In a previous series of 100 patients with PTCA immediately after thrombolysis a vessel occlusion by PTCA occurred in three patients (3%). Therefore the risk of an artificial reocclusion of the reopened vessel by PTCA in experienced hands is within the range of that in stable and unstable angina [18–20]. In all cases of an artificial reocclusion by PTCA the infarct-related vessel could not be reopened by further streptokinase treatment nor by mechanical maneuvers with the guide or with the dilatation balloon. An intimal dissection with subsequent total mechanical obstruction of the vessel was probably the pathophysiological mechanism.

A complete coronary angiography was strived for at the control study after four weeks. Because of the age and the clinical status of the patients such a restudy was not possible in all of them. In those, however, in whom a restudy was possible the luminal diameter of the coronary arteries at the site of the previous occlusion was measured. While the rate of obstruction before lysis and immediately after lysis were not significantly different, they were highly significant at the end of the four weeks interval. By PTCA the degree of stenosis was significantly diminished ($78.0 \pm 15.2\%$ vs $31.9 \pm 24.4\%$, $p < 0.0001$). While the mean stenosis of 78 % of luminal diameter clearly will impede the coronary flow a residual stenosis of only 31.9 % is hemodynamically not important [5–7].

The differences with respect to the improvement of wall motion between both groups were not very striking. There was, however, a significant improvement of delta-EF after post-extrasystolic potentiation in the group with successful PTCA.

After four weeks the death rate between both groups did not differ significantly from each other. The reasons for the lethal outcome, however, were different. While in group I there were seven cardiac deaths, in group II only two pts. died from cardiac origin. We have no explanation why a shock lung developed in three patients on day 2, 9, and 13. No hemodynamic deterioration had occurred prior to the shock lung syndrom.

Despite the total numbers in both groups are still small, there is the impression, that successful PTCA may prevent a reocclusion and by this a reinfarction in some patients. The rates of cardiac deaths and of vessel reocclusions are remarkably lower in patients with successful PTCA than in those without PTCA.

The study will be continued in order to further analyze the question, whether the PTCA procedure may lower cardiac mortality and reocclusion rate. The results in larger series, the analysis of the wall motion changes, the clinical and angiographical outcome after six months will show, whether this procedure will gain a definite place in the treatment of the acute myocardial infarction.

References

1. De Wood MA, Spores J, Notske R, Mouser LT, Burroughs R, Golden MS, Lang HT: Prevalence of total coronary occlusion during the early hours of transmural myocardial infarction. N Eng J Med 303:897–902, 1980.
2. Meyer J, Merx W, Schmitz H, Erbel R, Kiesslich T, Dörr R, Lambertz, H, Bethge C, Krebs W, Bardos P, Minale C, Messmer BJ, Effert S: Percutaneous transluminal coronary angioplasty immediately after intracoronary streptolysis of transmural myocardial infarction. Circulation 66:905–913, 1982.
3. Meyer J, Merx W, Dörr R, Lambertz H, Bethge C, Effert S: Successful treatment of acute myocardial infarction shock by combined percutaneous transluminal Coronary recanalization (PTCR) and percutaneous transluminal coronary angioplasty (PTCA). Am Heart J 103:132–134, 1982.

4. Serruys PW, Wijns W, Van den Brand M: Is transluminal coronary angioplasty mandatory after successful thrombolysis? Quantitative coronary angiographic study. Br Heart J 50:257–265, 1983.

5. Bache RJ, Schwartz JS: Effect of perfusion pressure distal to a coronary stenosis on transmural myocardial blood flow. Circulation 65:928–935, 1982.

6. Gottwik MG, Siebers M, Kirkeeide R, Schaper W: Hämodynamik von Koronarstenosen. Z Kardiol 73/II:47–54, 1984.

7. Schaper J, Schaper W: Reperfusion of ischemic myocardium: Ultrastructural and histochemical aspects. J Am Coll Cardiol 1:1037–1046, 1983.

8. Harrison DG, Ferguson DW, Collins SM, Skorton DJ, Ericksen EE, Kioschos JM, Marcus ML, White CW: Rethrombosis after reperfusion with streptokinase – Importance of geometry of residual lesions. Circulation 69:991–999, 1984.

9. Meyer J, Merx W, Schweizer P, Erbel R, Dörr R, Helfenberg R, Messmer BJ, Effert S: Advantages of combining transluminal coronary angioplasty (PTCA) with selective coronary thrombolysis in acute infarction. Circulation 66/II:261, 1982.

10. Hartzler GO, Rutherford BD, McConahay DR: Percutaneous transluminal coronary angioplasty: Application for acute myocardial infarction. Am J Cardiol 53:117–121, 1984.

11. Erbel R, Pop T, Meinertz T, Kasper W, Rückel A, Pfeiffer C, Schreiner G, Meyer J: Rapid recanalization in acute myocardial infarction by combined mechanical and medical therapy. Circulation 68/III:326, 1983.

12. Meyer J, Erbel R, Schmitz HJ, Pop T, Meinertz T, Schreiner G, Henkel B, Henrichs KL, Rupprecht HJ, Effert S: Transluminale Angioplastik – Unstabile Angina, Frischer Infarkt. 50. Jahrestg. Dtsch. Ges. Herz- und Kreislaufforsch., Mannheim, 1984, Z Kardiol 73/II:167–176, 1984.

13. Rogers WJ, Smith LR, Oberman A, Kouchoukos NT, Mantle JA, Russel RO, Rackley CE: Surgical vs nonsurgical management of patients after myocardial infarction. Circulation 62/I:67–74, 1980.

14. Mathey DG, Rodewald G, Rentrop P, Leitz K, Merx W, Messmer BJ, Rutsch W, Bücherl ES: Intracoronary streptokinase thrombolytic recanalization and subsequent surgical bypass of remaining atherosclerotic stenosis in acute myocardial infarction: Complementary combined approach effecting reduced infarct size, preventing reinfarction, and improving left ventricular function. Am Heart J 102:1194–1201, 1981.

15. De Wood MA, Spores J, Berg R Jr, Kendall RW, Grunwald RP, Selinger SL, Hensley GR, Sutherland KJ, Sheilds JP: Acute myocardial infarction: A decade of experience with surgical reperfusion in 701 patients. Circulation 68/II:8–16, 1983.

16. Messmer BJ, Merx W, Meuer J, Bardos P, Minale C, Effert S: New developments in medical-surgical treatment of acute myocardial infarction. Ann Thorac Surg 35:70–78, 1983.

17. Walker WE, Smalling RW, Fuentes F, Gould KL, Johnson WE, Reduto LA, Sterling RP, Weiland AP, Wynn MM: Role of coronary artery bypass surgery after intracoronary streptokinase infusion for myocardial infarction. Am Heart J 107:826, 1984.

18. Grünzig AR, Senning A, Siegenthaler WE: Nonoperative dilatation of coronary artery stenosis: Percutaneous transluminal coronary angioplasty. N Engl J Med 301:61–68, 1979.

19. Meyer J Böcker B, Erbel R, Bardos P, Messmer BJ, Effert S: Treatment of unstable angina with transluminal coronary angioplasty (PTCA). Circulation 62/III:160, 1980.

20. Meyer J, Schmitz HJ, Kiesslich T, Erbel R, Krebs W, Schulz W, Bardos P, Minale C, Messmer BJ, Effert S: Percutaneous transluminal coronary angioplasty in patients with stable and unstable angina pectoris: Analysis of early and late results. Am Heart J 106:973–980, 1983.

INDEX